A History of Diabetes in Pregnancy

Harold Kalter

A History of Diabetes in Pregnancy

The Impact of Maternal Diabetes on Offspring Prenatal Development and Survival

Springer

Dr. Harold Kalter
Ring House, Apt 432
E. Jefferson Street 1801
20852 Rockville Maryland
USA
kalterh@gmail.com

ISBN 978-94-007-1556-1 e-ISBN 978-94-007-1557-8
DOI 10.1007/978-94-007-1557-8
Springer Dordrecht Heidelberg London New York

Library of Congress Control Number: 2011932789

Printed on acid-free paper

Springer is part of Springer Science+Business Media (www.springer.com)

Preface

A happy chance led to my interest in the subject of this book, an invitation out of the blue from the editors of the New England Journal of Medicine to write a review of the causes of congenital malformations in human beings as they were then known. Years earlier Josef Warkany, a pioneer in the field of teratology, and I had reviewed the same subject in the same journal (Warkany and Kalter 1961), and feeling it would lead to a stronger statement I asked him to join me in its writing.

The work that emerged rested on a critical reading and analysis of the biomedical literature of the previous several decades that dealt with congenital malformations and their causes, known and supposed (Kalter and Warkany 1983). These primary sources–reports of individual cases, hospital series, population surveys, vital statistics, and the like–contained many suspicions and allegations as well as some clear evidence about the origins of these abnormalities. Our task was to consider this body of evidence and come to an assessment of them for the purpose of estimating the likelihood of preventing such conditions.

The causes had earlier been broadly categorized into genic, chromosomal, environmental, and complex or unknown. About the first two generally there was little theoretical that was not settled, but about the others there was little that was certain. Thus the environmental origins of congenital malformations would get most of our attention, especially as that was where the controversies lay. A considerable number of such agents had been found to be teratogenic in laboratory animals. But no more than a handful had been unquestionably identified as having caused congenital malformations in human beings. These were ionizing radiation, already identified by the 1920s; the rubella virus, revealed in 1941; later some other infectious agents; and afterward several therapeutic substances, environmental contaminants, and a miscellany of others–cytotoxic, anticoagulant, and anticonvulsant drugs, thalidomide, organic mercury, and so forth.

In addition some noninfectious maternal illnesses were thought to cause or be associated with fetal maldevelopment; most of them seldom occurring however–except for one, insulin dependent diabetes mellitus. Years of study had made ever more firmly entrenched the belief that children of women with diabetes had an increased frequency of serious congenital malformations. This disease was intriguing. First, it was common in populations generally, and hence diabetic pregnancy was common as well. Next it appeared to be a constant feature of the human constitution, not waning and waxing as did infectious diseases. And last it seemed to me that the long-held belief in its teratogenicity had not been closely scrutinized and needed further looking into.

Writings on the subject of pregnancy in diabetic women, beginning with those from the decades before the discovery of insulin in 1921, were voluminous and needed becoming acquainted with. Reading these pages, sometimes opaque and fragmentary, led to the report presented here.

Contents

Chapter 1
Introduction

Long accepted beliefs are difficult to challenge. What are accepted as medical truths may not be as fiercely adhered to and as vigorously championed as are religious convictions or even political philosophies; but long-held scientific orthodoxies can be zealously defended and anyone foolhardy enough to question them must be sure of his position.

What is in question here is the generally held belief that the babies of women with insulin dependent diabetes mellitus are congenitally malformed more often than babies of nondiabetic women.

How did this idea get started and what has maintained it? Before the middle of the twentieth century the major question diabetologists and obstetricians caring for pregnant diabetic patients asked was why so many of their babies were born dead or died soon afterward. Congenital malformations did not seem to be part of the answer, so were given little attention. Only as the death rate of infants of diabetic mothers began to subside, with improving control of the disease, in tandem with the rate in the general population, did malformations become more conspicuous and a problem.

Congenital malformations are not rare. In the general population malformations of a serious nature are present in the astonishingly high frequency of about 3% of newborn children. While in the births of diabetic women this has usually been said to be about doubled or even trebled. From such observations the belief followed that vigorous management of the disease early in pregnancy would counteract this tendency.

One is permitted nevertheless to remain unconvinced. My hesitancy stemmed from the fragmentary knowledge mentioned earlier of the known causes of human congenital malformations; which left many uncertainties, including those about the teratogenicity of diabetes. And a feeling that a reading of the medical literature regarding the outcome of pregnancy in diabetic women was needed to look into the prevailing belief.

The pages below outline, discuss, and analyze this literature. The approach taken has been to scrutinize the numerous and varied sources of information—hospital and clinic surveys, case histories and population studies of individual malformations, etc.—in order to examine the hazards besetting the conceptus in diabetic women,

H. Kalter, *A History of Diabetes in Pregnancy*,
DOI 10.1007/978-94-007-1557-8_1, © Springer Science+Business Media B.V. 2012

regarding viability and development, spontaneous abortion, perinatal death, and congenital malformation. Scrutiny that led in the end to question this belief—that congenital malformations occur more frequently in the children of diabetic women than of nondiabetic women.

How, then, to account for the judgment that the opposite seemed to be the case? Is it to be explained in part by loose application of the term malformation, a problem often besetting teratology generally? To its being based on pregnancies unrepresentative of the disease in the overall population? Would judgment have been tempered by comparison with nondiabetic pregnancies, seldom made?

The task undertaken was to examine the written record and come to a judgment as to its findings. If it led only to a reexamination of the facts and a rethinking of the subject it will have been beneficial. Let us see.

Chapter 2
The Framework

In the history of medicine major advances promising new-found health paradoxically have sometimes led to emergence of new disease. A significant instance of this advance and retreat is seen in the annals of diabetes mellitus, a record of human success in whose train there emerged tough new questions. Questions presented by our subjects, the embryos and newborn infants of pregnant diabetic women. The focus here is on the hazards faced by them, introduced by a main concern, death of the newborn.

Early Childhood Death

One of the much trumpeted social and medical achievements of the twentieth century is the great reduction in the rate of deaths of children under the age of 1 year—by which the standard of civilization is customarily judged. Years ago it was declared that "a low rate…indicates a healthy community, a high rate the reverse" (Newman 1906) and "infant mortality is the most sensitive index we possess of social welfare…" (Newsholme 1910), a criterion that still reigns (Shapiro et al. 1965; Yankauer 1990).

Extraordinary progress thus shines forth from the precipitous decline in the mortality rate of children under 1 year of age, e.g. in the US, which went from 99.9 to 7.0 per 1000 children born alive—greater than 90%—in the 80 years or so following the end of the First World War (U.S. Bureau of the Census 1960; National Center for Health Statistics 1998). And the same great achievement was realized in many countries in Europe and elsewhere (Chase 1967; Thomson and Barron 1983). [It must be noted with curiosity that the US ranking in this statistic vis-à-vis the nations of the world is hardly better in 2010 than it was 100 years ago, in 1911, as noted at that time by S.W. Newmayer (Brosco 1999).]

The first month, but especially the first week, is the most perilous time of life, since that is when the most weak and damaged babies die. It is death in these first 7 postnatal days, plus that in the last weeks of pregnancy—together known as the perinatal period—that is of great relevance here. These earliest deaths also greatly

H. Kalter, *A History of Diabetes in Pregnancy*,
DOI 10.1007/978-94-007-1557-8_2, © Springer Science+Business Media B.V. 2012

participated in the great decline, falling in the US from 32.5 per 1000 live births and fetal deaths in 1950 to 6.6 in 2005 (Powell-Griner 1986; MacDorman and Kirmeyer 2009).

This reduction was largely brought about by the virtual elimination of many public health problems and pediatric diseases. But advance was most uneven. At the same time that many widespread causes of neonatal and infant death, disability, and distress—hygienic, nutritional, infectious—were so impressively ameliorated barely any headway was made with others.

The Role of Diabetes

The momentous discovery of insulin in 1921 (Banting and Best 1923) and its wide availability afterward (Wrenshall et al. 1962; Bliss 1982) soon had profound effects, loosing a cascade of consequences. First the barrier to reproduction by women with this disease was greatly lowered. But then, as the number of pregnancies of diabetic women increased, it was seen that many of their infants did not survive long. Which abated as some of the reasons for the perinatal deaths were discovered and successfully managed.

But with this ongoing decline a shift occurred in the cause of the deaths that continued to occur, this residue in fact growing in importance. What soon became, and has continued to be, among the chief causes of this offspring death were congenital malformations. And as these proved to be largely unpreventable they received increasing attention—especially as suspicion arose that maternal diabetes itself may be their cause.

Diabetes mellitus when present in early pregnancy profoundly affects the viability, growth, and development of the unborn. This work will trace the ideas and practices that have evolved over the years in the attempt to manage these difficulties. It will consider some of the most perplexing of the imperfectly answered or still unanswered of these problems, most prominent among them: whether diabetes causes or is associated with spontaneous abortion, retarded prenatal growth, and congenital malformations, whether such malformations form distinctive patterns, the relation between malformation and perinatal death, whether the form and degree of the maternal disease or its presymptomatic stages are related to these phenomena, and whether control of the disease from before or early in pregnancy can lessen these hazards.

For reasons to be seen the decade of the 1950s can be taken as a watershed in the ongoing progress in the treatment and outcome of diabetic pregnancy. Thus the events and problems encountered in dealing with these pregnancies before insulin was discovered and those emerging in the years between this discovery and the 1950s will introduce the subject.

[Methodological and conceptual matters must be noted. The definition of congenital malformations followed by diabetologists, obstetricians, and pediatricians has not always been clear or uniform; ascertainment of pregnant diabetic women (i.e. avenues of their selection for study and treatment) was often biased; no controls or poorly matched controls were usually the case (Rubin and Murphy 1958; Wilson 1960; Simpson 1978; Mills 1982). Such considerations make it necessary first to deal with definition and classification of congenital malformations, diabetes in pregnancy, etc.]

Data Sources

The main source of information used here were reports of pregnancies of diabetic women by hospital-based physicians in the US, Canada, and many European countries. They were identified by searching the medical literature, using the Quarterly Cumulative Index Medicus for older ones, Internet sources, and, most usefully—however biased they may have been—the citations in the reports themselves, providing the trail to older and older publications. Consulted also were reports of multicenter, population, and epidemiological surveys, and public-health matters with respect to the births of diabetic women.

The advantages of hospital-based reports compared with vital-statistics and other such data are that they are more complete (judging from the underreporting public records commonly suffer from; see e.g. Greb et al. 1987; Snell et al. 1992); usually providing information otherwise lacking, such as detailed descriptions of individual pregnancies and offspring, and are more informative, especially sometimes being supported by autopsy records.

Hospital-based studies however also had their drawbacks, requiring cautious interpretation of their findings. An important problem was that the composition of the patients served by different hospitals varied, demographically, medically, and so on, some of which were without doubt relevant here. For example, some hospitals were primary-care facilities, whose patients were drawn from their immediate communities and for the most part were representative of the disease picture of its population. Other reports were from larger hospitals or specialized medical facilities many of whose patients were referred from hospitals in the area or from outside the area altogether. These patients were no doubt less representative of the spectrum of the illness present in the entire population. How must the facts from such different sources be handled? The problems of procedure and interpretation that these and other uncertainties presented will be considered below.

Definition

A full definition of diabetes in pregnancy will be detailed below. Here only a few general remarks are necessary. Diabetes mellitus is the omnibus term given to what are probably several etiologically distinct disorders of carbohydrate metabolism, characterized by chronic hyperglycemia, in which there is usually an absolute or relative deficiency of insulin or its reduced secretion or impaired action. The disease predominantly occurs in two generally distinct forms, denoted type 1, insulin dependent, mostly of juvenile onset, and type 2, noninsulin dependent, mostly of maturity or adult onset, further discussed below (National Diabetes Data Group 1979; World Health Organization 1985).

In addition to the general classification another exists for diabetes in pregnancy. This also has two broad categories: diabetes that antedates pregnancy, often called pregestational diabetes, and diabetes that first occurs during pregnancy, called gestational diabetes. These also will be elaborated upon below. Both forms may be either insulin dependent or independent, but the former is most often dependent and the latter most often independent. [Exceptions—there are always exception—to general pronouncements, which will emerge as the writing progresses.]

The untoward outcomes of diabetic pregnancy that are the main concern here—spontaneous abortion, fetal and neonatal death, and congenital malformation—are associated almost entirely with insulin dependent pregestational diabetes. For the sake mostly of developing the historical picture of the subject gestational diabetes and related topics will also be considered. But the main focus will be on the pregestational insulin dependent variety, and hence when the unqualified term 'diabetes' is used it will refer to that variety.

Chapter 3
The Early Years

Diabetes mellitus is an old disease, mentioned in ancient and medieval sources (Barach 1928)—though the validity of even that contention is disputed nowadays (Bottazzo 1993). Despite this antiquity the first instance of pregnancy in a woman with diabetes was only recorded less than 200 years ago (Bennewitz 1824). Which in fact may not have been an instance of the type of the disease this work is mainly concerned with (Hadden and Hillebrand 1989). So you see we have already encountered some doubts.

What is certain is that the story of diabetes in pregnancy began toward the end of the nineteenth century. The reason for this late appearance in human history is understandable. Before the modern age such occurrences could have happened only exceedingly rarely, because diabetic women of reproductive age virtually did not exist, the form of the disease that occurs at younger ages—the kind this work will focus on—having been responsible for a high toll of infertility and early death.

Maternal Mortality

In the pre-insulin years a very high death rate was common in the small minority of diabetic women who became pregnant. Duncan (1882) noted that of the 16 cases collected by him 10 died soon after or within a year of delivery; such devastating percentages also noted later, 54% by Eshner (1907), 25% by Williams (1909), 23% by Joslin (1915), and 25–55% reported in publications in 1894–1908, cited by Lambie (1926). These may actually have referred to less serious instances of the disease; Parsons et al. (1926) doubted that "patients with severe diabetes ever survived pregnancy in the pre-insulin era."

Outcomes in the years just preceding the discovery of insulin seemed to reflect a possible improvement in this dismal record, although even in the first years of the insulin era the diabetic maternal death rate still far exceeded that occurring generally. The literature of the early period recorded six deaths in 73 pregnancies, 8.2% (Bowen and Heilbrun 1932); but a summary of the years from then to midcentury already noted improvements that had made "pregnancy relatively safe for diabetic

H. Kalter, *A History of Diabetes in Pregnancy*,
DOI 10.1007/978-94-007-1557-8_3, © Springer Science+Business Media B.V. 2012

women" (Gilbert and Dunlop 1949), improvements that compared favorably with contemporary nondiabetic rates (Kyle 1963).

A compilation of reports of diabetic pregnancies surveyed in the 1940s and 1950s shows that maternal diabetic death had declined to about 1.0–1.2% in the US and Europe, which was still about 10 times the overall rate in white women in the US during those years. Although the decline continued, a gap still remained near the end of the century (National Center for Health Statistics 1992).

The diabetic maternal mortality rate no doubt declined even further in most recent years, as it had for pregnancies generally, if only judging from the infrequency of its being mentioned in publications of the last several years. A report from Finland confirmed this scarcity, there having been five deaths during pregnancy or the postpartum period in 972 type 1 diabetic women in 1975–1997, i.e. 5.14 per 1000, which still somewhat exceeding that for nondiabetic women—none of which however was associated with diabetic complications (Leinonen et al. 2001).

Fertility

Before the discovery of insulin it was the rare diabetic woman who became pregnant, the rarity due to physical impairment and reduced life expectancy. Physicians of the time with wide experience had seldom or never seen such pregnancies (Bouchardat 1887; Lecorché 1885; Taylor 1899).

This dearth was commented on by Duncan (1882), in noting that he heard from colleagues how seldom they had seen such occurrences in women with the disease. Collecting the small number of instances he had personal or other knowledge of he prophesied that "attention being called to the subject, the list of cases will soon be augmented." Indeed the scarcity continued in the years leading up to the 1920s and even later (van Noorden 1909; Wiener 1924; Gray and Feemster 1926; Walker 1928; Skipper 1933).

An early explanation of the infertility, uterine atrophy, was given by Graefe (1898), as perhaps due to amenorrhea (Herman 1902), its basis lack of ovarian follicles (Parisot 1911). The structural and functional changes in the reproductive system of diabetic women that possibly underlaid the infertility were summarized by Lambie (1926). But even years later not much more was understood of its underlying basis (Eastman 1946), no doubt because the problem by then having all but disappeared its solution was not pressing.

The problem slowly lessened with the discovery and increasing availability of insulin, with reports soon appearing of the efficacy of this new panacea in restoring menstruation and supporting pregnancy (Lambie 1926). During the earliest years few pregnant diabetic women were treated with it however (Reveno 1923; Graham 1924, see Wilder and Parsons 1928), and even in medical centers its use continued to be uncommon (Parsons et al. 1926). From this handful of instances a mere hint of the capability of the new ingredient to promote the fertility of diabetic women could be guessed. But, as foretold, and not long in fulfillment, "the incidence of pregnancy in diabetic women is likely to rise" (Wilder and Parsons 1928; Randall 1947; Gilbert and Dunlop 1949). Worldwide at least 55 diabetic pregnancies were recorded in the medical literature in 1923–1927 (Wilder and Parsons 1928). In the London Hospital alone 15% of 177 diabetic women admitted in 1923–1931 were pregnant (Skipper 1933).

As insulin led to regular and normal menstruation, ovulation apparently proceeding normally, and pregnancy no longer the oddity it had been not long before, there followed a continual increase in the prevalence of diabetic pregnancy (Kramer 1936; Koller 1953); soon approaching that of diabetes itself in women of reproductive age in the US during that period (Spiegelman and Marks 1946) and afterward (Marks et al. 1971). This frequency depended on the overall rate of diabetes in women of reproductive age and the increasing prevalence of early-onset diabetes (Mather and Keen 1985; Bingley and Gale 1989; Levy-Marchal and Czernichow 1992).

The findings though were sometimes discordant. The fertility of diabetic women may still have been impaired, as indicated by the many instances of delayed menarcheal age (Bergqvist 1954; Post and White 1958; Knorre 1969; Sutherland et al. 1983; Kjaer et al. 1989a, b) and the frequency of diabetes in women of reproductive ages being greater than the mean rate of their pregnancies (Drury and Powell 1987; Harris et al. 1987). Also, not to be discounted, the increasing frequency may have been partly due to the disproportionate number of the pregnancies reported by referral centers (Randall 1947).

Nevertheless, while conception in diabetic women was much improved, before 1985 they had fewer pregnancies and fewer births than nondiabetic women (Kjaer et al. 1992b; Pedersen et al. 1994). Fertility is said to have become normal later, at least in those in whom the disease was uncomplicated and strict metabolic control was exercised (Zarzycki and Zieniewicz 2005; Jonasson et al. 2007).

Chapter 4
Spontaneous Abortion

Spontaneous abortion is defined as death of the embryo before attaining viability, i.e. prior to the period when it becomes able to maintain independent life. This viability was once held to be reached at 28 weeks of pregnancy following the first day of the last menstrual period (Hook and Porter 1980). But as now defined, in keeping with the success of medical technology in keeping younger fetuses alive (Anon. 1988), spontaneous abortion is death of the conceptus before 20 weeks of pregnancy.

During the early insulin years, with the other problems caretakers had to contend with, whether the frequency of spontaneous abortion was increased in diabetic pregnancy was never a major matter of disagreement, though even then there were differences of opinion about it. Skipper (1933) said it was "relatively uncommon," and White (1935) called it "relatively…frequent." Others conceded that at best "the effect is small" (Moss and Mulholland 1951).

Such differences were perhaps expected of a medical generation for the most part not well aware of how frequent spontaneous abortion usually is. Today it is well established that abortion in recognized pregnancies (i.e. in women with a missed menstrual period) is quite common, varying from 10 to 25%, depending on the type of study and analysis. The lowest estimates, of about 10%, were obtained by prospective surveys of already pregnant women in clinical settings (Jansen 1982), those of 12–15% by retrospective investigations of pregnancy histories (Warburton and Fraser 1964; Naylor 1974; Leridon 1976), and 15–25% by the use of life-table probability procedures (Harlap et al. 1980; Leridon 1977).

The etiology and epidemiology of spontaneous abortion have been much studied. While a great deal of the blame for such events has been implicitly directed at the great frequency of chromosomal and morphological abnormalities in abortuses, there is little understanding of the connection between these aberrations and embryonic death. Nor are the reasons well understood for the many such deaths not accompanied by such phenomena (Boué et al. 1975; Porter and Hook 1980; Carr 1983; Roman and Stevenson 1983; Rushton 1985).

H. Kalter, *A History of Diabetes in Pregnancy*,
DOI 10.1007/978-94-007-1557-8_4,

Early Studies

The frequency of spontaneous abortion noted in the earliest studies of diabetic pregnancies was usually low, owing no doubt to women commonly first being seen by physicians in later months of pregnancy. This limitation and other methodological inadequacies of many inquiries led to underestimates of the abortion frequency, as pointed out by Combs and Kitzmiller (1991). Knowlege of the actual frequency of spontaneous abortion thus obviously required that women be seen from early in pregnancy.

My reading of relevant publications taking this limitation into account—following the preliminary lead of Gellis and Hsia (1959)—resulted in a review of over 50 reports from US and European hospitals appearing from 1950 to 1986, which included more than 8000 diabetic pregnancies probably observed from specifically stated relatively early periods (Kalter 1987). In such pregnancies the mean frequency of spontaneous abortion was 12.7%, i.e. approximately the rate found in studies of general clinic populations (Warburton and Fraser 1964; Naylor 1974; Leridon 1976). Which thus indicated that diabetes was not associated with an excess of spontaneous abortion in recognized pregnancy.

The review also found that the diabetic spontaneous abortion rate was substantially the same before and since 1960; in conspicuous contrast with the later great decrease in the perinatal death rate in diabetic pregnancy, a contrast that pointed to the two entities being of separate etiology.

To some authors it seemed, on the contrary, that embryonic and perinatal death should have common roots, so that if diabetes were associated with death in late pregnancy it should also be associated with death in early pregnancy, i.e. abortion, an idea not easily relinquished (e.g. Eastman 1946).

Later Studies

The assertion that spontaneous abortion is not increased in diabetic pregnancy has been challenged; calling for the question to be reconsidered. It must be recalled that determining the frequency of spontaneous abortion has often been hindered by confusing and intruding factors common to retrospective inquiries. These include faulty maternal recall, biased detection of spontaneous abortion, vagaries of the sampling method, innumerable demographic, social, and biological confounding variables, and possible environmental influences—aspects that have been fully discussed (Harlap et al. 1980; Kalter 1987). (It must be noted that such aspects have seldom been considered in studies alleging that spontaneous abortion is increased in diabetic pregnancy.)

Reproductive loss also occurs before pregnancy recognition, hence to discover its full extent pregnancies must be monitored from soon after conception. Studies that have done so entailed women enrolled in diabetes programs from early in pregnancy, allowing surveillance over the entire gestation period, including the earliest weeks.

Such early study was necessitated by finding that various harmful reproductive outcomes appeared to be associated with high levels of maternal blood glucose early in pregnancy (Leslie et al. 1978; Miller et al. 1981; Ylinen et al. 1981). But following this new track would have been problematic had it not been for the discovery of a novel blood component, glycosylated hemoglobin, and new methods of measuring it.

Glycosylated Hemoglobin

The diagnosis and management of diabetes depend on knowledge of the concentration of glucose in blood. Traditionally this was measured by the oral glucose tolerance test. But a number of difficulties—including reproducibility, individual variability, and confounding factors—made the test an unreliable measure of glycemic state and indicator of effectiveness of metabolic control of pregnancy outcome (O'Sullivan and Mahan 1966; Hadden 1975).

A more convincing indicator of the glycemic state was found to be the level of glycosylated hemoglobin, HbA_1, a minor component of hemoglobin A, comprising about 4–5% of the total hemoglobin in normal persons (Mayer and Freedman 1983). The importance of HbA_1 to the care of diabetics consisted in its being the product of a nonenzymatic nearly irreversible process by which glucose is bound to hemoglobin (Bunn et al. 1976), and—considering the protracted lifespan of red blood cells—thus represented an average of the plasma glucose concentration during the several weeks preceding its determination.

The relevance of these facts to studies of diabetes became apparent with the discovery that the level of one of the fractions of hemoglobin, HbA_{1c}, may be two to three times greater in diabetic than in nondiabetic individuals (Rahbar et al. 1968), and that its concentration in the former was proportional to the blood glucose level, falling with metabolic management of the disease (Koenig et al. 1976a, b).

It is the relation of diabetic status early in pregnancy, as gauged by the level of HbA_{1c}, to the frequency of spontaneous abortion that is to be considered here. Its relation to congenital malformations will be considered below.

Glycosylated Hemoglobin and Spontaneous Abortion

Study began in the late 1970s of the relation of spontaneous abortion risk and maternal blood glucose level as denoted by glycosylated hemoglobin. The primary purpose was to lessen the harmful outcomes of the diabetic state by allowing its management from early in pregnancy.

Such studies soon enabled various comparisons of spontaneous abortion: in diabetic aborters and nonaborters; in aborters with glycosylated hemoglobin levels above and below the group mean; in women intensively and conventionally managed; in preconception clinic attenders and nonattenders; in insulin dependent and nondependent pregnancies; and, where controls were included, in diabetic and nondiabetic pregnancies. In fact however few of the comparisons were statistically significantly different from eachother.

The studies varied regionally in the span of years surveyed and in the number of patients sampled, but were similar in almost all other ways: all were prospective; patients were seen consecutively and were predominantly pregestational insulin dependent diabetics; all were metabolically managed from before or soon after conception; all or almost all patients were white; all pregnancies were confirmed; spontaneous abortion was defined fairly uniformly; standard methods of measuring glycosylated hemglobin were employed.

The following is an overview of such studies from the time of the first reports in the early 1980s through the present.

Birmingham

Wright et al. (1983) were among the first to consider the question. They found the frequency of spontaneous abortion in weeks 9–12 of gestation in insulin dependent women enrolled in a diabetic clinic in 1979–1981 to be 17.2%. The glycosylated hemoglobin level ranged widely, from 6.1 to 16.9%, with a mean of 11.5%. [For comparison, in a group of nondiabetic women in the early weeks of pregnancy the range was 4.1–6.9% with a mean of 5.6%—Morris et al. 1985].

The range was similar in women that aborted and in those that did not, and the spontaneous abortion frequency, though greater in those with levels above the group mean than below, was not statistically significantly different. These findings were nevertheless taken as indicating that prolonged poor glycemic control in the weeks preceding pregnancy or during early in the first trimester contributed to the likelihood of spontaneous abortion. The question remained whether 17.2% was an excessive spontaneous abortion frequency for women enrolled in a study of pregnancy in its earliest weeks. It is considered below.

Cincinnati

An early report from this center noted 29.5% spontaneous abortion in clinically apparent insulin dependent diabetic pregnancies in 1978–1983, suggesting a substantially greater risk than in the general population (Miodovnik et al. 1984). The next communication, whose focus was association with glycemic level, noted a smaller spontaneous abortion rate, 22.4% before 20 weeks in about these same years, with no explanation of the difference (Miodovnik et al. 1985).

The subjects were two groups of women, one in 1978–1980 and the other in 1981–1984, and in both groups those that aborted had a mean glycemic level greater than those that did not (11.2% vs 9.9% and 12.8% vs 11.3% respectively). Within each group the spontaneous abortion increase was not statistically significantly different at levels of less than 12% from that at levels above; but in both combined it was statistically significant—an unacceptable procedure, especially as different methods were used to gauge the level (Rosenn et al. 1991). The cutoff used was 12%, but with no reason given for the choice. Wright et al. (1983) had used 11% for the comparison because that was approximately the mean in the study group; had 12% been chosen the spontaneous abortion frequency in those above and below that level would not have been significantly different.

Subsequent reports noted lower spontaneous abortion frequencies before 20 weeks, 21.4%, and then a still lower one, 17.7% (Miodovnik et al. 1986, 1988), the latter not too different from the 12–15% in recognized pregnancies in general (Hertz-Picciotto and Samuels 1988). But in an apparently later study the spontaneous abortion rate in women with glucose concentration above 12–13%, said ambiguously to have been enrolled before 9 weeks of gestation, was again elevated, to 24.2% (Rosenn et al. 1994).

Matters of ascertainment and representativeness of the diabetic women constituting the study groups were not clarified, especially with respect to race and ethnicity, factors related to abortion frequency of relevance here (Porter and Hook 1980), since the study came from a municipal hospital largely serving an inner-city population. Nor explained was the exclusion of pregnancies that continued beyond 20 weeks and ended in a congenitally malformed infant, which would have overestimated the calculated spontaneous abortion frequency.

Studies from this center continued to the end of the century, with outcomes of preconception care programs compared in three intervals from 1978 to 1993, spontaneous abortion data not included however (McElvy et al. 2000). Early glycohemoglobin concentration decreased from interval to interval, as did perinatal mortality and congenital malformation rates, the last dipping from 14 to 3.6 to 2.2%, the reductions attributed to glycemic improvement, discussed further below.

A Multicenter Study

An inquiry into these questions in several US centers found the spontaneous abortion frequency in diabetic and control women to be virtually identical, 15.7 and 16.2% respectively (Mills et al. 1988a). Though the mean glycosylated hemoglobin level was significantly higher in the diabetic women the finding seemed to indicate that elevated blood glucose level by itself was not a risk for abortion.

The data were collected at five centers, the diabetic subjects ascertained by "public appeals as well as through the medical system" and the control group mostly by solicitations through mailings (Mills et al. 1983). Although the control and diabetic women closely resembled eachother in characteristics indicative of abortion risk, the centers no doubt varied in ascertainment and composition of patients.

It must be noted that the spontaneous abortion frequency in both groups, though monitored from about the time of conception, was smaller than has usually been the case with such early initiation of pregnancy monitoring (see e.g. Hertz-Picciotto et al. 1988; Wilcox et al. 1988; Steer et al. 1989; Modvig et al. 1990).

Other Studies

Other earlier studies had inconsistent findings. In some the relation was examined by comparing the glycosylated hemoglobin level in aborters and nonaborters, in others by comparing the fraction of aborters and nonaborters above and below the mean for the entire group. In those including controls the total spontaneous abortion frequency was not different in diabetic women than in controls, or the glycosylated hemoglobin level was elevated in diabetic aborters but not in controls (Mills et al. 1988a; Hanson et al. 1990).

In some the spontaneous abortion frequency was not different in women with glycemic levels above than in those with levels below the mean (Sheridan-Pereira et al. 1983; Lucas et al. 1989), while in others it was significantly greater in the former (Wright et al. 1983; Miodovnik et al. 1985; Key et al. 1987; Greene et al. 1989). In studies that monitored women from before conception it was lower than in cases seen later (Dicker et al. 1988); whereas in others it was no lower than in the controls (Mills et al. 1988a); i.e. a thoroughly mixed bag.

Dose Response

The findings may also be considered from the dose-response standpoint. The toxicological principle that the magnitude of an adverse effect is proportional to that of the cause is subject to the proviso that there may be a threshold, an amount of the causal factor below which an effect is not demonstrated. If it is postulated that glycohemoglobin level beyond the usual one is associated with an increased spontaneous abortion frequency, and if this adverse effect is subject to the toxicological principle enunciated, it follows that only beyond the threshold may there be a response whose degree may be proportional to its magnitude.

After this long-winded introduction the anticlimax is that in only a few instances was it possible to examine the data in this manner. Some gave evidence of a dose-response relation (Key et al. 1987; Rosenn et al. 1994); while in others the evidence, though equivocal, was negative, since the spontaneous abortion frequencies associated with the two greatest levels were not significantly different from eachother (Wright et al. 1983; Mills et al. 1988a; Greene et al. 1989).

An Interim Comment

It is notable that studies declaring that the spontaneous abortion frequency was significantly increased in diabetic pregnancy seldom included investigations into the pathology of the abortuses. One might have thought it necessary to look into the basis of the alleged increase, to determine e.g. whether there might have been an increased malformation frequency, especially as this was thought to be significantly raised in diabetic pregnancy.

Pathology studies that were made had negative results. Mills et al. (1988a) reported equal numbers of grossly malformed diabetic and control embryos, and Bendon et al. (1990) found no histological feature different in abortus tissue from diabetic than nondiabetic women. And last, an amniocentesis study determined that chromosome abnormality was not increased in fetuses of diabetic women (Henriques et al. 1991).

Tentative Conclusion

It is clear from this overview that the studies presented no consistent evidence of an increased spontaneous abortion frequency in diabetic pregnancy; as was independently concluded in a review of insulin dependent diabetic women (Smith 1989), or was at "worst elevated only slightly above that in the general population" (Combs and Kitzmiller 1991); nor that spontaneous abortion frequency is correlated with glycosylated hemoglobin levels in early pregnancy.

Two matters especially weakened such studies. Few of them included nondiabetic pregnant controls; and only when such a group is as closely and thoroughly monitored and from as early in pregnancy as the index women can a convincing answer to these questions come forth. The biases in retrospective as well as in various forms of prospective studies of the complex phenomenon of spontaneous abortion have been extensively noted (e.g. Leridon 1977), and ignoring them diminishes the value of a work.

The greatest difficulty remained in explaining the low spontaneous abortion frequencies in diabetic women with glycohemoglobin levels below the means for their groups, frequencies far smaller than those generally occurring in pregnancies monitored from soon after their onset. At the same time it must be recognized that such frequencies in the women with far greater than normal glycohemoglobin levels fell within the range previously often found in overall early-monitored pregnancies, and thus can hardly be considered unusual.

The essential question therefore was whether the apparently increased frequency of spontaneous abortion found in some of the studies was to be imputed to the maternal disease state or to monitoring the pregnancies from or almost from their onset. The danger of neglecting the latter possibility was clearly pointed out by an overall population study that found a total frequency of spontaneous postimplantation abortion of 31% (Wilcox et al. 1988).

Recent Studies

The very few articles of relevance published most recently are considered chronologically.

In a later report from Cincinnati, apparently summarizing all pregnancies seen up to that point, those bearing major congenital malformations were disregarded, resulting in the spontaneous abortion frequency being overestimated (Rosenn et al. 1994). It requires no further comment.

In pregnancies of women with pre-existent diabetes seen in 1990–1994 in several maternity units in an area of northwest England the first trimester spontaneous abortion frequency was 16.4% (Casson et al. 1997). This it seemed was not thought unusual since it was not further considered.

In studies of the glycosylated hemoglobin level in diabetic women in a region of Denmark in 1980–1992 the overall spontaneous abortion frequency was a low 10.3%, but whether related to the glycemic level was left unclear (Nielsen et al. 1997). A similar frequency, 9.8%, was previously noted in diabetic pregnancies, in the partly overlapping years of 1976–1990 (Nielsen and Nielsen 1993). Extraordinarily, in later pregnancies in the encompassing years 1985–2003, a greatly increased spontaneous abortion frequency was noted, of 21.6%, a leap for which no explanation was forthcoming (Nielsen et al. 2006a). Nor was the relation of spontaneous abortion to glycemic level specifically noted, the major concern being congenital malformation.

In a similar but limited study of such women in Italy the overall spontaneous abortion frequency was 21.4%, and not statistically significantly different from that in those whose glycemic level was less or greater than 10.0 (Mello et al. 1997).

In Norwich, England the spontaneous abortion frequency in first pregnancies of women with type 1 diabetes in 1991–2000 was compared in those with fair or poor glycemic control, the frequency being 3.6% at a glycemic level of less than 7.5 and 14.5% at 7.5% and above, a statistically significant difference (Temple et al. 2002). It is not clear why only first pregnancies were scrutinized. Nevertheless something was incongruous here, since as commented above the lower frequency was far less than that predominantly found in the general population, while the higher frequency approximated the usually noted one.

In prospectively identified pregnant type 1 diabetic women in 1998–1999 in Scotland 7.3% ended in spontaneous abortion, the glycemic data undisclosed however (Penney et al. 2003). The same nondisclosure was true of a report of pregnancies of diabetic women in 1999–2000 in the Netherlands, with 11.3% spontaneous abortion frequency (Evers et al. 2004); low levels in both instances.

A study in Sofia of type 1 pregnancies in 1998–2004, its findings presented in untranslated Bulgarian, hence not fully analyzed, noted mean first trimester glycemic values of 10.1% vs. 7.0% in aborters and nonaborters respectively, the overall spontaneous abortion frequency of 17.2% was disclosed but not that in each group separately (Todorova et al. 2004).

A Polish study of diabetic women in whom intensive and conventional insulin treatment was compared found no significantly different spontaneous abortion rate between them, both with similar low first trimester glycemic levels of 7.8 and 7.5% (Cypryk et al. 2004).

A study from Madrid also failed to give specific information about glycemic values in aborters versus nonaborters, noting only that in prospectively collected diabetic women the overall spontaneous abortion frequecy was a modest 7.9% (Galindo et al. 2006).

A close reading of these reports of the outcomes, of those of the more recent as well as the older studies, despite the inconsistencies, made it clear that they did not support the belief that type 1 diabetes is abortigenic.

Chapter 5
Perinatal Death

The most tenacious and demanding difficulty presented by the pregnancies of diabetic women is the toll of fetal and neonatal deaths they experienced. The very high rates that prevailed in the years before the discovery of insulin continued little improved for some time after the advent of this miraculous panacea; and even appeared to worsen as the therapy enabled many diabetic women to live long enough to become pregnant. Though with the passing years these deaths steadily diminished their frequency was still manyfold increased in the late twentieth century and even in the early years of the twenty-first century (Hawthorne et al. 1997; Vääräsmäki et al. 2000; Penney et al. 2003; Melamed and Hod 2009; Persson et al. 2009). This chapter will examine their associated features. But first the general nature and attributes of such deaths will be considered.

Definition and Classification

Early offspring death includes several components differing from one another in various ways. The need to consider them individually was realized when, given increased attention in the 1920s, it became necessary to consider when viability begins during prenatal life.

A legal decree regarding this question was promulgated in Great Britain in 1926 with the passage of an act that formally defined stillbirths as intrauterine deaths occurring after 28 weeks of pregnancy (Armstrong 1986). At about the same time it was recognized that stillbirths and the earliest neonatal deaths shared in the prenatal origin of many of their causes, and that these largely differed from the causes of death of older infants, which were mostly of postnatal origin (Crosse and Mackintosh 1954; Bakketeig et al. 1984).

Hence it was suggested that the first two, stillbirth and early neonatal death, be considered a unit and given a separate name—perinatal death (Peller 1923, 1948). This called for neonatal death itself to be divided into early and late, defined quite arbitrarily as those in the 1st week and the 2nd through 4th weeks after birth, respectively. These terminologies have been useful and among other things enabled

H. Kalter, *A History of Diabetes in Pregnancy*,
DOI 10.1007/978-94-007-1557-8_5, © Springer Science+Business Media B.V. 2012

clinicians, public health workers, demographers, epidemiologists, and other investigators to compare their findings.

While these definitions have largely endured, that of stillbirth underwent a change. Its original delimitation, 28 weeks of gestation, began to shift as medical advance made possible the increased survival of prematurely born infants, resulting in a lowered age of viability and a necessary modification in its definition. Thus today the widely accepted definition of stillbirth is intrauterine death after 20 weeks of pregnancy. Which in its turn led to stillbirth, like neonatal death, being subdivided, for the reason given below, into early and late, the former from 20 through 28 weeks and the latter after 28 weeks of gestation.

These intervals, needing a foundation, were to be based on the method of dating gestational length from the first day of the last menstrual period before pregnancy onset; which is the practice of most clinicians and epidemiologists, and is convenient—but biologically incorrect. To obtain the more correct figure, 14 days—the usual time between the first day of the last menstrual period and presumed conception—must be subtracted from the conventionally derived age.

But like everything biological this rule also had its caveats (Berg 1991; Moore 1991; Saunders and Paterson 1991), since whatever starting time is used there is bound to be uncertainty of the length of gestation. To attempt to obviate this difficulty, and "to eliminate national idiosyncracies," the World Health Organization (1977) recommended that weight of the conceptus be used as the preferred criterion of stillbirth classification, with—at least for international comparison—the minimum of 1000 g or certain fetal measurements (equivalent to 28 weeks of gestation) continue to indicate the attainment of viability. Details of this topic were given a lucid exposition by Hook and Porter (1980).

Perinatal Death in Diabetes

Perinatal death has steadily decreased in the developed countries of the world since statistics regarding them were first widely gathered 90 or more years ago (e.g. US Bureau of the Census 1960; Chase 1967; Hirst et al. 1968; Powell-Griner 1986, 1989). Their causes—direct and indirect—are many: medical, demographic, social, cultural, environmental (Woolf 1947; Butler and Alberman 1969; Thomson and Barron 1983; Bakketeig et al. 1984; Golding 1991; Emanuel 1993).

Perinatal death also declined in diabetic pregnancy, sharing no doubt the features associated with their improvement generally, e.g. racial, ethnic, socioeconomic, though these were rarely mentioned in reports of such pregnancies. Others, such as nationality, region, time, etc., were sometimes inherent in the reports themselves.

Details of these matters were sometimes sparse in older reports of hospital-based material, though sometimes compensated for by the richness of many other aspects. On the whole however only a few of the many features listed above that are related to mortality were reported often enough and in detail enough to judge their association with the rate and temporal trend of perinatal death, making analysis of their roles often only suggestive.

Gestational and Neonatal Age

Important in considering perinatal death are age divisions late in gestation: the number of perinatal deaths reported, greater when both mortality segments, stillbirth and neonatal death, were included, less when one or the other was not. With respect to diabetic births these matters did not present much difficulty. As regards stillbirth, most investigators were orthodox in their views about the onset of viability, limiting reporting to the late stage. This was especially true in Europe, and in particular in Great Britain, where this standard was first adopted. Fewer than half of the reports explicitly provided this information at all, but it is probable that the conservative precept was adhered to by most physicians. As for neonatal deaths, many articles only reported early ones; but even when left unsaid, since these far outweighed late ones it is likely that the great majority reported were early.

Maternal Age

The most often mentioned maternal feature in diabetic pregnancy was mean age or its range, but even this was noted infrequently. Maternal age is important because, as has long been known, it is closely associated with the background perinatal death rate, being slightly increased before about age 20, reaching a low at 20–24, and then rising ever more steeply with further advance of age (Sutherland 1949; Thomson and Barron 1983; Bakketeig et al. 1984; Golding 1991).

The same was no doubt true of pregnancies of diabetic women, and therefore the average maternal age at conception must be taken into account. If advanced it may have been due to the reduced fertility and increased menarcheal age once occurring widely in diabetic women. Infertility, known to be especially true of women with onset of diabetes at young ages, persisted into the early decades of the insulin era (Bergqvist 1954; Worm 1955; Post and White 1958), and was still being remarked upon in more recent years (Pinget et al. 1979; Burkart et al. 1989; Gens and Michaelis 1990; Kjaer et al. 1992a, b; Livshits and Seidman 2009).

Analysis of the responsibility of maternal age for perinatal death in diabetic pregnancy would no doubt benefit by considering the possible effects of change in age-specific birth rate, of the sort that occurred in US and west European populations, which was credited with some share in the decreased overall infant mortality rate (Gendell and Hellegers 1973; Morris et al. 1975; Meirik et al. 1979). Unfortunately this could not be evaluated in diabetic pregnancy because of the poverty of the reported data.

Analysis of parity or birth order, also known to be associated with perinatal death, was more successful. While parity is closely tied to maternal age its separate relation to perinatal death has been debated (Golding 1991). Nevertheless I examined its possible role by using the infrequently given parity data—proportion of women who were primigravid—in reports of diabetic pregnancies.

Information regarding maternal age at conception was reported more often in older than more recent publications. But at all times was limited and fragmentary, and consisted of age range, mean age (stated or calculated from the data given), or gravidity proportions.

Data regarding age range revealed little that was definitive, but perhaps pointed to a slight shift to a younger span over time. Those concerning age, stated in a fair number of reports, gave a clearer, but puzzling picture. Mean age hardly changed over the first 50 years of the insulin era, hovering at about 28–29 years. Later a small change seems to have occurred, with a decrease to about 27 years. This small reduction can scarcely be credited with any but the most minor part in lowering the diabetic perinatal death rate (which in any case began earlier than did the maternal-age shift). A direct indication of the apparently negligible effect of maternal age was given by a few comparisons of younger and older women (Andersson 1950; McCain and Lester 1950; Möllerström 1950; Jokipii 1955; Gellis and Hsia 1959; Malins 1968).

The difference between the earlier noted mean age of diabetic women at conception, 28–29 years, and a later overall population one, 25.7 years in 1962 (Anon 1963), may partly clarify the excessive mortality rate; while the closeness of the later diabetic mean of 27 to the overall 26.7 in 1992 (Ventura et al. 1992) perhaps said something about the mortality rate having approached the population level.

Two reports compared mean maternal age in diabetic and overall births, 31 and 23 years respectively, in 1936–1946 in Pittsburgh (Rike and Fawcett 1948), and 32 and 24 years, in 1940–1949 in a New York City hospital (Frankel 1950). Such information was sparse in later reports, controls seldom being included. These few bits of information pointed to an older mean age of pregnant diabetic women, but whether this contributed to the greater perinatal death rate is impossible to say.

Primigravidity, a possible measure of average conception age, was even less informative, its rate varying haphazardly over time and without correlation with maternal age. One analysis for example found the perinatal death rate no different in multiparous diabetic women than in primiparous ones (Gellis and Hsia 1959).

The indication thus was that insulin-dependent diabetic women, in the past and perhaps even more recently, did not became pregnant as readily as women generally, and hence their mean age was greater. These disparities however, as already surmised, probably accounted for little of the increased perinatal death rate in diabetic pregnancies; and it may be concluded that any effect of advanced maternal age of diabetic women on perinatal survival was obscured by that of the diabetes itself.

The Early Insulin Era

The rate of offspring death in the few diabetic pregnancies in years before insulin was discovered was incredibly high—about 50% dying in utero and during labor and 80% of the remainder in the first days after birth (Lambie 1926). The deaths were ascribed to various causes including excessive fetal size, making for difficult labor (Lambie 1926), and even generations later: "…a considerable proportion of the increased fetal loss in diabetic pregnancies is due to dystocia which results from fetal oversize" (Ross et al. 1952).

Although insulin soon improved the fertility of diabetic women it did far less to reduce the high perinatal death rate, which continued quite high for years (Henley 1947).

The first reports of insulin given to pregnant diabetic women came from physicians describing the course of the illness and pregnancy in their patients. A summary of many of the earliest pregnancies illustrated the continuing seriousness of the disease for the offspring. In 28 cases lasting to the later months of pregnancy the perinatal death rate was 39.3% (Wilder and Parsons 1928), an appreciable improvement over the preinsulin record, but far short of the level in the overall US population, which was 7.7% in the 1920s (U.S. Bureau of the Census 1960, p. 25).

The number of diabetic pregnancies grew rapidly during the following 20–25 years, as did the number of hospitals and centers caring for pregnant diabetic women. But the new medical facilities failed to make a substantial dent in the mortality rate. The poor record ["simply dreadful" Brandstrup and Okkels (1938) called it] persisted into the 1940s, being about 25% in US series and 35% to over 40% in European ones. It was not till about 50 years later that the mortalities nearly reached the population level. This great accomplishment was recapitulated and the roles of several causes of it that came into play especially since the 1970s were enumerated in an excellent review (Kitzmiller 1993).

The Two Forms of Diabetes

Most of the diabetic pregnancies reported in the early decades of the insulin era concerned diabetes of pregestational onset. Later reports increasingly included diabetes that first occurred or was diagnosed during pregnancy, i.e. gestational diabetes, but often without presenting the outcomes for the two forms separately. Which is unfortunate because with time the perinatal death frequency in them, not very different in the earliest years, greatly diverged, improvement in the pregestational form greatly lagging behind the other. Thus the failure to separate their progressively differing outcomes further complicated study of trends in the mortality rate associated with the pregestational disease.

Facility Size

The diabetic perinatal death rate was much reduced in the larger medical facilities, as might have been expected with their excellent maternal care. And indeed they invariably had better outcomes than the smaller ones. But even this advantage largely faded away after the 1960s, as the steady reduction in the perinatal death rate all but wiped out this differential.

The lower mortality frequency in the larger facilities nevertheless was surprising, because the better care they offered would have been offset to some extent by their patients largely being referred and hence more severely ill. As was recognized, the larger centers were attended by selected patients but who were "cooperative and superbly supervised" (Jones 1952), all in all, a puzzling situation.

Stillbirth and Neonatal Death

Reports presenting analyzable data made it clear that the rate of stillbirth in the early years was always greater than that of neonatal death, being 60–65% of all perinatal deaths; contrasted with 50–55% in overall hospital pregnancies during these decades. Time however brought the diabetic stillbirth picture into line with the background.

Neonatal deaths overwhelmingly occurred within a week of birth, mostly in the first couple of days of life (Peel and Oakley 1949; Oakley 1953; Neave 1967). In the early insulin years it was over 80%. But this figure was also more or less true of neonatal deaths in the general population (Powell-Griner 1986), despite the overall reduction in the neonatal mortality rate over time. All told, perinatal death in diabetic pregnancies in these years was about 8–12 times greater than in overall births.

Causes Generally

The persistently high perinatal death rate in diabetic pregnancy in the earliest insulin decades was baffling. Its supposed determinants were numerous and each had its own advocates.

It should be remembered that not much was known of the causes of perinatal death even in the overall population. An early attempt at delineating them divided stillbirths and 1st week deaths into those of maternal, placental, and fetal origins, but found that the main one, fetal trauma, fit into none of them (Tingle 1926). Deaths in Baltimore, beside those attributed to syphilis, were largely due to toxemia with the others of unknown cause (Dippel 1934). Other contemporary reports were equally vague. The Registrar-General's report for Scotland for 1939 noted that 37% of stillbirths were of ill-defined or unknown cause, 14% due to difficult labor, 13% to fetal deformities, and the remainder to hemorrhage, toxemia, and general diseases (Baird 1942). Another concomitant of many perinatal deaths was prematurity, i.e. birthweight less than 1000 g, though prematurity was itself not regarded as "a cause of death," and in such instances the lethal factors were the same as in mature babies, asphyxia, trauma, infection, and congenital malformation (McNeil 1943).

The same theme recurs repeatedly in publications during that era (Potter and Adair 1943; Labate 1947; Arey 1949; Sutherland 1949). Namely, that many deaths were due to toxemia and other maternal illnesses; but essentially were attributed to vague and ill-defined "physiological" conditions (Sutherland 1949; Duncan et al. 1952), autopsies failing "to reveal the cause of stillbirth and first week death in a large proportion of cases" (Baird et al. 1954).

Causes in Pregnancy

The causes of perinatal death in diabetic pregnancy were equally perplexing even in midcentury. Some saw the main problem to be fetal overgrowth, due it was thought to growth hormone excess, neonatal hypoglycemia, maternal toxemia, and congenital malformations (Lawrence and Oakley 1942). Others emphasized poor care in regulating the maternal disease (Miller et al. 1944). An influential group of investigators at first pointed to "...a direct agent, active in the last four weeks of pregnancy," then to a defective ovum, which included congenital anomalies, disturbed chemistry of diabetes, and later hormone imbalance and obstetrical and placental causes, with the picture summed up as follows: "...poor control of maternal diabetes...congenital defects...maternal vascular disease...prematurity... duration of diabetes...age of inception...imbalance of the sex hormones of pregnancy" (White 1935; 1946, 1949; White and Hunt 1943). In some of these ideas great foresight was shown, while others were off the mark.

Consensus coalesced in the 1950s as increased numbers of diabetic pregnancies allowed for broader overview. It was well understood by then that stillbirth often followed numerous maternal diseases, vascular and others, plus fetal anomalies (White 1950; Jones 1958), but most remained without satisfactory explanation. Even extensive postmortem examination (e.g. Warren and LeCompte 1952) did not clarify the problem [a full account of the results of such examinations will be presented below]. All told little progress was made, and even much later the "precise cause of the excessive stillbirth rate" in diabetic pregnancies remained unknown (Landon and Gabbe 1995).

Better knowledge of the proximate causes of neonatal death was helpful. Most were characterized by some combination of chronological but not developmental prematurity, i.e. of date but not size, respiratory difficulties, pulmonary atelectasis (these three all associated with each other, of course), generalized cardiac enlargement, overall excessive size, often followed by traumatic injuries secondary to difficult delivery, congenital defects, etc. (Given et al. 1950; Hall and Tillman 1951; Hagbard 1956; Miller 1956).

There was little that was really new in most of these observations, e.g. poor maternal care had early been voiced to be a factor in the high mortality rate, and the frequent presence of the triad of prematurity, asphyxia, and atelectasis had been noted earlier (Sisson 1940); and even much later respiratory distress continued to be a problem (Robert et al. 1976; Bye et al. 1980; Cunningham et al. 1982; Piper and

Langer 1993; Piper 2002). Near the end of the past century, and even early in present one, assigning causes of perinatal death remained rudimentary (Golding 1987; Pauli and Reiser 1994; Incerpi et al. 1998; de Reu et al. 2009).

As noted various elements were thought of relevance in the high rate of perinatal death. One of them, quality of prenatal maternal care, had been considered to be important since the 1930s. It was an enduring belief that the care the pregnant diabetic woman received in regulating her disease, through medical and dietary management, was the most important ingredient for lessening the harmful effects of diabetes on the fetus and infant. Some felt it was efficacious "especially if it be instituted early" (Ronsheim 1933), while others thought care was most important in the last months of pregnancy (Skipper 1933).

The quality of the care given to pregnant diabetic women has continued to be regarded of great importance; the topic of care in its modern guises will be returned to below. Another aspect of care and its relation to perinatal death—control of the maternal disease by insulin treatment—is discussed below under the head of disease severity in offspring death.

Macrosomia

A feature continually implicated in poor fetal survival in diabetic pregnancy was macrosomia, i.e. significantly increased neonatal length and weight, usually defined as 4.0 kg or more, owing not to prolonged gestation but to fetal overgrowth, especially in the last trimester of pregnancy, producing babies large for gestational age.

This was frequently true in the past (Hsia and Gellis 1957), affecting as many as one-third of births (Pedowitz and Shlevin 1952). Newborns of diabetic mothers in Copenhagen e.g. were 18.1% heavier and 2.9% longer than a matched control group (Pedersen 1954b). Even more recently large centers reported big babies in 25–42% of the pregnancies (Kitzmiller 1986). Yet paradoxically, according to certain developmental criteria, such infants could be considered growth retarded (Pederson and Osler 1885; Gruenwald 1966).

Many reports noting giant infants were summarized early (Fischer 1935). Time reduced its frequency. In 1932–1947 diabetic mothers had excessively large babies nine times as often as mothers generally (Nathanson 1950); 30–40 years later diabetes only doubled the risk of infant macrosomia (Boyd et al. 1983); but it is still happening (Schwartz and Teramo 2000; Taylor et al. 2002; Johnstone et al. 2006; Persson et al. 2009; Weindling 2009).

Heavy babies usually had a difficult birth and were subject to skeletal and neurological injuries and sometimes death (Given et al. 1950; Pedowitz and Shlevin 1952); and still are (Das et al. 2009). But the question remains whether big babies are at increased risk of stillbirth. There is evidence that the perinatal death rate of excessively large babies in general is at least twice that of normal-sized ones (Stevenson et al. 1982). But the answer is uncertain so far as diabetic births were concerned (Kitzmiller 1986).

In the past macrosomia was even found in "cases with excellent control of diabetes throughout pregnancy" (Lavietes et al. 1943; Gilbert and Dunlop 1949), and occurred later even in well controlled pregnancies (Knight 1983; Dandona et al. 1986; Berk et al. 1989; Hunter et al. 1993; Hare 1994; Silva et al. 2005), and is still not well understood (Kitzmiller 1986; Fenichel et al. 1990).

Like other problems the question has been sidestepped by the great decrease in the perinatal death rate in diabetic pregnancies, and the lowered risk of trauma in diabetic births (Mimouni et al. 1992). Macrosomia is further dealt with below in its relation to prediabetes and gestational diabetes.

Sex Hormone Imbalance

An early theory, taken seriously by clinicians for 20 years or more, proposed that maternal sex hormone imbalance, often found in toxemic pregnant diabetic women (Murphy 1933; Smith and Smith 1935), was responsible for increased perinatal death (White et al 1939). The expectation thus was that replacement therapy would reduce the incidence of toxemia and lead to improvement in offspring survival rate. The results of such therapy, when applied with other more usual sorts of management of the disease in pregnancy, appeared to support the belief (White and Hunt 1943; White 1949; Nelson et al. 1953; White et al 1956).

The theory began fading away when skepticism set in following recognition of the imprecision of the means of assaying the hormones (Reis 1956); noting that hormone therapy provided no significant advantage, and that as good results were obtained simply by careful supervision of pregnancy (Medical Research Council 1954; Miller 1956; Reis et al. 1958; Gellis and Hsia 1959). Thus cruel facts, as they will, rapidly vanquished a long and widely held theory. Despite these considerations belief in the efficacy of hormones persisted locally a while longer (White 1965).

Disease Severity

The problem seemed to be clarified by relating perinatal death to severity of the maternal disease. But there was disagreement about what constituted severity and how it was to be classified (Jones 1956). A conflict arose about whether it was to be judged by historical or by metabolic criteria. The one based judgment on age at onset of the disease, its duration at the time of pregnancy, and degree and extent of maternal vascular pathology; and the other on the metabolic state of the diabetic patient as indicated by insulin requirement during pregnancy, i.e. difficulty of management (Given et al. 1950; Tolstoi et al. 1953; White 1949; Nelson et al. 1953). Classification was confused however because of the poor correlation of these criteria with fetal loss (Hurwitz and Higano 1952; Oakley 1953).

Regarded from the neutral standpoint of a present-day observer these approaches can be seen to have had complementary features, both being indicators of mortality risk—if severity in fact were associated with that risk. They might especially have been useful because they were quantitatively classifiable and statistically evaluable, plentiful unambiguous relevant data having been accumulated during the previous couple of decades.

To summarize, severity was estimated or classified by two criteria: duration and extent of vascular disease, and insulin requirement. My assessment of the extensive data from the 1930s to 1950s found earliness of onset, duration, and insulin dose not conclusively related to offspring survival. Adding to the difficulty, disease duration and insulin dose were barely correlated, which was not always true for onset age and duration.

In contrast with these negative or ambiguous relations, that between perinatal death and the quality of control of diabetes was decidedly positive. Although control or supervision of the disease was not always explicitly defined, what it meant for one group can be taken as typical (Lawrence and Oakley 1942): completeness of supervision referred to the earliness and regularity of being seen during diabetic pregnancy, and treatment being adjusted as needed. It was such individualized management of pregnancy, apparently not in itself equivalent to insulin dose, that my appraisal found associated with the markedly improved perinatal death rate; though so happy an outcome was not invariable (e.g. see Given and Tolstoi 1957, for disappointing results).

Nevertheless, what for the most part were good auguries, which guided and foreshadowed the future emphasis on maternal glycemic control (Kitzmiller 1993; Hare 1994).

Other Alleged Relations

Numerous other elements, especially intrauterine ones, were alleged to be involved in offspring death: a direct lethal factor perhaps associated with the toxemia and preeclampsia experienced in the last 4 weeks by many diabetic women (White 1935); as well as various other maternal and fetal dangers—ketoacidosis, hydramnios, premature labor, macrosomia, hypoglycemia, developmental immaturity, and congenital malformations (Eastman 1946; Bachman 1952; Miller 1956; Stevenson 1956). But the association of these features and perinatal death was illusory or often far from consistent (Kyle 1963).

For example, extensive studies indicated that toxemia was not important; but others found mortality rate to be significantly greater in pregnancies of insulin-treated women with various complications than in those without them, while there were no such differences in those not requiring insulin (Miller et al. 1944). Clearly the relation if any was complex and no doubt was made even more so by variable standards and definitions of toxemia (Lawrence and Oakley 1942; Peel and Oakley 1949; Hagbard 1956). Even later, though there had been much improvement, the survival rate of infants from diabetic pregnancies complicated by nephropathy, preeclampsia, and so on did not always reach that of the general population (Garner et al. 1990; Kitzmiller and Combs 1993).

The reader must have noted that congenital malformations were repeatedly mentioned in this recitation of the causes or concomitants of perinatal death, though often merely as an afterthought. In early studies these were one of the few consistently identified elements of significance. And this became increasingly more conspicuous, as the perinatal death rate decreased with the passing years, many of their causes—infectious, nutritious, social, etc.—weakening or disappearing; while congenital malformations, still undiminished, came to be an increasingly larger proportion of them (Edouard and Alberman 1980; Kalter 1991). Their possible importance in the high diabetic perinatal death rate will be considered below.

Preventing Stillbirth

As we saw, the greatest challenge in the study of diabetes in pregnancy in the early insulin era was the terrible rate of stillbirths, which comprised about two-thirds of all perinatal deaths. Since there seemed to be potential ways of averting these deaths, attention became concentrated on them and the neonatal mortality problem for the moment was largely set aside.

Intrauterine death being predominantly a phenomenon of the last weeks of pregnancy (e.g. Peel and Oakley 1949; Pedowitz and Shlevin 1955), it seemed that many stillbirths could be prevented, or rather circumvented, by performing elective cesarean delivery before they could occur. This was the strategy advocated especially by obstetricians but also by others (Nothmann and Hermstein 1932; Ronsheim 1933; White 1935; Titus 1937); hence it soon became the widespread practice to deliver pregnant diabetic women by cesarean section 4–5 weeks before expected parturition (Eastman 1946).

At the same time there was much skepticism of the necessity and benefits of this practice (Peckham 1931; Skipper 1933; Hurwitz and Irving 1937; Herrick and Tillman 1938; Shir 1939; Mengert and Laughlin 1939; Hall and Tillman 1951; Sindram 1951; Miller 1956). For example, it was noted that a large proportion of deaths had already occurred by the end of the 36th week (Hurwitz and Higano 1952), and very few additional ones thus would have been prevented by early delivery.

Sometimes the rescued prematurely delivered infants died at birth and added to the neonatal death toll, an unexpected drawback to realizing the supposed full potential of the practice. As it was put, "…early termination does not alter the outcome of pregnancy, but merely changes the death-bed of the foetus…" (Barnes and Morgans 1949). Such deaths were the product of the difficulty of striking a balance between the need to deliver babies before most intrauterine deaths occurred and not doing it early enough to deliver babies that might die neonatally because of respiratory immaturity (Hurwitz and Higano 1952; Gellis and Hsia 1959). To thwart most of the intrauterine deaths and also minimize the neonatal problem the compromise selected was delivery at about 35–38 weeks of gestation.

This strategy appeared to have the desired outcome. A summary noted that it reduced the stillbirth rate by half or more, and that the one untoward by-product, a slightly increased neonatal mortality rate, did not tarnish the overall improved result (Bachman 1952). It was noted later however that this optimistic appraisal was marred by statistical nonsignificance (Miller 1956). My summary of the reports of an even larger number of pregnancies mostly during the 1930s and 1940s supported the optimism respecting stillbirths, and found no worse neonatal mortality rate.

These favorable results were weakened, however, by several flaws. The first, patient selection. Women chosen for cesarean section presumably were those with indications of impending intrauterine death—obstetrical history, fetal oversize, uncontrolled diabetes, etc. (Kyle 1963). In some instances cesarean section was also made at or near term when emergencies necessitated it (McCain and Lester 1950). Many such indications however were not helpful in identifying women at risk (Whitely and Adams 1952); and factors that "influenced the obstetrician to induce labour or await spontaneous onset rather than deliver by cesarian section are not always clear…" (Stevenson 1956). Also women selected for the procedure probably received medical attention earlier in pregnancy and more frequently and ongoing than those delivering at term; maternal care being an important element in mitigating the cesarean rate, this may have been a source of some of the improved stillbirth record in these deliveries.

The results were also made more rosy by allowing fetuses already known to be dead in utero to be delivered at term. The proportion of deaths in such deliveries could not be compared with that of cesarean-section deliveries (Reis et al. 1950). Only by excluding the stillborns could this be done, and as pointed out, when the recognized intrauterine deaths were omitted from the calculation the fetal loss in vaginal deliveries was reduced to a level that would not have been bettered by additional cesareans (Jones 1952).

But there was a possible countervailing situation as well. Comparing neonatal deaths in vaginal and cesarean-section deliveries, several studies reported a slight but statistically significant advantage of the latter (Gellis and Hsia 1959). This was influenced however by misleading data from deliveries prior to the 33rd week, which when excluded revealed no significant difference in the rate of neonatal death in the two types of delivery. This plus the good results that were achieved simply by diligent care during the last weeks of pregnancy (Nelson et al. 1953; Pedersen and Brandstrup 1956) confirmed the opinions of those who throughout had regarded the routine cesarean section practice skeptically.

The White Classification

What had to some extent hampered the study and management of diabetic pregnancy in the first 25 years or so of the insulin era was the lack of an objective system of grading the seriousness of the disease state. Such a system might also have found use as an indicator of the extent of fetal risk, and if predictive would have aided in instituting preventive measures. Some of the need for a new focus also came perhaps from the growing recognition that the beneficial effects of close management of pregnancy, which were beginning to be realized, meant that at least some of the causes of the excessive prenatal mortality rate resided in the maternal organism.

Such considerations may have been the rationale of a new system of classification of diabetes in pregnancy (White 1949). The devising of this system was undoubtedly one of the most important, and certainly the most durable, of White's many contributions to the study of diabetes in pregnancy. It consisted of an integrated method of grading the "pre-pregnancy" maternal state—disease onset age and duration plus intensity of vascular pathology—according to level of severity, denoted as classes A through F. The scheme will be described and discussed in detail below.

The White system, though soon accepted by many investigators, at first had its critics. For example the difficulty was noted of applying a system based on pre-pregnancy criteria to patients first seen during pregnancy (Long et al. 1954). It was also complained that it "did not take into account insulin amount needed or ease or difficulty of maintaining control" (Dampeer 1958). These complaints were not widely shared, and the White system was soon broadly applied and indeed said to have been accorded "virtually semiofficial status" (Jones 1956), at least in the US.

In Europe the White system was felt to be unsatisfactory, because of the inconsistency of the relations between the relevant variables proposed by the system and pregnancy outcome (Oakley 1953; Pedersen 1954a). A suggested alternative, which was believed would improve the prediction of diabetic pregnancy outcome (Pedersen and Mølsted-Pedersen 1965), was an individualized scheme that relied on "prognostically bad signs" appearing during pregnancy (Pedersen et al. 1974). Which never caught on, and was rarely used outside of Copenhagen. A simplified scheme was proposed later, whose purpose was less to predict harmful fetal outcome than to aid in management of pregnant diabetic women (Essex et al. 1973).

The White system increasingly demonstrated its usefulness in relating disease severity to perinatal death, hence in estimating fetal risk prenatally or early in pregnancy and helping avert the threat, a close relation which continued even as the latter greatly decreased; usefulness furthermore that has continued into the new century (Cormier et al. 2010).

There were always exceptions. The overall correlation was not seen everywhere. For example the Lying-in Hospital in Providence, Rhode Island had less severe cases but a higher perinatal death rate (Jones 1958); while patients seen at the Joslin Clinic in Boston were more severely affected but had a smaller mortality rate (Gellis and Hsia 1959). The reasons for such disparities were perhaps many, subtle, and nonspecific.

Chapter 6
Prediabetes

The term prediabetes once upon a time referred to two separate areas of study, similar yet different, an earlier one now largely forgotten and a current one. Nevertheless both were similar in their focus, the period preceding the onset of overt diabetes, and in their purpose, the discovery of elements leading to the development of full-blown disease, in order to forestall its manifestation. They differed however in the phenomena studied, the older area, adverse outcomes of earlier pregnancies, and the later area, preceding pathophysiological processes (Leiva 1996). Who could possibly have forseen how it would all turn out?

In any case, what should not be neglected is that this was an old quest. Joslin noted in 1928 that "He [Naunyn] sees in heredity the common bond which unites the different forms, or as he said, 'to speak more exactly, the heredity of the diabetic tendency.'…Almost any illness or injury…may serve as the cause." An area of conjecture also not resolved even years later (Friedman and Fialkow 1980).

Prediabetes, whatever its focus, is a chapter virtually forgotten in the story of diabetic pregnancy. Recounted here are years of intense study of what came to be realized was a disease that did not exist, or as it was put "…a unique disease. No one has ever suffered from it" (Pyke 1962).

What its students studied were adverse outcomes of pregnancy in the prediabetic period, i.e. of diabetic women before the disease became manifest; whose study it was hypothesized would yield understanding of the processes leading to it (Jackson 1959; Conn and Fajans 1961; Camerini-Davalos 1964). As stated by Krall (1965), "Diabetes doesn't occur overnight but starts at birth or earlier…"

The adverse outcomes were the familiar ones of perinatal death and congenital malformation, plus one other (Jackson 1959). In fact it was the last—namely, excessive offspring birthweight or macrosomia—that was considered the hallmark of prediabetes, and whose belief as an indicator of potential diabetes was most durable.

This macrosomia was an old phenomenon. It was present in the very first documented instance of a birth to a diabetic woman (Bennewitz 1824), the subject of a thesis in which the comment appeared—as a translation from the Latin text puts it—that there had been a "child…Hercules weighing twelve civil pounds…" (Hadden and Hillebrand 1989). Fifty-eight years later, in a survey of the few diabetic births that had been recorded in the interval, another such outcome was noted by

H. Kalter, *A History of Diabetes in Pregnancy*,
DOI 10.1007/978-94-007-1557-8_6, © Springer Science+Business Media B.V. 2012

Duncan (1882) who was impressed by a "dead foetus...described as enormous... its weight...extraordinary...." Death it seems was generally the fate of these large babies, so much so that they were expressively depicted (Fournier, cited by Lambie 1926) as "giant babies with feet of clay, unfit for life" (my translation).

As pregnancies of women with overt diabetes became commoner during the early insulin years large babies born to them became more common, 15–25% of births in one report (Eastman 1946) and even more frequently, 45–75%, in another (Bachman 1952).

Macrosomia in Prediabetic Pregnancy

But diabetic women it was soon discovered often had very large babies even before developing the disease. A discovery enabled by the mounting number of them living to mature ages, leading to knowledge of the outcome of their prediabetic pregnancies.

It began with a report of 155 women in Vienna who had developed diabetes in middle or later life who recalled the birthweights of 608 of their babies of earlier pregnancies—nearly 11% weighed 5 kg (11 lb) or more in contrast with only 0.3% in a large group of births overall (Bix 1933). Earlier inconclusive reports of excessive neonatal weight were cited by Skipper (1933), who nevertheless said "it is no exaggeration to state that the birth of a child of excessive size always suggests the advisability of investigating the mother for diabetes."

It was then noted that giant babies were often born years before, as long as 10 years before, clinical diabetes became manifest, whose dimensions became clearer when corroborations started pouring forth (Allen 1939). The first of these, which set the pattern for its successors, noted that 3.9% of 256 prediabetic births weighed over 5 kg (a much lower frequency than Bix had noted, perhaps because it was not maternal memory but hospital records that were relied on), but even so, much greater than the control 0.07% (Miller et al. 1944), the latter close to the 0.13% of full-term infants born in 1932–1947 in a New York hospital (Nathanson 1950).

Another important point, whose meaning was not immediately appreciated, was that its frequency seemed to increase with closeness to the time of onset of the diabetes. Many articles backed up these findings (e.g. Kriss and Futcher 1948; Reis et al. 1950; Kade and Dietel 1952; Marquardsen 1952; Moreau et al. 1955); but confirmation was not universal, sometimes no difference being found between the mean birthweight of children of prediabetic women and the control or usual one (e.g. Barns and Morgans 1948).

The positive findings varied in several ways, especially in frequency of the big babies. This was not only because of variable weight criteria and uncritically accepted maternal memory, but mainly because of differences in various maternal attributes, whose association with birthweight was not yet well recognized.

The trend also differed. Big babies sometimes occurred only in the years immediately preceding diabetes onset (Paton 1948; see Pirart 1955 for further references); or in an increasing frequency throughout the prediabetic years (Moss and Mulholland 1951; Jackson 1952; Hagbard 1958); some the opposite, the frequency generally decreasing (Peel and Oakley 1949; Malins and FitzGerald 1965); or there was an elevated but constant level over most of the prediabetic period (Futcher and Long 1954; Rolland 1954; Pirart 1955).

In fact it was the last pattern that led to the suggestion that macrosomia was a constitutional feature of the prediabetic period, calling attention to the role of other factors as well as or even rather than the potential diabetes in its occurrence. One of which was frequent maternal obesity, thought by some to be irrelevant (Miller 1945), but definitely associated in retrospective studies (Futcher and Long 1954; Pirart 1955; Pomeranze et al. 1959); and in others of a different variety.

Prediabetes Pregnancy Mortality

Prediabetes was also associated with increased perinatal death. This was first noted in an incidental tabular entry to the effect that 19% of 142 pregnancies had ended in stillbirth "prior to the onset of diabetes," in contrast with 6% in a contemporary series of consecutive births (White 1935).

Numerous such reports followed over the next 25 years (Mengert and Laughlin 1939; Miller et al. 1944; Barns and Morgans 1948; Rike and Fawcett 1948; Patterson and Burnstein 1949; Peel and Oakley 1949; McCain and Lester 1950; Zilliacus 1950; Moss and Mulholland 1951; Jackson 1952; Pedowitz and Shlevin 1952; Rolland 1954; Jokipii 1955; Moreau et al. 1955; Hagbard 1958). Increased mortality appeared years before the onset of diabetes, as much as 15 or more years before, though it was most evident in the preceding 5 years (e.g. Malins and FitzGerald 1965). Others however continued to find mortality frequencies in the prediabetic years similar to population levels (Palmer and Barnes 1945; Herzstein and Dolger 1946; Imerslund 1948; Reis 1956; Kade and Dietel 1952; Marquardsen 1952; Pirart 1955).

Interestingly, it was agreed by all, even by some reporting an increased perinatal death rate, that spontaneous abortion defied this hazard, that its frequency was unaffected in prediabetic pregnancies. Much of the literature on these and other facets of the subject were fully reviewed (see Bachman 1952; Kyle 1963; Pedersen 1977).

What became obvious was that any analysis of the association of prediabetes and harmful pregnancy outcome must address the question of the possible confounding role of numerous variables. But of far greater importance was the fundamental question of what was meant by prediabetes. Authors addressing this matter usually agreed that the term referred to the period preceding "known" diabetes or the "discovery" or the "clinical manifestation" or the "recognition" of diabetes. But it was not long before it was widely admitted that time of disease onset defined in this manner was far from precise.

Furthermore, all of this paralleled the frequent occurrence of macrosomic babies in the years just before the onset of diabetes, whose story will be told below.

What Did it All Mean?

This murkiness had been alluded to even during the first decades of the insulin era. For example it was admitted that some prediabetic pregnancies probably included cases of undiagnosed diabetes (White 1935), and others not only conjectured that there was an "inability to determine the exact date of onset of diabetes," but also reasoned that this "probably led to the inclusion of instances of existing diabetes…." (Herzstein and Dolger 1946); a supposition soon echoed by others (Reis et al. 1952; Hagbard 1961; Kyle 1963; Malins and FitzGerald 1965).

Understandably this fatally weakened the legitimacy of the concept of prediabetes, and made doubtful its supposed effects on pregnancy outcome. In fact the conclusion became inescapable that the evidence gave very little support to the notion that the prediabetic state produces untoward effects on the fetus or infant, and that all of the infelicitous outcomes attributed to prediabetes must actually be imputed to association with very early as yet unrecognized stages of diabetes itself. But this was not the whole story.

Insidious Form of Diabetes

Studies of prediabetes were all made retrospectively, as they could not have been otherwise. Starting with frankly diabetic women adverse events occurring before the onset of the disease were looked back to. But the significant fact noted in nearly all these reports was that the diabetes onset occurred at advanced maternal ages (Miller 1945; Herzstein and Dolger 1946; Kriss and Futcher 1948; Paton 1948; Gilbert and Dunlop 1949). That is, most instances of the disease appeared near the end of the reproductive years or even postmenopausally; and furthermore were not insulin dependent. As was later realized the form of diabetes that followed this precursory span was what came to be known as noninsulin dependent or type 2 diabetes, a form, at the time, mostly of later adult onset. Even then it was understood to become "manifest over a longer period" (Kirk et al. 1985) and frequently to have an "insidious or asymptomatic onset" (Knowler et al. 1983).

Great changes in the incidence of type 2 diabetes later in the century as well as further remarks concerning it will be noted below.

The distinction between the late-occurring form and the insulin-dependent early-onset variety, although explicitly enunciated only later (Larsson et al. 1986; Orchard et al. 1986), was already recognized more than a century ago, when Lecorché (1885) wrote "Le diabète s'observe surtout chez elle au deux périodes extrême, avant la puberté, après la ménopause," and two generations later when Barns (1941) reiterated "…diabetes is much commoner in women during the latter part of the child-bearing period…which is largely responsible for the comparative rarity of pregnancy in the diabetic." For late thoughts on the subject see Srinivasan et al. (2008).

A Summary

What can be called the initial phase of the story of prediabetes can be summarized as follows. It came to be widely believed that the prediabetic period was characterized by several untoward outcomes of pregnancy, especially excessive birthweight and increased perinatal death (Malins and FitzGerald 1965). But it was soon perceived that the bad outcomes happened mostly or only in the years immediately preceding diabetes onset, at a time in fact when it might already have been present but as yet undiscovered. This made for the realization of the virtual impossibility of establishing the end of the prediabetic period, which combined with the accumulating negative evidence regarding the impact on perinatal death led to abandoning further attempts to associate prediabetic pregnancy with increased perinatal death.

More persistent however was the belief that babies born during this period were often very heavy. That such occurrences were auguries of, or as they would be termed today, risk factors for potential diabetes, was much weakened however, not only by the difficulty of clearly establishing the time of diabetes onset, but also by early indications of the complex entanglement of giant babies and potential diabetes with other factors—maternal predisposition to obesity, etc. (Futcher and Long 1954; Pirart 1955; Pedersen 1977). It was only later that these confounding elements were to some degree disentangled. But explanation of the births of these big babies during the prediabetic period was still called for.

Prospective Approach

This long-winded preface to the subject of prediabetes might seem far removed from the main strands of this work, pregestational and gestational diabetes. Nevertheless it is considered because by a trail we shall follow it eventually led to areas that are directly relevant.

First, doubt about the validity of retrospective studies led to the use of a new approach, one in which women were glucose-tolerance tested whose reproductive history indicated a risk of developing diabetes and an abnormal response taken as possible evidence of this potentiality. The first risk factors thought to be relevant were perinatal death and macrosomia, because they had been noted in prediabetic studies—although by then this simplistic notion had already begun to be discounted. In many studies the women were pregnant or recently pregnant. This was an important point.

A new fashion—the prospective approach—was then turned to, and many prediabetic pregnant women, 20-40%, especially those that had had big babies, when glucose tolerance tested, responded abnormally (see Engleson and Lindberg 1962). Even in the first such study certain maternal attributes were associated with big babies (Gilbert 1949), one of the major ones, as suspected, being obesity; though of course the analysis was confounded by many later discovered variables (see Larsson et al. 1986).

To put it all in a nutshell: many mothers of big babies were obese and obese mothers often had typical diabetic glucose-tolerance responses. That is, big babies, maternal obesity, and abnormal carbohydrate metabolism were all closely correlated—but their causal relations were uncertain, since none of its parts was able to predict diabetic outcome individually (O'Sullivan et al. 1966; Lubetzki et al. 1973; O'Sullivan and Mahan 1980).

There was little doubt, however, that bigness alone was a poor predictor of the risk of developing the noninsulin dependent form of the disease (Larsson et al. 1986). Which means that although prospective study of risk factors was able to characterize populations it was unable to predict the fate of individuals.

Despite the fruitlessness of these numerous studies something of positive value emerged. The glucose tolerance testing of pregnant women with the mentioned risk features inadvertently led to the discovery that a considerable proportion of all pregnant women had aberrant responses. [In all fairness, this revelation was preceded (but not appreciated) by a study that noted frequent abnormal responses in normal pregnant women, a study that was prompted by recalling that preexisting diabetes may be worsened by pregnancy (Hurwitz and Jensen 1946).] This discovery opened up a new area of investigation, carbohydrate disturbance exhibited during pregnancy, or gestational diabetes, to which a later chapter is devoted.

Prediabetes and Congenital Malformation

A number of reports mentioned births of congenitally malformed children during the prediabetic period, which it was inferred were due to this state. Except that the malformations were totally without pattern and the pregnancies producing them preceded the onset of diabetic symptoms by months to years.

The following are examples of the former. Earliest was a child with congenital heart disease born 6 months before the clinical onset of diabetes (Barns 1941). Another was hydrocephalus in a big baby whose mother was identified as prediabetic either because she had previously had a big baby or an abnormal glucose tolerance response in the index pregnancy (Lund and Weese 1953).

A woman with three infants with spina bifida and meningocele was considered to have been prediabetic at the time of the pregnancies because three months after the third one she displayed a typical abnormal glucose tolerance curve; which was indubitably corroborated by the fact that her grandmother was a diabetic and had six neonatal deaths in 14 pregnancies, and that in her fourth pregnancy she received insulin and had a perfectly normal child (Hoet 1954; Hoet et al. 1960).

Further cases concerned mothers of children with various skeletal abnormalities who became diabetic six or more years after the births; were discovered to have a high blood glucose level a year after the birth; had an abnormal glucose tolerance on the second day postpartum (McCracken 1965; Kalitzki 1965; Thalhammer et al.

1968). And the same allegations were made much later, viz. that women with children with various defects who had "slightly elevated blood glucose levels" and a family history of type 2 diabetes were "at risk for diabetes" (Van Allen and Myhre 1991; van der Wal and Mulder 1993). [Incidentally the skeletal defects were almost certainly brought to attention by reports of similar abnormalities in children of diabetic women (Lenz and Meier 1964; Kučera 1965; Passarge 1965), discussed below.]

Survey studies having such outcomes were examples of erroneous deductions based on gross underestimate of the background malformation frequency: a report of 3.2% malformations in offspring of prediabetic pregnancies contrasted with 0.5% in nondiabetic pregnancies (Kade and Dietel 1952); 4.0% of "serious" malformations compared with 1.7% in controls (Hagbard 1958)—the latter given the logical veneer that they were probably due to "transient unrecognized diabetes during pregnancy"; and another making the interesting comment that the findings were similar to Hagbard's, about 4%, but only if minor malformations were also considered (Carrington 1960). It should be recognized that the malformation frequencies reported in these prediabetic pregnancies were close to that of major malformations ordinarily noted in the general population (Kalter and Warkany 1983).

Turning things around, other studies examined the frequency of prediabetes (i.e. of the features usually considered indicative of diabetes risk) in mothers of infants with specific malformations or malformations in general. Cardiac defects were found in 20–30% of children with immediate family members with diabetes, but not in any of their mothers, who were considered latent diabetics (Downing and Goldberg 1956a, b). Controls were lacking, whose need was indicated by a study that found no difference in the frequency of diabetes in the relatives of children with and without congenital heart disease (Fraser 1960).

Surveys of infants with various malformations were similarly misleading (López-Quijada and Carrion 1974; Goldman 1976), including a bizarre report claiming that 75% of children with Down syndrome had mothers with evidence of prediabetes (Navarette et al. 1967). Like indication, in the form of increased immunological antagonism to insulin, in otherwise asymptomatic individuals, was seen in many mothers of children with defects (Wilson and Vallance-Owen 1966; Vallance-Owen et al. 1967). In later studies of insulin immunogenicity in pregnant diabetic women and their fetuses higher anti-insulin antibody level was not associated with spontaneous abortion, perinatal death, or major and minor congenital malformation (Mylvaganam et al. 1983).

And last, also deserving mention, were surveys with negative findings. The malformation frequency in children of mothers with abnormal glucose tolerance and control mothers was not significantly different (Wilkerson 1959; Barnes 1961); nor was there a difference between controls and infants of mothers diagnosed as diabetic after 35 years of age and thus prediabetic when pregnant (Neave 1967, 1984).

This chapter can appropriately be closed with a quotation from Hadden (1979): "Untreated asymptomatic diabetes does not often progress to frank diabetes. This… casts some doubt on the whole concept of a pre-diabetic phase…."

Chapter 7
Gestational Diabetes

Gestational diabetes was discovered only 50 years ago—in the sense that it was not until 1961 that it was given a name and became a definite entity. This late emergence onto the stage is surprising, since the condition was noted well over 100 years ago. But its long relegation to the sidelines was understandable because only later did the demanding problems presented by overt diabetes in pregnancy begin to relent and attention allowed to turn elsewhere.

Compensating for this neglect the several following decades saw a surge of interest in it and an outpouring of writings devoted to it. So much so that this minideluge was derided by a long-time worker in this vineyard. Using the then current jargon in a paper that appeared soon after his death he commented, "Studies relating to gestational diabetes constitute a growth industry and the many publications flowing therefrom have done little to clarify our thinking" (Drury 1989). So this chapter will open by asking how this proliferation came about and why clarification had been long frustrated.

What Is Gestational Diabetes?

It had long been known that diabetes and pregnancy could be associated in two ways: pregnancy can occur in a woman who is already diabetic, and diabetes can occur in a woman who is already pregnant. This distinction, then newly recalled, was an important one.

The latter, diabetes appearing or discovered for the first time during pregnancy, the subject here, was given the name gestational diabetes by O'Sullivan (1961). He explained that it referred to an asymptomatic condition signaled by blood glucose concentrations lying between a borderline area at the upper reaches of normality on the one hand and unequivocal diabetes on the other.

[An aside: Before the new name was introduced diabetic pregnancies of pregestational origin not requiring insulin were denoted class A (White 1949). Calling them as such continued after 1961 but less and less so until it was replaced by the new term. Here regardless of how named in the various publications all pregnancies

H. Kalter, *A History of Diabetes in Pregnancy*,
DOI 10.1007/978-94-007-1557-8_7,

that could possibly be identified as such are subsumed into the category gestational diabetes.]

The fundamental necessity for studying this phenomenon was to define normality for the purpose of knowing where to draw the line separating it from that which lay beyond. The primary task—agreement about definition and classification—took time to accomplish, and even later was not fully resolved. But in the beginning there was another problem.

Early Questions

In the beginning there was skepticism that diabetes could have an onset during pregnancy. Though it had been enunciated long before by Duncan (1882), summing up the cases of diabetes associated with pregnancy he had knowledge of, that "diabetes may come on during pregnancy…[and] pregnancy may occur during diabetes." The first of these possibilities was brought to light by about half of them apparently being of intragestational origin.

But questions about this interpretation soon arose. It was suspected that in some instances of diabetes developing during pregnancy it was only its "earliest manifestations [that] were discovered during that condition" (Stengel 1904). Also it was reasoned that when recognized in the first half of pregnancy the diabetes may have existed before it was recognized (Eshner 1907).

It was even proposed that its apparent infrequency was deceptive, the result of failure to detect preexisting mild or inapparent instances (Williams 1909); a contention supported by a collection from the literature of 66 "definite" cases of diabetes in pregnant women, 55 of which were considered to be present before conception and to have persisted afterward. The disbelief, that diabetes frequently arose during pregnancy, stemmed from the difficulty of distinguishing between diabetes and the physiological glycosuria of pregnancy.

Before turning to this glycosuria, which confused early students of diabetes, a brief account must be given of a common feature of the diabetes that first appeared during pregnancy.

Maternal Age in Diabetic Pregnancy

It was reasoned that diabetes in pregnancy was scarce for the most part "because diabetes occurs as a rule at a later period of life than pregnancy usually takes place" (Eshner 1907), or "because the disease usually occurs after menopause" (Williams 1909). Diabetes appearing in later age was already known years before, when Lecorché (1885) remarked that in his experience of 114 cases of diabetes in women 70 of them developed after menses had ceased; and furthermore he described these instances—again with a foresight that would not be advanced upon for several generations—as having [translating as literally as possible] a static manner, an attenuated form, and a slow course; characteristics of what was later recognized as non-insulin dependent type 2 diabetes, in distinction to the type that occurs at younger ages, which is overt and serious.

Glycosuria

This mixture of diabetes types—predating or occurring during pregnancy—was further complicated by questions raised by the phenomenon of glycosuria. It had been shown half a century earlier that appreciable amounts of sugar may be found in the urine of pregnant women (Blot 1856), but the nature of its presence there was uncertain. Various interpretations had been given, some regarding it as indicative of mild diabetes or even presaging worse (Williams 1909), a long continued dire outlook (Allen 1939; Hoet 1954).

One of the lesser sources of the confusion was just semantics. For example, in an article obviously misnamed "glycosuria gravidarum" the symptoms found in this supposed condition included polyuria, great thirst, emaciation, vulvar pruritus, maternal mortality of nearly 50%, frequent fetal and neonatal death, as well of course as sugar in the urine (Ruoff 1903). This list makes it clear that what had been encountered was true diabetes. Nevertheless the author persisted in ignoring the significance of his knowing of relatively few pregnancies with such symptoms.

It was understood that there could be no mistaking the diagnosis of diabetes if the glycosuria was excessive, accompanied by definite diabetic symptoms, or persisted after delivery. But otherwise glycosuria still presented a puzzle, and despite considerable study in the ensuing decades (Eastman 1946) some could still ask at a relatively late date "is it diabetic or non-diabetic?" (viz. King, discussion following Selman 1932).

On the whole, by the mid-1920s, this uncertainty was dissipating. It had been well established that trace amounts of glucose were frequently found in urine during uncomplicated pregnancy (Wiener 1924; Crook 1925; Lambie 1926). And it was accepted that it occurred most often in the absence of elevated blood glucose levels, appeared first during the last trimester of pregnancy, and disappeared abruptly soon after delivery. These features were later further substantiated especially by the use of chromatographic methods (Rowe et al. 1931; Flynn et al. 1953; Davison and Lovedale 1974).

This state has been called nondiabetic mellituria (Marble 1985), a term used as early as 100 or more years ago (Stengel 1904) affirming the realization that it was asymptomatic and unrelated to the disease diabetes. At present there seem to be different opinions about its basis—that it may be due to the markedly increased glucose load presented to the kidneys by the increased renal plasma flow that normally accompanies some pregnancies, or to increased glomerular filtration together with impaired tubular reabsorptive capacity for filtered glucose (Cunningham et al. 1993).

Diabetogenicity of Pregnancy

There is another kind of spontaneous or physiological glycosuria as well. Late in the 19th century it was discovered that glycosuria came about in almost all pregnant women upon ingesting a large amount of carbohydrate (Höst 1925). Study of this artificial state led to finding that it was preceded by hyperglycemia (Ehrenfest 1924).

In the light of this finding it can be appreciated that a blood-glucose test devised some years earlier was soon adapted to the diabetes question. [The oral glucose tolerance test was simultaneously introduced by Hamman and Hirschmann (1917) in the US and by Jacobsen (Lundbaek 1962) in Denmark.]

And at a time when difficulty of differentiating glycosuria from diabetes still lingered it was found that it could be managed by determining the glucose content of blood—whose aid in this diagnosis, it was said in the heartfelt words of another age, "conduces to peace of mind" (Joslin 1923). So that not long thereafter it could be asserted that the ability to make such estimations had eliminated diagnostic uncertainty (Walker 1928).

Side by side with the application of this newly devised tool for the diagnosis and care of pregnant diabetic women were numerous attempts to characterize and quantify blood glucose level during pregnancy in general. Many such efforts were made over the following 20 years or so, but were judged to be "confusing" in their inconsistent findings overall and especially in describing variations at particular times during pregnancy (Cobley and Lancaster 1955). Many critics found no evidence of hyperglycemia in their unselected samples of pregnant women; but did find that blood glucose elevation following glucose ingestion was sometimes delayed in returning to the basal level, especially during the last months of pregnancy.

Earlier signs of disturbed carbohydrate metabolism first appearing during pregnancy and disappearing after delivery were also interpreted as indicating that pregnancy had a diabetogenic effect (Berkeley et al. 1938; see Hagbard 1956 for additional reports of like observations).

Such findings soon led to questions about carbohydrate metabolism during pregnancy. For example Hoet (1954) in reviewing the then current understanding of the "disturbances in carbohydrate metabolism" that can appear during pregnancy, especially late pregnancy, offered the explanation that pregnancy imposed a "functional burden," which was further intensified by a diabetic tendency. To this Jackson (1961) added the qualified concurrence that there was no evidence that normal pregnancy was "diabetogenic," except temporarily when combined with a situation such as prediabetes. This was a twist on his earlier view that increased blood glucose level late in pregnancy was a "warning of prediabetes" (Jackson 1952).

A cautionary note was injected into all this by Burt (1960) who suggested that the unusual glucose tolerance response noted in some pregnant women may have been related to variables introduced by the intestinal absorption of the orally administered glucose. Nevertheless he believed that pregnancy was diabetogenic, at least as expressed by a loss of reactivity to insulin in late pregnancy (Burt 1956), a fact well established later (Cousins 1991a).

The evolution of the disputatious question of the so-called diabetogenicity of normal pregnancy was intertwined with the even more contentious one of prediabetes, which must be returned to briefly. After years of fruitless interpretation of records of earlier pregnancies of women who later developed diabetes it became clear that the widespread belief that so-called prediabetic pregnancies were prone to adverse outcomes was erroneous. But before this became entirely discredited it was discovered almost fortuitously that disturbances of carbohydrate metabolism were common during normal pregnancy.

In time this disturbance—i.e. mild glucose intolerance—was accepted as "part of normal pregnancy" (Freinkel et al. 1985). The question then followed, as these authors framed it, "how intolerant does the pregnant women have to become to be deemed abnormal?" However this excess blood glucose level is defined—which was and apparently has remained undecided (West 1975; O'Sullivan 1980; Schwartz and Brenner 1982; Naylor 1989)—such an excess labels a women as having gestational diabetes.

How common is this gestational diabetes? Depending on the limits assigned to normality it was quite limited, with about 1–5% of unselected pregnant women found to be hyperglycemic during the last half or third of pregnancy (Sepe et al. 1985; Cocilovo 1989; Dornhorst and Beard 1993; Pedula et al. 2009).

Blood Glucose Standards

It was known in the 1940s and 1950s that carbohydrate metabolism is frequently mildly disturbed during pregnancy—the so-called diabetogenic effect of pregnancy—but it was unclear whether the disturbance was not merely a physiological by-product of pregnancy itself.

Thus, as noted above, it remained unclear when the entity gestational diabetes was first discovered, especially since earlier investigators may not have had the same idea in mind as O'Sullivan (1961) had when coining the term. For example, Hurwitz and Jensen (1946) called the diabetes that often began during late pregnancy "true diabetes," though the blood glucose curve in some of their patients returned to normal some time after delivery (Hurwitz and Irving 1937).

It was also noted that the elevation in blood glucose that sometimes occurred after glucose ingestion was present only 2 h afterward (Hurwitz and Jensen 1946); which led to the proposal that high levels be considered diagnostic only if they persisted for 3 h (Hurwitz and Higano 1952). This was an early hint of the complexities that would necessitate the establishment of arbitrary criteria for the diagnosis of this entity.

[Time and again one finds that older studies have been forgotten and that their findings were echoed later as novel revelations. Conspicuous in this respect were unknowing or unacknowledged repetitions of many of the findings described just above, e.g. by Lind et al. 1991.]

A stab at setting up such diagnostic standards was made by O'Sullivan (1961) in the first of his many influential papers. The merit of his approach was that he clearly spelled out what he considered gestational diabetes to consist of, beginning with the subtitle of his paper, "Unsuspected, asymptomatic diabetes in pregnancy." Two criteria for this judgment were specified: first a concentration of blood glucose must be present that "removes it from the borderline areas that are subject to disagreement;" and second as the term indicated, not only must it arise or first be detected during pregnancy, but be "temporary" or "transient," i.e. disappear when pregnancy ended.

That this sort of diabetes was indeed overwhelmingly transitory was shown by a very large proportion of cases reverting to normal soon after delivery (e.g. O'Sullivan 1979). Although postpartum remission was considered a sine qua non (e.g. Hadden 1979; Hare 1989) it will be seen below what difficulties arose with this principle when attempts were made to modify it.

Vagaries of Blood Glucose Level

Since the glucose tolerance test has played so major a role in the story of gestational diabetes what it consisted of and what its shortcomings were must be noted. The need for a clinical test to evaluate carbohydrate tolerance led about 90 years ago to devising such a procedure. Over the years several variations of the test were introduced, most commonly oral and intravenous ones, which vied for acceptability despite both being flawed (Moyer and Womack 1950). In time it was the oral test that became accepted [see earlier and succeeding conferences on gestational diabetes—Metzger et al. (2007).]

Nevertheless the test was controversial and complicated by a number of uncertainties, namely the procedure itself, the criteria for selecting those to be tested, and defining abnormality. Attempts were made to deal with the first, the second though paid much attention was unresolved, and the last remained in dispute.

The Procedure and the Subjects

The purpose of the test was to determine how quickly an induced hyperglycemia was reversed as a gauge of the presence and degree of a disturbed carbohydrate metabolism. It was done by measuring the glucose content of blood first after an overnight fast (the fasting or basal level) and then at several intervals after oral ingestion of a specified amount of glucose.

Many variables influenced the outcome—the length of the fast, the blood component tested, etc. (Schwartz and Brenner 1982; Naylor 1989; Keen 1991; Schmidt et al. 1994; Schwartz et al. 1994), with variable impacts on glucose determination. A standardized procedure for comparison thus became required, leading over time to promulgation of newer versions, especially for some of the more important variables, e.g. the fasting period (Meinert 1972; American Diabetes Association

Workshop-Conference on Gestational Diabetes 1980; Freinkel et al. 1985; Metzger et al. 1991, 2007).

[A poignant moment: "pregnant women are apparently considered to be far less frail today than they once were when it was found impracticable to make the patients report fasting from the night before, as many pregnant women cannot starve long without feeling faint"—Williams and Willis 1929].

(For the numerous details see Diabetic Pregnancy Study Group of the European Association for the Study of Diabetes 1989; Metzger et al. 1991.)

Other significant and less controllable variables concerned the subjects themselves and how they were selected for testing. The earliest selection criteria were the supposed clinical indicators of potential diabetes, adopted with little modification from the expiring concept of prediabetes, with the one addition of a preliminary blood glucose test (Wilkerson and Remein 1957).

Since most of the clinical indicators were of little use in identifying individual pregnant women as at risk for gestational diabetes it was recommended that screening be limited to the most indicative one, the preliminary blood glucose test (O'Sullivan et al. 1973), and this was widely accepted (Carpenter and Coustan 1982; American Diabetes Association 1987; Metzger et al. 1991).

The maternal feature consistently affecting glucose tolerance was age, advance in which was associated with increased frequency of gestational diabetes (O'Sullivan et al. 1973), as it was for glucose intolerance generally (Wilkerson and O'Sullivan 1963; West et al. 1964; Krall 1965; Davison and Lovedale 1974; Harris 1988). Although the association was noted frequently (Macafee and Beischer 1974; Granat et al. 1979; Marquette et al. 1985; McFarland and Case 1985; Coustan et al. 1989; Jacobson and Cousins 1989) it was often confounded by coexistent maternal obesity (Macafee and Beischer 1974), whose separate impact proved difficult to evaluate.

Especially important was the need to give the glucose tolerance test at the time during pregnancy that would identify most gestational diabetics. Important because the blood glucose level varied over the course of pregnancy, generally increasing during the last trimesters (Lind et al. 1973; Merkatz et al. 1980; Jovanovic and Peterson 1985; Benjamin et al. 1986).

Other inherent sources of variability that made identification of those with aberrant blood glucose levels problematic were race, ethnicity, geography, and the like (Hadden 1985; Sepe et al. 1985; Cocilovo 1989; Jacobson and Cousins 1989; Berkowitz et al. 1992), and not least of all emotional factors and other intraindividual variability (West et al. 1964; McDonald et al. 1965; O'Sullivan and Mahan 1966; Campbell et al. 1974; Yudkin et al. 1990; Beischer et al. 1991; Dooley et al. 1991; Harlass et al. 1991; Campbell et al. 1992).

In the end, as O'Sullivan et al. (1973a) confessed, "there is no perfect way of screening for chronic disease entities. Economic, pragmatic, and individual factors are always the final determinants…." Nor has the question as yet been agreed upon of how wide the screening of pregnant women for impaired glucose tolerance or gestational diabetes should be, the underlying difficulties seeming to a neutral observer mostly to do with pragmatic considerations (Jarrett 1993).

The Definition and its Mutations

But the ultimate difficulty was definition. And that was because of the nature of the blood glucose value itself, its range in a random sample of individuals in most populations consisting of a single unbroken array from low to high (O'Sullivan and Mahan 1964; Gaspart 1985; Neilson et al. 1991; Tchobroutsky 1991)—much as was true e.g. of blood pressure (Roccella et al. 1987) and other physiological characteristics. And so no point on this curve could be designated as the absolute border between the upper limit of normality and the lower one of abnormality.

Thus the diagnosis was unclear for any given person with a blood glucose level within the region of this vaguely defined borderland (Stern et al. 1985). As was said years ago, while every diabetic has a high prolonged glucose tolerance curve not every such curve is indicative of diabetes (Mosenthal and Barry 1950), and the same was true of gestational diabetes.

This murkiness meant that the blood glucose level in most supposedly gestational diabetic women lay at the upper end of its normal distribution (Hadden 1975, 1979; Lind 1984; Buchanan 1991). A way of dealing with this question was to partition gestational diabetes into degrees of severity (Beard and Hoet 1982), and seeing whether the frequency of any associated fetal morbidity or mortality was similarly graded. [For many epidemiological aspects of gestational diabetes see Keen 1991; Metzger et al. 2007, among others.]

Soon thereafter, based on evidence of such differences, glucose tolerance response was divided into lesser and greater degrees, the former consisting of levels that could be restored to normal by dietary means alone and the latter a small minority requiring in addition insulin (Pedowitz and Shlevin 1964), which was itself sometimes subdivided according to degree and insulin need (Dolger et al. 1966; Zarowitz and Moltz 1966; Stallone and Ziel 1974; Pedersen 1977, pp. 63 et seq., Mestman 1980; Beard and Hoet 1982; Freinkel et al. 1985). Questions later arose about the benefits and safety of insulin therapy in mild cases of gestational diabetes (Hare 1991; Jarrett 1993).

Still the cardinal feature in the majority of cases was the reversion to normality of glucose tolerance in both forms soon after pregnancy ended. This was the earliest exercise in dividing gestational diabetes into different forms according to expression, severity, natural history, and etiology; and in recommending different courses of medical and obstetric care for each.

After standing for more than 20 years the basic definition began to undergo change. The first sign of discontent dealt with an assortment of terminological questions (Hadden 1979). While accepting the two fundamental attributes of the condition—onset or recognition during pregnancy and reversion to normality afterward—the definition was broadened by allowing the condition to be symptomatic as well as nonsymptomatic (Hadden 1979). Which seemed to me to exaggerate the importance of the few trivial signs that appeared.

This was a minor alteration compared with the modifications introduced next. The summary of American Diabetes Association Workshop-Conference on Gestational Diabetes (1980) omitted what had up to then been considered one of the two hallmarks of the condition—return to normal of the blood glucose level after parturition. No reason was given for this radical change, but the guess may be hazarded that it had a practical basis, namely to obviate the diagnostic quandary that ensued from patients very frequently not returning to be seen by physicians after giving birth. The Second Workshop (1985) went further and made this explicit by adding the phrase "whether or not…the condition persists after pregnancy." (A participant in the meeting told me that the supposition made above was correct: the purpose of the addition was to eliminate having to wait till after the delivery to be sure of the diagnosis.) The Third Workshop retained this version without further change (Metzger et al. 1991). Nor to be overlooked were other down-to-earth reasons: that it would eliminate "obfuscating variables" and facilitate "worldwide standardization" (Freinkel et al. 1986).

It was inevitable that the upshot of these modifications would be to expand the concept of gestational diabetes and thus gather within its folds a heterogeneous assortment of conditions. For example, not surprisingly, very soon after these changes were made the inference was drawn that if the condition did not return to normal after delivery it probably was of the sort that predated pregnancy (Oats and Beischer 1986). And in fact the conferences had anticipated this step by stating that the definition "does not exclude the possibility that the glucose intolerance may have antedated the pregnancy."

Even earlier Lind (1984) had predicted that such loosening of the definition would lead in this direction, permitting inclusion of instances of glucose intolerance etiologically different from that of the majority. These might consist of forms more strictly endogenous and hence more likely to be persistent. Gestational diabetes—if little else about it can be agreed upon—is understood typically to be a disorder of late gestation (Hare 1989). On the other hand examples of the disorder included under the enlarged rubric were those usually first detected early in pregnancy (as was noted long ago by Williams 1909), such as mild glucose intolerance predating pregnancy, unmasked or precocious type 2 or noninsulin-dependent diabetes, and slowly evolving type 1 diabetes (Freinkel et al. 1986; Harris 1988; Buchanan 1991; Hare 1994).

It is a wry comment on the sluggish development of ideas about this phenomenon that some of the same confusion about terminology, classification, and definition that investigators not surprisingly were attempting to sort out 100 years ago seemed still to befuddle their latter-day counterparts. It can only be gratifying that the definitional aggrandizement being promulgated was ignored (e.g. Philipson et al. 1985).

A late American Diabetes Association and World Health Organization definitions of diabetes, which departed from classification based on extent of insulin requirement, recommended a pathogenesis-based one, and continued to insist that the definition did not exclude the possibility that the glucose intolerance may antedate pregnancy (Wareham and O'Rahilly 1998). The present American Diabetes Association statement, as given on the Web, says that "a diagnosis of gestational diabetes (during pregnancy) doesn't mean that you had diabetes before you conceived, or that you will have diabetes after giving birth; a continued ambiguous way of putting it".

The White Classification

The division of gestational diabetes by severity suggested by Pedowitz and Shlevin (1964) was followed by further subgroupings with labels such as classes I and II, A_1 and A_2, A and AB, etc. It was partly such categorization that led to the confusion between the mildest degree of gestational diabetes and the category of minimal abnormality of carbohydrate metabolism that White (1949) in her system of classification called class A. What was this system? Its purpose was to grade the severity of ostensibly overt diabetes according to its chemical, clinical, and pathological features. The mildest degree, called class A, consisted of and was identified by a response to the glucose tolerance test that deviated but slightly from normal and required no insulin and very little or no dietary regulation for its management.

As originally formulated class A, as did all the more severe grades of White's classification, explicitly postulated the existence of the condition in the nonpregnant state. In this respect therefore class A was clearly distinct from the mild, nonsymptomatic condition arising or diagnosed during pregnancy known as gestational diabetes. (What brought nonsymptomatic individuals to White's attention in the first place was never clarified.)

White was able to devise and use such a prepregnancy classification because she worked in the specialized Joslin diabetes clinic, which was attended by patients from very early age and very early in the course of the disease. For example 60.5% of the 525 patients seen at the clinic in 1936–1951 had the disease from childhood or adolescence and 53% of the females were nulliparous (White 1952). Other investigators working most often in public maternity hospitals only saw women who were already pregnant and might not know their prepregnancy status.

This pre- and intrapregnancy distinction was soon blurred or lost since many physicians classified their patients class A even though they may not have known whether they had been diagnosed prior to pregnancy. This confusion was encouraged by White herself since she soon weakened her definition by omitting the prepregnancy stipulation or stating that the condition could be diagnosed before or during pregnancy (White 1952, 1974).

Others failing to recognize the distinction called attention to the increasing frequency of class A among their patients (e.g. Ayromlooi et al. 1977; Corwin 1979; Mølsted-Pedersen 1984; Olofsson et al. 1984a), the increase clearly illustrated by contrasting the 5% of White's (1935) patients of childbearing age with onset of diabetes during pregnancy with Gabbe's (1986) finding that "gestational diabetes… constitutes 90% of all diabetes in pregnancy…." The upshot was a continuing increase in the proportion of pregnant diabetic women who were put in class A; a trend much more prevalent in America than in more conservative Europe.

The blurring of class A and gestational diabetes is unfortunate. In my opinion the distinction was not merely an academic one, because although sharing secondary metabolic features the differences between the two were meaningful. Thus gestational diabetes was a response to the pregnant state regardless of what it may or may not have presaged, whereas class A diabetes was presumably endogenous and independent of pregnancy.

To get out of this sometimes semantic thicket Pedersen (1977, pp. 61, 64) suggested that the term class A be considered a comprehensive one, subsuming all "diabetes of such a mild degree that treatment with insulin was not felt necessary," and thus comprised cases diagnosed before as well as during pregnancy. Even with this there was disagreement. Hadden (1979) in his explication of the classification of asymptomatic pregnancy in diabetes averred that White's class A was not identical with asymptomatic diabetic pregnancy, but did not clearly explain his demurral.

The class A designation has outlived its usefulness. The White system as a whole right from the beginning was felt to be confusing and difficult to apply (Pedersen 1954a; Jones 1956). Because the term gestational diabetes was taken to be equivalent to and used interchangeably with class A (e.g. Gabbe et al. 1977; Mølsted-Pedersen 1984) the former less equivocal expression has largely displaced the latter.

A recent proposal returning it to its original signification may still rescue it. Hare (1989) to ease the confusion categorized class A separately from gestational diabetes, stipulating that it should refer to diet-managed diabetes of pregestational onset. But then Hare (1994) expressed the opinion that the separate categorization of gestational and pregestational diabetes "diminished the utility of class A," based on the fact that since 1980 no class A patient had been seen at the Joslin clinic—because women with pregestational diabetes invariably needed insulin during pregnancy. As for the White scheme generally it too may still be clinically useful e.g. for alerting physicians to the possibility of hypertensive complications and the need for preterm delivery (Greene et al. 1989).

Pregnancy Outcome

The final matter in this chapter, to the arrival of which it has been inexorably leading, deals with the belief—once almost intuitive—that elevated blood glucose levels indicative of gestational diabetes must threaten harm to the conceptus. Initially the most serious of these perceived risks was perinatal death, but this faded away as their prevalence progressively abated (Kalter 1991).

Congenital malformation, also said to result from gestational diabetes, was invalidated from the start. Its story was nevertheless instructive and is detailed below. Other conditions, fetal overgrowth and neonatal hypoglycemia, still frequently occurring despite their satisfactory management (Metzger et al. 1991), are subjects not relevant here (except perhaps cardiomegaly) and are discussed elsewhere in this work.

As for spontaneous abortion, it was never seriously claimed to be associated with gestational diabetes, because it was soon realized that this form of diabetes occurred predominantly in the later months of pregnancy, beyond the time it could be responsible for embryonic loss. A possible exception was class A diabetes, which having a pregestational onset could affect early stages of pregnancy. But it was clearly established that neither was associated with a frequency of spontaneous abortion beyond that expected (Kalter 1987).

The prevailing belief that prediabetes was associated with increased perinatal death and congenitally malformed offspring was unhesitatingly transferred to the newly conceived and poorly defined gestational diabetes (Dandrow and O'Sullivan 1966). It must be recognized that these questions were complicated, first by the diagnostic and terminological variations that were applied over the years to the phenomenon of disturbed carbohydrate metabolism associated with pregnancy; and second by the ubiquitous socioeconomic, demographic, etc. variables often inextricably raveled together with perinatal death and abnormalities of prenatal development (Leck 1972; Chung and Myrianthopoulos 1975a; Saxén 1983; Bakketeig et al. 1984; Kiely 1991).

Even before the term gestational diabetes was invented and interest in the new phenomenon had grown, increased perinatal death was noted in big babies of glucose tolerance-tested women; but without evidence of a relation to abnormal maternal metabolism (Hosemann 1950; Nathanson 1950; Saugstad 1981; Wilcox and Russell 1983). Hoet (1954) even quantified it, saying that "the fetal loss rate progresses from 20 to 50 percent in proportion to the increasing severity of the disordered glucose metabolism."

Routine study had identified many occurrences of diabetes with onset during pregnancy (Hagbard and Svanborg 1960). About half had "transitory" symptoms, i.e. metabolic abnormalities that disappeared after delivery and nursing, while in the remainder, called "permanent," the symptoms persisted and insulin was required. Perinatal death was only noted in passing—the overall frequency was about 41% and little different in the transitory and permanent forms. Although it did not go this far, an early summary of the then sparse class A data confirmed that impression (Kyle 1963).

Surveys of American and European hospital births in the 1950s noted that perinatal death in pregnancies with intragestational onset of diabetes was significantly more frequent than occurred overall, but less than in the births of overtly diabetic women (Kalter 1991).

Substantial improvement in the perinatal death rate in gestational diabetic pregnancy began as early as the 1960s, and soon approached the background level. Its full extent was obscured by underreporting, from which it would appear that these deaths had become of so little concern that their absence or scarcity was not thought important enough to record (e.g. Bacigalupo et al. 1984; Algert et al. 1985; Widness et al. 1985; Kitzmiller et al. 1988; Pastor et al. 1988; Mazze and Krogh 1992; Hod et al. 1996).

What was the reason for this gratifying achievement? Was it, as Beard and Hoet (1982) and many others thought, because of normalization of blood glucose? This is not the impression gotten from the results of a study that found no significant difference in perinatal death between untreated and insulin-treated gestationally diabetic women; which led to the conclusion that hyperglycemia was not the factor responsible for the increased fetal loss in gestational diabetic pregnancy (O'Sullivan et al. 1974a, b). On the other hand perinatal death was scarcer in insulin treated pregnancies than in previously untreated ones of the same women, an example perhaps of a risky comparison with a noncontemporaneous control (Roversi et al. 1975).

Later analyses of untreated and insulin-treated women with glucose intolerance examining the possible benefits of therapy on macrosomia and other persistent undesirable pregnancy outcomes came too late to do the same for perinatal death, since its overall rate had by then become so low (Coustan and Lewis 1978; Kalkhoff 1985; Lurie et al. 1992).

A more probable explanation of the temporal decrease is simply that gestational diabetic women shared in the steadily falling perinatal death rate that pregnant women in general came to enjoy throughout the western world, a view shared by Hadden (1980) and others.

Did Gestational Diabetes Ever Cause Them?

Just as failure to record perinatal death in gestational diabetes may have led to underestimate its frequency later, so it may be that an unsuspected type of selection led to its overestimate earlier.

Older studies of gestational diabetes finding increased perinatal death rate often had as its subjects pregnant women with various risk criteria. Features that had originally been discovered retrospectively through their association with pregnancies anteceding the development of diabetes—in the so-called prediabetic period—and were thus thought to foreshadow its development.

Even after the prediabetes concept was repudiated and these features as presages of the overt disease had become doubtful, they nevertheless were thought to identify women who were candidates for developing diabetes ("potential diabetes," as it was called by Hadden and Harley 1967), and long afterwards continued to be used to select pregnant women for glucose-tolerance testing.

Ironically these supposed foretellers of diabetes were some of the same features that were linked to increased perinatal death in the general population, some as much so today as in the past: maternal age, multiparity, and obesity, repeated stillbirth and neonatal death, and fetal macrosomia (Nathanson 1950; Stevenson et al. 1982 Boyd et al. 1983; Bakketeig et al. 1984; Hansen 1986; Kitzmiller 1986; Cousins 1987; Naeye 1990). And it is just these features that were excessively present in gestational diabetes, and may have contributed to the excessive perinatal death apparently characterizing it. Additionally complicating the situation, certain features—maternal obesity, large babies, abnormal glucose tolerance—were associated with one another (Lund and Weese 1953), as were maternal age and obesity correlated with glucose intolerance (Wilkerson and O'Sullivan 1963; Gillmer et al. 1980; Spellacy et al. 1985).

But the possible consequences of these intertwined features on perinatal death were rarely taken into consideration; and to top it all, the studies rarely included a control.

One group of investigators that did examine them found that maternal weight and age were of undeniable influence (Dandrow and O'Sullivan 1966; O'Sullivan et al. 1966, 1973). The findings were suggestive, but how, at that late date, could such suspicions be tested? Perhaps some circumstantial or even negative bits of evidence might have been useful in this regard. One possibility would have been to compare the pregnancy outcomes of women found to be gestationally diabetic following selection for the supposed risk criteria with those of women of the White class A designation discovered through an overall diabetes program. The former would be expected to be older, heavier, etc. than the latter, and to have experienced more detrimental outcomes. There is no way of proving this supposition however, since such features with regard to class A women were rarely if ever recorded. It happens though that the frequencies of perinatal death in pregnancies of these groups of women in the 1950s and 1960s in America hardly differed (4.2% vs 4.5%), so nothing can be proved one way or another by such comparisons.

Control data, scarce though they were, might have been helpful. During the earlier years of the study of this condition hardly any, appropriate or otherwise, were obtained, and this was little improved over time. Without the critical appraisal enabled by well chosen control material a spurious or overblown relation would go unchallenged. This is especially so because of the close correlation among most of the confounding variables associated with perinatal death. It is especially regrettable that this question was not raised during the years when the considerable mortality frequency prevailed that may have yielded helpful clues.

Fortunately among the reports of diabetes with onset during pregnancy made in the last 50 years or so that considered perinatal death a handful were identified that included control (i.e. nondiabetic) subjects of some sort. They showed that the frequency of perinatal death in the group supposedly at risk was not greater than in the controls. If these studies were representative it may be argued that gestational diabetes never significantly augmented the background level of perinatal death, and that concern with this purported outcome was largely misdirected.

A case might still have been made for this untoward outcome if, as Ales and Santini (1989) remarked, insulin could be shown to have had a rescuing effect, which again would have been most apparent in the earlier years. But this door, too, was shut by the lack of evidence of perinatal death being different in insulin-treated and untreated gestationally diabetic pregnancies.

Gestational Diabetes and Congenital Malformation

An early study of this likelihood surveyed births to gestationally diabetic women (called class A) in Copenhagen in 1926–1965 and found three of 62 congenitally malformed (Mølsted-Pedersen et al. 1964). The abnormalities were not named, nor were they included in a detailed list I obtained soon after the article was published.

Obviously it was lack of such details in most writings that complicated the task of analyzing whether congenital malformations were associated with the maternal condition. The greatest difficulty was the practice of merely stating the number malformed without naming the defects, making it impossible to determine their admissibility as abnormalities considered medically serious, those known as major congenital malformations. A total of 83 articles from 1964–1994 was identified that contain information regarding the occurrence of congenital malformations in gestational diabetes (see Kalter 1998 for a summarization).

The nine that appeared in the 1960s may be taken as illustration. In these 11.4% named and unnamed malformations were noted, a greater frequency than the approximately 3% of major congenital malformations usually found in well-examined newborn children (Kalter and Warkany 1983). Allowing only the ones clearly called major malformations reduced the frequency to the usual background level. The malformations in perinatal death, presenting no such uncertainties, yielded a frequency not significantly different from that in overall perinatal mortalities in that period (Kalter 1991). The frequency in later years continued at about the background level (Sheffied et al. 2002).

Thus the recorded data of over 30 years of almost 9000 offspring of gestational diabetic pregnancies clearly revealed that this form of diabetes did not cause an excess of major congenital malformations. Indeed, if these frequencies are unusual in any way it is that they were on the low side, ranging, in articles in which the malformations were all named, from 1.3 to 2.1%, which probably indicated that the offspring were as a rule not well examined (Kalter 1998). The exceptions, again, were the generally more closely examined perinatal mortalities, whose malformation frequency was about 26 to 33%, closely matching that found in contemporary overall mortalities (Kalter 1991), again supporting the nonassociation with the maternal illness.

I conclude this section with a word about a study that claimed to find a threefold frequency of renal malformations in diabetic women, including those with gestational and type 1 and type 2 diabetes, without discriminting between them, and so was a totally useless effort especially egregious at this late date (Davis et al. 2010),

Carbohydrate Metabolism and Pregnancy Outcome

Concern with the risk of adverse outcomes in gestationally diabetic pregnancy will now be reversed and consideration given to impaired carbohydrate metabolism in pregnancies with these outcomes. Since such metabolic disturbances during pregnancy were considered harbingers of the development of overt diabetes the discussion can be taken as related to the similar one devoted to prediabetes.

It was often found, in the days when the original formulation of the concept of prediabetes was extant, that perinatal death was excessive in previous pregnancies of women who in their then current pregnancies were judged to be gestationally diabetic. But it was ignored that in many cases one of the criteria by which the women were selected for glucose tolerance testing was that they had unexplained stillbirths.

In the latter days of this concept, and even after its demise, an increased frequency of abnormal glucose tolerance was noted in women whose past pregnancies had ended with offspring death. Some deaths had even occurred many years previously and the glucose testing usually done long afterward (e.g. Salzberger and Liban 1975; Sutherland and Fisher 1982). A similar pattern was noted for women delivering congenitally malformed children (Navarrete et al. 1967; López-Quijada and Carrion 1974; Goldman 1976). Only later was it objected that "retrospective analyses of data collected in this way with the object of identifying any association between gestational diabetes and reproductive failure is a temptation to be resisted" (Farmer and Russell 1984) except perhaps when combined with matched controls (Maresh et al. 1989).

It was also noted that congenital malformations were more frequent in offspring of women with elevated blood glucose levels (Farmer et al. 1988). This was not restricted to the diabetic end of the distribution, implying that abnormal blood glucose was a common factor in the etiology of malformations generally. But other studies of this sort yielded no such finding (Weiner 1988; Little et al. 1990; Berkus and Langer 1993); nor were perinatal mortalities or congenital malformations associated with blood glucose level in nondiabetic pregnant women, in studies made to examine the usefulness and practicality of universal glucose tolerance testing (Abell and Beischer 1975; Jacobson and Cousins 1989). And with this another set of ideas bit the dust.

That a recent thorough coverage—as its title indicated—of the consequences to mother and child, of gestational diabetes, devoted not one word to the subject of congenital malformations, must mean that it had been conceded that this form of diabetes was not teratogenic (Kaaja and Rönnemaa 2008).

Finale

This topic must end by asking—as has been done more or less explicitly during the last 20–30 years—whether there was in reality a clinical entity gestational diabetes at all (Jarrett 1981, 1993; Beard and Hoet 1982; Drury 1989), and if it did exist whether it had any of the unfavorable pregnancy outcomes laid at its feet. At its most elemental the argument for there being no such entity held that glucose intolerance first discovered during pregnancy was not a unique phenomenon but was no more than a temporary disturbance of glucose metabolism associated with pregnancy—regardless of whether or not it foretold a noninsulin dependent diabetes.

If this was so can it be that the imputed undesirable effects of gestational diabetes were largely attributable to confounding factors, just as maternal obesity and age were implicated in garden variety impaired glucose tolerance? The points in defense of this possibility were succinctly set forth by Jarrett (1993); but the final word may have been spoken by Harris (1988) who argued that impaired glucose tolerance was no more common in pregnant than in nonpregnant women.

Chapter 8
Pregestational Diabetes Type 2

Now let's now turn to the real thing: diabetes present during pregnancy. This takes three forms. One, gestational diabetes, already mentioned, can be further disregarded. The second, which was and continues to be the main concern of the patient, physician, and investigator, is the insulin dependent variety, called type 1, which will be returned to below.

The third, known as type 2, differs from type 1 in being noninsulin dependent, usually having a mean onset age considerably greater than that of type 1, is often associated wih obesity, occurs excessively in minority ethnic and racial groups, designated indigenous peoples, and most significantly has greatly increased in frequency in recent years (Naqshbandi et al. 2008).

References to this form were mentioned here and there above. In recent years, especially since the advent of the present century, type 2 diabetes for no clearly understood reason seems to have leaped in frequency, often far exceeding that of type 1 diabetes. This has been widespread, happening throughout the world, e.g. Amsterdam, Toronto, New Zealand, Great Britain, and elsewhere (Dabelea et al. 1998; Weijers et al. 1998; Feig and Palda 2002; Holu et al. 2004; Pavkov et al. 2007; Anon. 2009). And, as of old, in the American Indian group the subject here.

It is well to note again the cardinal difference between the two pregestational forms: type 1 is insulin dependent and juvenile in onset; whereas type 2 has varied and heterogeneous features. It is usually noninsulin dependent, is mostly of maturity or adult onset, or was so at least until recently, frequently has an "insidious or asymptomatic onset" thus becoming "manifest over a longer period," is often obesity related, and occurs disproportionately in minority groups and native peoples (Kirk et al. 1985; National Diabetes Data Group 1979; World Health Organization 1985; Dyck et al. 2010).

Especially, "what is clear is that the rapid appearance of type 2 diabetes particularly among…indigenous and developing populations has been precipitated by environmental rather than genetic factors," in essence changes in lifestyle, namely obesity and sedentariness (Tuomilehto et al. 2001b; McDermott et al. 2010); features supported by "parallel epidemics of obesity and type 2 diabetes…." (McIntyre et al. 2009).

H. Kalter, *A History of Diabetes in Pregnancy*,
DOI 10.1007/978-94-007-1557-8_8,

Type 2 Diabetes in Pima Indians

Long before this it was noted that the Pima Indians of the Gila River Indian Community in southern Arizona had at the time the highest known prevalence of noninsulin dependent diabetes in the world (Knowler et al. 1978, 1983). This people were long the best studied of the ethnic and racial groups in which impaired glucose tolerance greatly exceeded the usual 1–5% and in whom the level of noninsulin dependent diabetes was often excessive.

The first striking feature of this "biologically unusual" people (Hadden 1986) was that contrary to the usual unimodal, fairly symmetrical frequency distribution of glucose tolerance levels, in them the distribution was distinctly bimodal, the right-hand curve consisting of values at ages 35 years and above (Rushforth et al. 1971). Also the disease often had a relatively early onset (Knowler et al. 1978), so that abnormalities of glucose tolerance often occurred in pregnant women (Comess et al. 1969). Because of this and because the effects of the condition upon pregnancy outcome were unusual, the findings in the Pima Indians are described in detail.

In 1965–1967 all 237 nonpregnant parous Pima women 25–44 years of age were glucose tolerance tested and found to consist of those who were nondiabetic (< 140 mg/dL plasma glucose), indeterminate (140–159 mg/dL), and diabetic (≥ 160 mg/dL), and to the last group were added 10 previously well-documented diabetic women. The indeterminates were not further considered. Medical records were available for the 1207 prior pregnancies of the diabetic and nondiabetic women exceeding 20 weeks of gestation. Children of the diabetics born before being diagnosed were considered offspring of prediabetic pregnancies and those born afterward offspring of diabetic pregnancies (Comess et al. 1969; Bennett et al. 1979; Pettitt et al. 1980, 1985).

Perinatal death, a subject uppermost in the minds of many investigators in those years, was at first barely alluded to. Aside from the remark that the births included stillbirths and that some of them occurred in the diabetic pregnancies this subject too was not further mentioned. Only in the second report, which appeared 10 years later, were a few more details imparted, rather perfunctorily however (Bennett et al. 1979). It was reported that in 1960–1965 the perinatal death rate was 25% in the diabetic pregnancies, decreasing to 7% in 1970–1975. The possible causes and meaning of this decrease were left unconsidered, except for a statement that implied that no difference in management of the diabetes had been instituted that could account for the improvement. The rate in the nondiabetics in these two spans of years was not stated. Concurrently pregnant women were glucose tolerance tested, mostly in the 3rd trimester, with a perinatal death of 2.6% in those with blood glucose levels of ≥ 140 mg/dL (Pettitt et al. 1985), indicating that it was not unusual.

Congenital malformation was the focus of the earlier reports, to which the matter of mortality was subordinated. It was originally found that the malformation frequency in the offspring of the diabetic pregnancies was about eight times that in those of nondiabetic and prediabetic ones, although the results presented in the second report modified this to about three times; thus indicating that the form of diabetes prevalent in this small population appeared to be teratogenic.

My analyis of these data conflicted with this conclusion. A striking fact concerned the relation of the malformation frequency to maternal age at diabetes onset. Of the total of 13 abnormal children born to the diabetic women nine were among the 42 whose mothers were in the younger onset age group, 15–24 years, while the other four were among the 72 children of the older onset group, a statistically significant difference.

Complementing this, 10 of the abnormal children occurred in the 46 births of the insulin-treated women and the remaining three in the 68 receiving oral glycemic drugs or no treatment, also a significant difference. Thus it is clear that the congenital malformations occurred almost exclusively in the children of a "small subpopulation" (Comess et al. 1969) of diabetic women whose disease had an early onset and in whom it was severe enough to require insulin; a severity also evidenced by the fact that in many of them vascular complications developed during their child-bearing years. Thus although childhood diabetes was apparently rare in these people (Bennett et al. 1979), what was probably a precocious and severe form of insulin dependent diabetes was quite prevalent, and this it seems had the same harmful effects on pregnancy outcome as had been reported for pregestational diabetes in other populations.

There is more however. Most of the detailed results were reported in the initial publication, where it was noted that the nondiabetic, prediabetic, and diabetic women had all together 53 malformed children and that over half of the malformations had been discovered postneonatally. But not stated was the number of the malformed children in each of the three groups diagnosed before leaving the hospital and how many after the neonatal period; crucial facts, as has been emphasized repeatedly here.

It is to be emphasized that comparison and judgment of frequencies of malformations must be limited to those discovered in the first days of life, and those appearing or discovered in later infancy and childhood are to be discounted for this purpose. The reasons for this are outlined in a later chapter. But, since the malformations discovered in the newborn period were not identified, and because the congenital nature of some of the abnormalities is uncertain, it must be questioned whether the offspring had an excess frequency of them.

Finally, attention must be directed to a misinterpreted malformation. One child of a diabetic pregnancy was diagnosed as having a "pattern of anomalies consistent with the sacrococcygeal syndrome reported to be associated with diabetic pregnancies." Yet the table listing the anomalies mentioned no vertebral malformation. Mentioned however were malformed femora, which apparently were equated with sacral dysplasia—in doing which the authors may be forgiven, since they were merely following the lead of a contemporary publication that made the same mistake (Passarge and Lenz 1966), as a recent analysis made evident (Kalter 1993), and as will be further explored below.

The diabetes in Pima Indians of this locality was abundantly studied in later years, but that of congenital malformations and other pregnancy outcomes had not advanced beyond where it left off decades earlier (e.g. Ravussin 1993; Franks et al. 2006; Pavkov et al. 2007, 2008).

Type 2 Diabetes in other Groups

A bimodal blood glucose concentration was also reported in several other noncaucasian ethnic and racial groups (Rosenthal et al. 1985; Dowse et al. 1994), and in some along with a high frequency of noninsulin dependent diabetes during pregnancy (Sicree et al. 1986; Doery et al. 1989; Benjamin et al. 1993; Murphy et al. 1993). Retrospective surveys revealed increased stillbirth rates in some groups (Balkau et al. 1985; Sicree et al. 1986), with the usual difficulties of interpretation; while no untoward or equivocal pregnancy outcome was noted in others with high levels of diabetes during pregnancy (Forsbach et al. 1988; Contreras-Soto et al. 1991; Hollingsworth et al. 1991).

Of interest were the pregnancy outcomes in the diabetic women in these populations, in whom the disease may have reflected the premature appearance of a severe expression of type 2 diabetes. Even the relatively sparse information available gave the impression that in the past women with the condition experienced an excess of stillbirth and neonatal death, though it would be difficult to prove the supposition (e.g. Contreras-Soto et al. 1991). Not so it seems more recently, where in a large Yorkshire district hospital in 1994–2002 Asian women with pregestational diabetes had an increased rate of perinatal death and undescribed malformation, the latter 2.6% in those on insulin before pregnancy and 0.3% in those not, obviously not a serious problem (Verheijen et al. 2006).

Type 2 and Gestational Diabetes

Before taking a look at the recent examples of type 2 diabetes its supposed connection to gestational diabetes should be considered, a connection discussed several times in preceding pages. The question was whether the latter presaged the former, as was recently presumed (Reece 2010). What is clear is that, as was succinctly expressed, there are "parallel epidemics of obesity and type 2 diabetes…." (McIntyre et al. 2009). That is, obesity is a significant feature of both, but whether that is sufficient to make them associated is problematic.

It has almost become a given however that that is so. In some reports outcomes of type 2 and gestational diabetes were so intertwined that the former was considered to include the latter as premonitory of it; so much were they unhesitatingly conflated that interpretation of pregnancy outcome had become impossible (Cundy et al. 2000; Schaefer-Graf et al. 2000).

There was a rash in recent years of literary excavations examining the purported association, as though a new fashion had appeared. Systematic reviews looked into the question by examining the factors in prior gestational diabetes that were associated with the risk for developing type 2 diabetes (Dornhorst and Rossi 1998); the conclusion being that the conversion of the one into the other varied with the length and diligence of the follow up (Kim et al. 2002; Bellamy et al. 2009), the tacit assumption in all this being, to quote an ancient source, post hoc ergo propter hoc. Others have followed the same trodden path (e.g. Baptiste-Roberts et al. 2009; Case et al. 2009; England et al. 2009; Simmons 2009; Langer 2010). We shall see where the trail led, if anywhere.

Type 2 Diabetes in Recent Years

Let's first repeat, type 2 diabetes is a noninsulin dependent form of the disease, and until recently was mostly of later adult onset. Also it is far more prevalent at present than it once was, due it is believed to an epidemic of overweight. It would seem therefore, that largely having an environmental basis, it should be largely preventable. But there is some intrinsic basis for the disease as well, since as seen it occurs more often in some segments of the population than in others, though this was not always explicit.

For example, in an early report from a Los Angeles hospital, offspring of women of undesignated ethnicity with pregestational noninsulin-dependent diabetes had an increased frequency of major and minor congenital malformations, which not being named prevented determining its validity (Towner et al. 1995).

As noted, in recent years type 2 diabetes in pregnancy has unaccountably increased in frequency, especially since the beginning of the new century, calling for an evaluation or reevaluation of its effects on the unborn.

Again, while increasing in prevalence overall it is apparently doing so far more in some groups than in others. For example in Birminghham in 1990–1998 while in whites 8.5% of pregestational pregnancies were type 2, in Indo-Asian groups it was 67.6% (Dunne et al. 2000). A differential seen in other areas of Europe as well (Vangen et al. 2003; Clausen et al. 2005). This disproportion has not always prevailed, as noted below.

The question here is whether the frequency of congenital malformations was increased in offspring of women with this form of diabetes.

This was found to be so in pregestational diabetic pregnancies in 1985–2000 in Auckland, New Zealand, the majority of which were type 2 (most peculiarly, without explanation, almost all were treated with insulin during pregnancy), and occurred predominantly in Maori and Pacific Island peoples, in distinction to the type 1 population which were mostly European (Farrell et al. 2002). The frequency of major congenital malformations was 4.4%, but except for half of the defects being cardiac none was named. A vital piece of information, the number of malformed perinatal deaths, was not stated. [An incidental notation in an earlier publication, regarding perinatal death in type 2 pregnancies in 1985–1997, mentioned that congenital malformations accounted for "only" 10% of the perinatal mortalities (Cundy et al. 2000).] With no discernable justification gestational diabetes was considered to include a subgroup of unrecognized type 2 diabetes, the reason being that newly recognized "they must have" been of that form.

A study of women with type 2 diabetes in 1990–2002 in a West Midlands English area also concluded that malformations were increased (Dunne et al. 2003). In itself unusual, three-quarters of the diabetic women were non-Caucasian, over 90% receiving insulin during pregnancy (once more, difficult to understand of a form of the illness ordinarily said not to require insulin). The outcomes however were presented in toto, not by ethnicity. Spontaneous abortion was 8.8%, not excessive; and perinatal death 4.3%. Information regarding congenital malformations was incomplete, but indicated an increased rate, being 9.9% in all births (the fraction in perinatal death was unstated), 44% of them cardiovascular, some number in perinatal death; others not named, leaving a big question mark. The ultimate question, the individual finding in survivors and nonsurvivors, thus was left unanswered.

Others contested such findings. In type 2 diabetics in Copenhagen in 1996–2001 perinatal death and congenital malformations were not significantly more frequent than in the background population (Clausen et al. 2005). In a nationwide prospective survey in 1986–1988 of noninsulin dependent pregestational diabetic women in several parts of France the spontaneous abortion, perinatal death, and congenital malformation frequencies were unexceptional (Anon. 1991). The overview continued in 2000–2001, with not unusual frequencies of perinatal death, 4.1%, and unnamed major congenital malformations, 3.4% (Boulot et al. 2003), the latter throwing into doubt the assertion of a relation of elevated glycemic status and malformation frequency.

Type 2 pregnancies in maternity units in East Anglia in 1999–2004 had a higher frequency of presumably major malformations than type 1 (12.3% vs 4.4%) as well as of perinatal deaths (6.2% vs 2.8%); the credibility of all this dependent on the details, of which there was a total absence (Roland et al. 2005). One possibly relevant detail was the ethnic difference between women with type 1 and type 2 diabetes: 96% of the former Caucasian, only 58% of the latter were so desgnated. How this may have been related to the malformations was not considered.

Details were sparse in a report of a small number of type 2 diabetic pregnancies in Nice, France in 1999–2002 (Hiéronimus et al. 2004). No sense could be made of the fetal outcome, since only the combined percent of major and minor congenital malformations was reported, with no indication of occurrence in perinatal death.

Type 2 diabetic women in the Netherlands in 1992–2006 were 52% white and 44% non-Dutch, Moroccan and Asian (de Valk et al. 2006). The spontaneous abortion rate was not unusual, 13.6%, perinatal death was within expected bounds, major malformations occurred in 3.5%, again not unusual (a sacral teratoma considered a major defect by the authors was disregarded by me; see Warkany 1971, pp. 1239–1247).

Type 2 pregnancies in 2002–2003 in England, Wales, and Northern Ireland were about one quarter of all diabetic pregnancies, with black, Asian, and other minority groups predominating (Macintosh et al. 2006). Congenital malformations called major were seen in 4.3% of births, almost half of them cardiovascular and neural tube, others unacceptable or of uncertain seriousness. Individual frequency in survivors and mortalities was not noted, precluding analysis. Also many anomalies were diagnosed prenatally, but whether electively aborted was not stated.

A study of type 2 diabetic pregnancies in Norway in 1988–1998 was also negative (Vangen et al. 2003). Of all births during this period 1.8% were of immigrants from North Africa and South Asia, whose outcomes being similar were combined, with perinatal death and congenital malformations not significantly associated; and this was so despite an elevated glycemic level in early pregnancy in the majority of the women.

As these publications have shown, and as an editorial pointed out (Reece and Homko 2005), inconsistencies have been common. The very definition of type 2 diabetes seemed to be unclear, the recent occurrence of the disease at younger ages in itself challenged the notion that it follows gestational diabetes rather than precedes it. The entire concept needs to be rethought.

Chapter 9
Pregestational Diabetes Type 1

We turn now to the form of diabetes that is the main concern of the patient and physician, insulin dependent diabetes of pregestational origin—and to the classifications of diabetes especially devised for diabetes in pregnancy (White 1949, 1965, 1974, 1978; Pedersen and Mølsted-Pedersen 1965; Brudenell 1975). Their main purpose was to attempt to predict fetal hazard, particularly mortality, which being foretold would alert caretakers to institute special management procedures. Other purposes were to afford understanding of the connection between the maternal disease and fetal risk, to allow geographic and temporal comparisons of patient samples, treatment regimens, pregnancy outcomes, etc.

Several schemes were devised. One, used for a time in parts of Great Britain, comprised a simple division—gestational diabetes and established diabetes, i.e. diabetes already present before pregnancy (Brudenell 1975). Another sought to make individualized prognoses of fetal outcome by identifying possible danger signs appearing during pregnancy. Its purpose was to predict and perhaps avert adverse outcomes of pregnancy by recognizing what were named "prognostically bad signs occurring during pregnancy" such as pyelitis, acidosis, and toxemia, as well as "neglecting" women (Pedersen and Mølsted-Pedersen 1965; Pedersen 1977).

Its appropriateness was supported by the three- to fourfold increased perinatal death rate in the infants of women with such signs. Its value was even greater when combined with the White system; the one relying on features preceding pregnancy and the other on those occurring during pregnancy. A major inadequacy was that it did not provide a graded estimate of risk, all the signs seeming to be about equal in indicating deleteriousness (Pedersen and Mølsted-Pedersen 1965). Perhaps for this reason, aside from some Danish and other centers, and that not for too long, it did not find continued favor.

By far the most widely used classification was that dividing diabetes existing before pregnancy into classes of increasing seriousness, according to several criteria (White 1949).

H. Kalter, *A History of Diabetes in Pregnancy*,
DOI 10.1007/978-94-007-1557-8_9,

White Classification

By 1949, when White introduced her scheme for evaluating maternal and especially fetal risk factors in diabetic pregnancy, study of the causes of its persistently high perinatal death rate—little changed over the 27 years since the discovery of insulin—had yielded little understanding of its basis and only vague insight into its prevention. Noting that age of onset of the disease, its duration, and the presence of certain pathological maternal characteristics were often correlated with fetal death, White integrated these features into a classification of seriousness of the disease—a brave attempt to give some order to the struggle of dealing with a major problem.

Strangely the system was first applied, not to gauge its relation to fetal death, but to indicate the doses of sex hormones to be used therapeutically. This oddity was partly remedied not long after, when a continuous decline in perinatal survival with advancing White class was noted (White et al. 1953).

Problems with the White System

Disagreement with the classification soon arose. Pedersen (1954a) found that fetal mortality increased with duration of diabetes, but not with age at onset or with severity of vascular complications, and recommended modifying the White proposal to address these inconsistencies. Also, he was prompted to formulate his own system, mentioned above. Oakley (1953) also disagreed with the White plan, but even more so, since he found that neither age nor duration was associated with fetal mortality.

A more fundamental question was what constituted severity of diabetes; or rather what correlated best with fetal mortality: historical factors and extent of maternal vascular damage, or clinical indicators, represented primarily by insulin dose requirements and difficulty of maintaining control, each view with its supporters (Jones 1956; Dampeer 1958). Pedersen (1952a), advocating the clinical approach, recommended that "alterations in the daily dose of insulin [be] used as a measure of alterations in the severity of diabetes." Jones (1953), finding a poor correlation between the historical and clinical indications, felt that the White grading was an inefficient predictor of fetal loss; but later, although concluding that insulin requirement and fetal loss were related, found the former less important than the historical features and vascular progression of the disease (Jones 1956). Nevertheless, while thought cumbersome, and needing modification to make its use practical, the White system was considered a major advance, and soon had "virtual semiofficial recognition" (Anon. 1954; Jones 1956).

The White System—Prepregnancy Based

Since White worked in a long-established clinic largely devoted to the care of juvenile diabetics from the time of onset of the disease she could assess the condition from an early age. Thus, and because she felt it was "best done" at that time, her system of clinically grading the severity of diabetes was "based upon the pre-pregnancy state…" (White 1949; White et al. 1952, 1953, 1971). Nevertheless, the pregestational basis of her system made for at least two problems: the difficulty of applying the criteria to patients usually not seen till they were already pregnant, and the tendency of investigators in later years to confuse the mildest degree of diabetes of pregestational onset and the usually mild diabetes of intragestational onset.

The system of grading diabetes severity she devised over 60 years ago (White 1949) has stood the test of time well (see Zazworsky et al. 2004). It consisted of steps of increasing degrees of severity, denoted by the letters A–R, according to age at onset, disease duration and severity, and extent of certain vascular and other complications. In time the system underwent several expansions and modifications, outlined below. Insulin was always required in the more serious of the classes, but usually not in the mildest.

This mildest degree, called class A, consisted of a slightly elevated blood glucose concentration, as gauged by the glucose tolerance test, but with fasting concentrations that were normal or near normal and a diabetic state that was asymptomatic. No criteria with respect to age at onset and disease duration applied to this class. Normalization of the glucose level was usually achievable by dietary means alone. The 'condition' may in fact have largely represented the upper end of the normal range of glucose tolerance in the population (Victor 1974; National Diabetes Data Group 1979). One puzzling thing, already alluded to, which to my knowledge was never explained, is why and how a nonpregnant person with a possibly borderline, asymptomatic state would have routinely come to the attention of medical personnel in a diabetes clinic.

Of all the White classes this one has been the most confused and confusing, since views of it and its definition shifted and altered over the years. The essential problem was whether mild glucose intolerance in a nonpregnant woman was to be equated with a similar state in a pregnant woman.

Recognition of the occurrence of mild degrees of glucose intolerance prompted new thinking about a number of things. It helped displace the concept of prediabetes by substituting for it the idea that there was a latent situation the stress of pregnancy could uncover. It followed, if this were so, that all women should be examined to detect this latent state, a prelude to the later advocacy of universal glucose tolerance testing of pregnant women. It also led to the later confusion between pregestational class A diabetes and the gestational form; exemplified by Peel and Oakley's (1949) assertion that "pregnancy in most cases increases the severity of an existing diabetes or, when latent, brings it to light."

Examining the effects on pregnancy outcome in true class A diabetics was made more difficult as the strict definition initially given by White (1949) was increasingly less often adhered to, and class A became ever more commingled with gestational diabetes. However, data that allowed separate examination of their consequences showed that neither of these mild degrees of glucose intolerance had discernible effects on spontaneous abortion or perinatal death (Kalter 1987).

It was noticed early that a small proportion of pregnant class A diabetic women had a fasting hyperglycemia that called for insulin administration. This required the creation of a separate category for this condition and for conditions satisfactorily managed by dietary means alone, the major rationale for which was the possibility that they might carry different prognoses. But so far as offspring were concerned this was not substantiated (see below).

A last word. The White classification was not ironclad. Occasionally the classification of a patient changed, either from pregnancy to pregnancy or during a pregnancy. For example, class A became B if otherwise uncontrollable abnormal blood glucose level occurred necessitating insulin or oral hypoglycemic drug administration.

Insulin Dependent Diabetic Pregnancy

While insulin has been a lifesaver for diabetic individuals, this great medical achievement had innumerable unintended consequences, as historians put it. For young diabetics the paradox was well phrased years ago, when it was said that "the problem of diabetic pregnancy was created by the introduction of the insulin treatment" (Andersson 1950); and "the advent of insulin has given rise to a new problem. The juvenile diabetic who has been helped to survive, mature, and marry and reproduce faces the problem of premature vascular sclerotic changes" (Reis et al. 1950).

These vascular effects formed part of the basis of the White classification, together with insulin need, onset age, and duration considerations. Diabetic women who required insulin were placed in classes B and beyond. The age at onset of the diabetes in these classes progressively decreased and the duration of the disease increased and presented increasingly more severe complications.

Class B features were adult onset (≥20 years), duration of <10 years, and clinical absence of vascular disease; in C and D respectively juvenile (10–19 years) and childhood (<10 years) onset, duration of 10–19 and ≥20 years, and no or minimal evidence of vascular complication; and classes beyond D (mostly F, H, and R) no age and duration criteria, but serious, often advanced stages of renal, coronary, and retinal pathology. (For other details and implications of the classes see, e.g. Kitzmiller et al. 1982 and Hare 1989, 1994.)

This scheme went through several modifications and expansions (White 1965, 1978). Classes C and D were subdivided, the first according to age at onset and disease duration, the second according to type of disease complication. In addition further classes were added to accommodate newer problems, but were not often used, and an older one was discarded (Hare and White 1980). Furthermore, as in time perinatal death decreased, distinctions between classes B, C, and D almost disappeared, and their definitions were sometimes no longer appropriate (Kitzmiller et al. 1981). The revised classification, as it stands presently, was described by Hare (1989, 1994). PubMed has yielded nothing further.

White Class Variation

Do the White classes vary geographically and temporally along with changes in demography and prevalence of insulin dependent diabetes? The reason for the question is to raise the possibility that such variation affected rates of perinatal death and congenital malformation, questions addressed below.

Aside from examining such matters, the inquiry revealed a conspicuous change. This was a shift, which happened very early, in distribution of the classes at the lowest end of the system, as class A was invaded, and it may be said corrupted, by its confusion with the concept of gestational diabetes, as was already mentioned. The upshot of this was an increase in the proportion of cases classified as A as the concept took hold and the practice grew of routinely testing pregnant women for carbohydrate intolerance (Beard 1976). This fashion caught on in America sooner and reached greater heights than in Europe; perhaps because of lack of enthusiasm about this latest American innovation.

In the same way, parts of Europe, particularly Great Britain, at first resisted adopting the White classification as a whole. To return to the question of whether variations occurred in the distribution of the advanced White classes, the distorting effect of class A first had to be discounted. Doing this, if interpretation be dared, seemed to point to there having taken place in Europe a continual increase in average severity of diabetes in pregnancy and in America a plateauing of severity. Can the former possibility be related even remotely to the widely reported growing prevalence of childhood diabetes in Europe and elsewhere (Levy-Marchal and Czernichow 1992; Gale 2002)?

The subjects of spontaneous abortion and perinatal death in White classes B and beyond are discussed below.

Chapter 10
Congenital Malformations—Questions

It is remarkable that prenatal development so seldom goes awry and that babies born malformed are so few. But congenital malformations happen, and with the increasing control of many medical problems of the newborn they emerged into conspicuousness. It is this topic we turn to, asking what are malformations, what causes them, how often do they happen.

What Are Congenital Malformations?

Various terms have been used to denote congenital malformations—congenital abnormality, congenital defect, congenital anomaly, birth defect, the last meant for easy consumption by the general public. Since there is no reason for this multiplicity except elegant variation it is 'congenital malformation' that usually will be used here.

For the purpose of this work attention will predominantly be focused on malformations evident in the first days of life, because that is when most medically serious ones are discovered, and because most reports of malformations in offspring generally, as in those of diabetic pregnancies, concerned neonatal infants. Later appearing or discovered malformations will be considerd below.

Defining malformation is the primary challenge. Broad definitions, such as "abnormalities attributable to faulty development" (McKeown and Record 1960), or "structural defects present at birth" (Warkany 1971), leave their key terms unsettled. Although abnormalities from the submicroscopic to the glaringly gross, strictly speaking, would be admitted by the term structural, in practice semantic quibbles have made for no difficulty, because the malformations predominantly the subject of clinical and epidemiological teratology are those discovered almost entirely by the unassisted eye or with the aid of standard clinical instruments. Such then are the conditions relevant to the subject discussed here; and abnormalities that did not conform to this limitation—molecular, cellular, metabolic, endocrine, functional, etc.—have been discounted.

H. Kalter, *A History of Diabetes in Pregnancy*,
DOI 10.1007/978-94-007-1557-8_10,

The term faulty development can also be reasonably dealt with, by limiting malformations to those resulting from disturbances of development of parts having to do with the laying down, early in prenatal life, of basic embryonic structures and the formation of organ systems. This excludes conditions such as tumors, nevi, angiomata, etc.

Also excluded were two other wide varieties of abnormality. First, because they are relatively common and scarcely of medical significance: minor defects, anatomic variants, trivial blemishes, abnormal biochemical and other functional states; and second, because they are of known or probable etiology exempting them from being attributed to maternal diabetes: defects of chromosomal, genic, and possibly exogenous or complex origin, such as trisomies, chondrodystrophy, cretinism, dwarfism, deafness, mental retardation, etc.

Many aberrant or unusual physical characteristics have their origin during prenatal life. Note that in this sentence the word abnormal to designate deviant was studiously avoided. The terms abnormal and abnormality indicate something beyond or different from normal, and easily told apart from it. But saying what is normal is itself not easily pinned down, because the word normal, presenting a philosophical dilemma, can mean so many things descriptive—regular, standard, usual, ordinary, symmetrical, healthy, common, typical, natural, average, expected, and so on.

The difficulties that grappling with this puzzle can lead to were inadvertently alluded to by a writer who held that "truly discontinuous phenomena in nature are excessively rare, particularly in biology" (Murphy 1966). What he may have meant is that in science the concept of abnormality is pointless since the location along a continuous distribution at which the normal is departed from is indeterminable.

On the contrary, in a critical phase of existence, embryonic life, discontinuities may be common; but be revealed only when developmental processes fail to surpass quantitative thresholds and give rise to outcomes that differ qualitatively from what would have eventuated otherwise (Fraser 1976). These are not outcomes that deviate in shape, dimension, relation, or any other manifestation of degree, or do not lie at the extremity of arrangements of finely shaded, progressively diverging appearances, but are species without link to what they are marked off from. Such phenomena, regardless of how the word is defined, it cannot be denied are abnormal.

But not all of what may be called developmental abnormalities have the same medical import. Thus what abnormal means for the purposes of this work calls for some distinctions to be made between those with different consequences for viability, health, and well being. The distinction most often made is that between what are called serious or major congenital malformations on the one hand and minor or inconsequential defects, aberrations, variants, etc. on the other.

There are good reasons for this distinction. The former are those that have dire consequences, that cause or are associated with embryonic or perinatal death, require surgical or medical care soon after birth, or are gravely physically handicapping. Understandably therefore they have been given much attention by the medical and biological world, as well as the lay public. And because of this they have long and widely been registered and thus form a body of record against which comparison and analysis has been made (Warkany and Kalter 1961; Kalter and Warkany 1983).

These, denoted major congenital malformations, ironically, are among the most frequently occurring of abnormalities of prenatal development, and include a large variety of malformations of numerous systems of the body, central nervous, cardiovascular, orofacial, gastrointestinal, urogenital, skeletal, etc. Parenthetically, considering that many of them, in the days of premodern medicine, were usually lethal or impaired reproduction, what this means as far as evolution is concerned would be an interesting topic for discussion, but not here egligably.

And then there are the many structural aberrancies that depart little from the typical or affect nonvital parts of the body. These, the so-called minor congenital malformations, usually entail only trivial medical or cosmetic impairment. [The instance of Ann Boleyn may be mentioned, one where such a defect, in her case the presence of "a rudimentary sixth finger on her left hand" (Mattingly 1941, p. 246), did not interfere, at first at any rate, with her attractiveness.]

However, saying what is a minor abnormality may not be easy; since, depending on the inclusiveness of the term (and there is little consensus here) and the assiduity of the search for them, the number of such conditions an infant may be discovered to possess can vary from few to many, and the proportion of the newborn population so affected can likewise vary greatly. Examples follow.

In an early foray into this uncharted field unselected newborn infants were examined for 26 different "minor anomalies" and one or more, mostly of the ear and hand, discovered in 14.7% of them; in addition 14.3% had one or more of 14 "normal phenotypic variants," again mostly affecting the ear (e.g. folding over of the upper helix) and face (hemangiomas) (Marden et al. 1964). In another, an expanded search, children not exposed in utero to certain drugs were examined for the presence of 104 unnamed physical features called minor malformations and 42.9% found to have one or more of them (Holmes et al. 1985). Other studies similarly found that some large fraction of infants had such minor physical features, in the absence of associated major congenital malformations (Méhes 1983, 1988; Merlob et al. 1985; Leppig et al. 1987).

Acknowledging the perplexity presented by this *embarras de richesses*, students of these phenomena attempted to put them into perspective by arbitrarily dividing them into those occurring in less and more than some proportion of infants (e.g. 4%), and calling only the less common ones defects, on the reasonable assumption that very common ones could not be "abnormal" (Smith 1971). But because there was no agreement about which features were relevant and meaningful such categorical measures could have hardly held promise of diagnostic or other usefulness (especially since most of them undoutedly were physical or morphometric variants and seldom had the least medical significance). Evaluating their heuristic significance was thus impeded by the absence of agreement as to which of the isolated nonvariants were to be accepted as minor defects and which not (Pinsky 1985; Leppig et al. 1987; Merlob 1994).

These controversial matters were of little concern in this work where it was necessary simply to recognize that there are two categories of congenital abnormalities, one the major congenital malformations, which are the principal focus here, and second the minor anomalies and trivial physical variants, which are considered only in relation to the others.

Studies made from about the middle of the twentieth century to the present will be examined to judge the widely held belief that congenital malformations occur excessively in the children of diabetic women.

Cause and Frequency

Congenital malformations and their causes have been intensively studied and their meaning pondered since these phenomena were first observed by humankind (Saint-Hilaire 1832; Ballantyne 1894; Warkany 1977). Their causation is obviously of great importance to the writing here, being integral to examining their association with diabetic pregnancy. First as to general aspects.

About 3% of newborn infants possess major congenital malformations, as shown by numerous surveys made during the past 70 or more years (e.g. Malpas 1937; McIntosh et al. 1954; Böök and Fraccaro 1956; Leck et al. 1968; Saxén 1973; Regemorter et al. 1984), though Birnbaum (1912) 100 years ago came close. There is in addition a similar proportion with medically relevant but less harmful abnormalities not usually evident until some time after birth (McIntosh et al. 1954; McKeown and Record 1960; Ekelund et al. 1970; Klemetti et al. 1978). If their scope is broadened by relaxing the definition or expanded by follow up it may be as large as the 7.4% noted in one study (Mellin 1966). But in the main only major malformations discovered in the neonatal period are dealt with here, since with very few exceptions that is when offspring of diabetic pregnancies were examined for congenital malformations. So much for their frequency.

As to the causes of major congenital malformations, to make a long story short, comparatively little is known with certainty at the present time, a gloomy assessment to be qualified over these pages. Time has shown their etiology to be multiplex, falling into a diverse catalogue, while yielding a rough order and classification. This consists of five broad categories: single mutant genes; chromosomal aberrations; interactions between hereditary susceptibilities and usually undefined nongenetic factors; discrete environmental factors; and all others—i.e. those still with no unambiguously identified origin. Of these categories a calculation assigned about 7.5% of major malformations to a monogenic basis, 6% to association with chromosomal aberrations, 5% to identified discrete environmental causes, 20% on the basis of various lines of evidence to the combined action of genetic and environmental components—the so-called multifactorial and ecogenetic defects—and the remainder, over 60%, still a terra incognita (Kalter and Warkany 1983); still the situation today well into the twenty first century. These categories will be recalled below, when the association of diabetic pregnancy with congenital malformations will be discussed, since those occurring in the infants of diabetic women that are unequivocally known to be of genic, chromosomal, or nondiabetic environmental origin must be discounted when assessing the association.

While hardly satisfactory this knowledge must be considered a vast leap beyond what was accepted by medical people in the past; when e.g. maternal impressions could be held responsible for deforming infants in utero (Gould and Pyle 1898, p. 81). [A humorous but perhaps semiserious example of this belief occurs in chapter 75 of Melville's Moby-Dick, where a "harelipped" whale is reported with a "fissure…about a foot across," whose mother "during an important interval was sailing down the Peruvian coast, when earthquakes caused the beach to gape." The author at least was rationally deterministic in timing the catastrophic event to an embryologically susceptible interval.]

Despite the general consensus mentioned above, the reported frequency of congenital malformations has varied. Which is not surprising, since in addition to variations of definition their frequency discovered has depended on numerous factors—demographic, environmental, temporal, geographic, surveillance practice and efficiency, observer skill and experience, birth registration and hospital record completeness and accuracy, etc. (Kennedy 1967; Klingberg and Papier 1979; Janerich and Polednak 1983; Leck 1984, 1993; Khoury 1989).

But studies that were aware of such difficulties and applied uniform criteria and ascertainment procedures, as noted, usually found a background rate of major congenital malformations of about 3%, a figure that has not varied in years (Warkany and Kalter 1961; Kalter and Warkany 1983; Rosch and Steinbicker 2003; Sípek et al. 2009).

Death and Malformation

The frequency of malformations in human embryos and fetuses is about six to seven times greater than the approximately 3% seen in newborn children (Sentrakul and Potter 1966; Poland et al. 1981; Shepard et al. 1988, 1989); the difference mostly accounted for by spontaneous abortion of malformed conceptuses (Warkany 1978; Shiota 1993).

The frequency is also greater in perinatal mortality—stillbirth and early neonatal death—than in surviving newborn infants. But while in the survivors it has remained fairly steady since its earliest determination, the relative rate in perinatal mortality has increased steadily over time—owing to the success in preventing many of the other causes of such deaths.

An example of this inverse relation is the contrast between findings of surveys in Vienna in 1934–1953 and in 1981–1983, which found that as the perinatal death rate fell the malformation frequency increased, from 5.6% in the earlier period to 23.4% in the later (Fink 1955; Huber and Reinold 1985). The relation was well supported by a recent comprehensive review of 50 years of hospital-based reports (Kalter 1991).

The trend however was arrested and perhaps reversed in some localities, by the practice first introduced about 40 years ago of aborting pregnancies in which lethal abnormalities were recognized prenatally (Powell-Griner and Woolbright 1990). In one area e.g. nearly half the decline in the perinatal death rate in a 9-year period was due to this practice, with the frequency of perinatal death due to congenital malformations thus declining from 23% at its beginning to 14% at its end (Northern Regional Survey Steering Group 1992).

Stillbirth and neonatal death differed from eachother in this respect however, the malformation frequency having increased over time far less or not at all earlier than later. Since the frequency was similar in both 60 years ago this divergence pointed at least partly to differential success in overcoming the causes or concomitants of death in them. Certain facts pointed to the reason for this, namely clear distinctions between the predominant types of malformations occurring in them, in stillbirths 75–85% being of the central nervous system (mostly failure of neural tube closure), whereas in neonatal deaths the commonest were cardiovascular defects, malformation types carrying very different prognoses for viability and well-being (Kalter 1991, 2007). How these facts impinge on the topic of the association of congenital malformations and diabetic pregnancy will be pursued below.

Chapter 11
Diabetes and Malformation

With the temporal waning of infant mortality, beginning as early as the 1930s and especially the 1940s, congenital malformations received ever more attention. This chapter and subsequent ones address whether malformations in general or certain ones have been more common in the children of diabetic than nondiabetic women. Opinion regarding this question differed however, the evidence being fragmentary, flawed, and ambiguous. Such failings and lack of appreciation of concepts regarding congenital malformations made approach to the question difficult.

Whether both diabetes that antedated pregnancy as well as the form that first occurred during pregnancy posed malformation risk only later became clarified. Earlier, both types of diabetes were considered together in many studies and outcomes of pregnancies were usually not reported separately. Which is understandable since the foremost problem then, the high perinatal death rate, was shared by both types of diabetes.

And finally, also often poorly appreciated at first was the impact numerous features can have on the diagnosis of malformation: infant age at examination, means of diagnosis, inclusion or omission of perinatal deaths, autopsy rate, thoroughness of postmortem examination, interests and experience of investigators, accuracy and completeness of records, representativeness of the pregnant women, etc.

The Prevailing Opinion

Opinion solidified about 60 years ago that the frequency of congenital malformations was increased perhaps threefold or more in the children of insulin dependent pregestationally diabetic women (Hagbard 1956; Gellis and Hsia 1959). And despite isolated demurrals and skepticism (Warkany and Kalter 1961) it has persisted and been widespread (Miller 1956; Farquhar 1959; Rubin and Murphy 1958; Simpson 1978; Neave 1984; Mills and Withiam 1986; Reece and Hobbins 1986; Greene 1989; Cousins 1991b; Landon and Gabbe 1995; Casson et al. 1997; Coustan 1998; Damti and Riskin-Mashiah 2009; Dunne et al. 2009).

H. Kalter, *A History of Diabetes in Pregnancy*,
DOI 10.1007/978-94-007-1557-8_11,

Nevertheless doubts lingered. To try to get a handle on this persistent question numerous matters were examined to determine its basis and credibility. The inquiry mostly hinged on hospital-based reports of the outcome of diabetic pregnancies, but public health and epidemiological records that were possibly pertinent were also considered.

A challenge to the undertaking laid in dealing with the various incommensurables in these publications, especially regarding ascertainment, definition, and diagnosis of congenital malformations. It is of little consolation to read that the struggle of making sense of the records of the past was not rare. For example see Morison's (1971, p. vii) exasperation at similar struggles. "All honest efforts to throw light on historical darkness…have my enthusiastic support. But it has fallen to my lot…to read some of the most tiresome historical literature in existence. Young men seeking academic promotion, old men seeking publicity, neither one nor the other knowing the subject in depth…write worthless articles, and the so-called learned journals are altogether too hospitable to these effusions." Morison was over 80 years old when he wrote and felt free to express himself as he pleased. As candid also was an editor of the British Medical Journal when he said "…much of what is published in peer reviewed journals is of very low quality" (Smith 1994).

Diagnostic Problems

Many of the difficulties of judgment and comparison this writer has had to deal with were present even in more recent studies, but some older ones were perhaps more vexing. The nature and sources of many of these problems were noted by Warkany (1971, pp. 124–125) when he lamented that "there exist many publications that contend that the incidence [of congenital malformations in the offspring of diabetic mothers] is definitely increased, but some of the statements rely on impressions that are not adequately controlled and suffer from lack of clear definition of the term 'congenital malformations.' Some include stillbirths and necropsies; others deal with surviving children. Some conclusions are based on single examinations, others on repeated examinations. It is also probable that infants of diabetic mothers often are more thoroughly examined than the controls. …The continued discussion of teratogenic effects of maternal diabetes illustrates the difficulties of ascertaining maternal factors in the etiology of congenital malformations."

Some commentators, noting these tendencies, explained the wide variation in malformation frequency reported in diabetic pregnancy in earlier decades as follows: some writers "include every trivial abnormality found on clinical examination, whereas others used technical aids to diagnosis or recorded only lethal malformations discovered at autopsy. Some have mentioned only those anomalies which are obvious in the first week whereas others have followed their cases and have added those malformations which were discovered later" Farquhar (1959). Most troubling, as Miller (1956) complained, was the fact that "few reports bother to list the kinds of anomalies encountered."

Clearly, reports that failed to enumerate malformations, or included trivial departures from normality, or commingled findings in newborn and older children, etc. could be of no help in determining whether the frequency of malformations in offspring of diabetic pregnancy was greater than that of serious malformations detected in the neonatal period in the general population. It is such ingredients in the numerous publications whose pages have yielded the data on which this work are based that had to be to judged.

A far-out example may be mentioned. White (1952), summing up her experiences with congenital malformations in the Joslin Clinic in Boston said that "congenital anomalies...have occurred in 80% of the infants of our diabetic mothers...and include defects of the skull and heart, cysts of the kidney, ovary, pancreas, mouth; angioma, syndactylism, claw hand, club foot, web toes, congenital hip, dwarfism, feeblemindedness, and Mongolian idiocy." Questioned as to how these entities had been discovered (Rubin and Murphy 1958), she replied, "Many of the abnormalities had been revealed by subsequent visits of these children, during x-ray examinations, etc. Every deviation from normal has been counted...and included are such slight abnormalities as a nevus, shovel rib, ear nodules and many other things.... The figure was based on a pilot study...conducted not only on the newborn, but on children of diabetic mothers up to age twenty." In Europe too there were such confusing practices. Koller (1953) e.g. not only reported serious malformations found at birth but also conditions dubiously labeled malformations as well as those found at follow-up examination of older children. Even in more recent years egregious examples of the looseness of the definition of congenital malformation are often found in the diabetes literature (Neufeld 1987).

Age at examination was influential. Results were distorted when abnormalities that only became expressed at older ages were reported; or when malformations fatal at younger ones were disregarded. Although extended coverage was perhaps needed for complete ascertainment, in studies made to determine the possible prenatal consequences of a discrete influence like maternal diabetes, it was necessary to set a limit as to the age of children to be examined; and it was most logical that this be the neonatal period.

It is not surprising then that when no uniformity of age of examination was adhered to, the already variable outcomes of potentially prenatally harmful situations were magnified and difficulties of comparison and interpretation made further problematic.

It may have been awareness of this possible source of error that led Hagbard (1956, 1959) to present defects observed in neonates separately from those discovered at later ages. This did not keep him from another fault however, i.e. aggregating the malformations discovered; since only a listing can enable judgment of the acceptability of the defects found. The same fault was committed by Stevenson (1956), who compensated a bit by observing that "an interesting feature of many of these cases is the high incidence of abnormalities of the limbs," anticipating some assertions of the next decade; and also by asking rhetorically why "if a metabolic disturbance does play a part in human development it should be limited to this particular time," i.e. of limb bud development.

By this remark he recognized that defective prenatal development occurred early in gestation, as did others of that generation, e.g. Corner (cited by Miller 1946) and Hagbard (1956), who stated "We are concerned mainly with the first trimester of pregnancy, as most deformities develop during the first 7–8 weeks of embryonic life…." Thus the startling revelation by Mills et al. (1979) that malformations in infants of diabetic women occurred early in gestation had been enunciated generations before. Still, to some such disclosure seemed "almost revolutionary" and again a "veritable revolution in biological thought" (Opitz 1994; discussion in Holmes 1994).

Jones (1952) was an innovator in reporting minor congenital malformations (which to him corresponded to those that were "correctable") separately from those that were severe or incompatible with life. But he did not name any defect, which forestalled insight into his method of classification.

In order to reach the primary goal of evaluating malformation frequency in neonates from diabetic pregnancies the present writer had to disregard reported abnormalities that did not conform to the standard usage of the term major malformation (as explained below) as well as those found later than the neonatal period. A final point, ending this litany of complaints, is to note the rarity over the years of control subjects, matched or not, obligatory for valid judgment of the relevant findings in the offspring of diabetic women.

The foundation of this work, because they comprised the basis of universal comparison, are the congenital malformations called major that: are present at birth, cause or are associated with perinatal death, need surgical intervention for continued life, or are a threat to health and well being. Excluded are malformations with a known or probable cytogenetic, genic, or environmental etiology. Other aspects of this problem are not ignored; minor malformations, as they are called, are discussed and developmental abnormalities discovered upon examining children during post-neonatal months are considered.

Early Observations

It is illuminating to read the earliest reports of the outcome of diabetic pregnancy mentioning a malformed child, and see the difficulties of interpretation they often embodied. This was true from the first one asserting that diabetes is teratogenic, a report of two children with hydrocephalus, one dead late in the neonatal period, the fate of the other uncertain at 10 months of age; but with the return to normality during pregnancy in one of the mothers casting doubt on the correctness of the diagnosis (Lecorché 1885). Remembering furthermore that hydrocephalus has a heterogeneous etiology, frequently arising postnatally as a result of infection or trauma (Russell 1949), the nature of such occurrences was often unclear. There seems not to have been another report of a defect during the pre-insulin years till the birth of a girl in 1922 (Rosenberg 1924). Although described as healthy at birth she died at

13 days of age with a congenital heart defect. Her mother died nine months later in a diabetic coma.

In the first two decades of the insulin era such occurrences were rare, despite the increasing commonness of diabetic pregnancy. In all, seven children with malformations of mothers with diabetes were reported (Gray and Feemster 1926; Nevinny and Schretter 1930; Peckham 1931; Skipper 1933; Hurwitz and Irving 1937; Allen 1939), but the circumstances of many of them were such that today they would not be ascribed to the maternal disease.

Other such observations came from a long-existing Boston diabetes center, the Baker Clinic (afterward the Joslin Clinic). Earlier ones are detailed here; those in later years noted elsewhere. The first report presented findings beginning with the earliest days of the clinic, 1898–1935, from 166 pregnancies of the preinsulin and insulin eras collectively (White 1935). Seven of the children were abnormal, which bore out the author's contention that "congenital defects occur frequently" in these cases. The condition of two of the children is hardly to be attributed to the maternal disease however—one, a "Mongolian idiot," now known to be due to a chromosomal abnormality (Lejeune et al. 1959), and the other, an achondroplasia, not further described, but known today to be largely gene-caused. The others were microcephaly, gastrointestinal atresia, two instances of congenital heart defect, and a "monster." Omitting the first two gives a frequency of 3.0%, corresponding to the one usually reported for the general population (Kalter and Warkany 1983).

There also were seven stillbirths, one with an unnamed abnormality, a frequency, compared perhaps for lack of any better, with congenital defects in stillbirths in a Baltimore hospital in approximately the same years (Dippel 1934); inappropriate for the task however, since the latter were mostly associated with infectious diseases, especially syphilis. A contemporary death-certificate report from that period in Philadelphia recorded a higher rate of malformed stillbirths (Murphy 1939). More to the point were hospital-based perinatal death studies made before 1959, a review of which found that 12.0% of stillbirths and 16.4% of first-week deaths were malformed (Kalter 1991). Thus White's (1935) finding of one abnormal in seven stillbirths is hardly remarkable.

Early publications from the Boston clinic presented the results of successively supplemented pregnancy numbers; the data were not consistent however and must be evaluated individually (White et al. 1939; White and Hunt 1943; White 1949). The first, regarding patients seen in 1936–1939, noted three children with congenital malformations in 35 deliveries—congenital heart defects, hand and foot abnormalities, and isolated bilateral dislocation of the hip.

The last requires a comment. First, to call it congenital, i.e. present at birth, though that is the conventional designation, is incorrect, since it is usually only the slight anomalies that predispose to dislocation that exist prior to birth while the defect itself is probably precipitated by later trauma. Next it is a relatively common defect (a fact known since its recognition by Dupuytren almost 150 years ago), but nevertheless presents diagnostic difficulties. Third it frequently has an appreciable genetic component. And last it very often undergoes spontaneous restitution (Hass 1951; Barlow 1962; Warkany 1971, p. 992 et seq., Anon. 1992; Rosendahl et al.

1992). For all these reasons it cannot be included in the toll of congenital malformations under consideration here as associated with maternal diabetes.

The next report, overlapping the one preceding, encompassed the years 1936–1945, and concerned 125 infants of whom, discounting the three noted above, 17 were said to have congenital anomalies (White and Hunt 1943). Among these were numerous conditions whose designation as malformation can be challenged: pancreatic rests, short tendon, ovarian cysts, angioma, cysts of the mouth, varices of the heart. Others of known etiology ("Mongolian idiocy" and cretinism) or heterogeneous states of unclear origin (dwarfism and mental retardation) the maternal disease cannot be held responsible for. Those more likely qualifying as congenital malformations were kidney cysts, an encephalocele in a child that died after the "second week," and two instances of skull defects not further specified.

The last of the publications, bringing the record to 1949, reported congenital anomalies in six of 439 deliveries, bilateral renal agenesis, anencephalus, "hemorrhagic disease," and the remainder unnamed; in a follow up of the survivors there was said to be a "high incidence of congenital defects most of which have been slight in character…" (White 1949).

The few findings from this clinic can be of little use in determining whether congenital malformations are present excessively in diabetic pregnancy generally. More definitive information started to appear in the 1940s when congenital malformation data began to be more regularly and more informatively presented, especially separately for perinatal death. The latter was in fact the only reliable indication of congenital malformation frequency for diabetic births of that time, since investigators being chiefly concerned with explaining the deaths paid great attention to them and on the contrary seldom mentioned the survivors with regard to malformations at all.

Malformations in Perinatal Death

Analysis of the association of congenital malformations and diabetic pregnancy must take into consideration a most consequential fact, namely that the frequency of perinatal death and the frequency of malformation in perinatal death are inversely related, and thus as the former decreased over time the latter increased—which of course is as true in diabetic pregnancy as in the general population. Because of this fundamental relation the frequency of malformations in perinatally dying infants must be considered separately from that in surviving infants.

It must also be noted that the frequency of congenital malformations in the fatalities is greater than in the survivors. Most past writers did not recognize or ignored this fact, and seldom presented findings in surviving and nonsurviving offspring separately, which obstructed valid examination of the relation of congenital malformations to diabetic pregnancy.

Even so, analysis of malformations in perinatal death may be hampered for a number of reasons: because some stillbirths, at times a significant component of perinatal death, may not be examinable, owing to autolysis following in utero retention (Keeling 1987); because many malformations are not inevitably lethal, especially as their prognosis has improved with medical progress; and because as noted the relative frequency of malformations in perinatal death has increased over time as the overall rate of such deaths has decreased (Kalter 1991); all of which made judgment vis a vis contemporary vital statistics even more necessary. This was true as much years ago, when Hagbard (1961) found the proportion of fetal deaths with malformations had increased from 9% in 1948–1951 to 20% in 1956–1960, as a result of decline in other causes of death.

Studying malformations in perinatal death had several advantages: it provided fuller information, since dead infants were usually autopsied and closely examined; and since most malformations in perinatal death were major ones, questions about major vs minor and other unsettled matters did not intrude. Some authors, especially earlier ones, actually confined the reporting of malformations to those found in mortalities, almost certainly because one of their main focuses was uncovering the causes of the then great perinatal death rate in diabetic pregnancy. In some instances in fact the only congenital malformations mentioned were those found in mortalities (e.g. Clayton 1956; Gellis and Hsia 1959).

Six publications of this sort cited by Miller (1956) reported malformation frequencies of 0–5.7% (including a private communication by Reid reporting 2.4% lethal malformations in infants of diabetic women compared with 0.75% in nondiabetics in the same hospital; a rare instance of such a comparison—even in later years). The significance of Reid's communication was that this 2.4% figure was found in the Joslin Clinic, the same institution in which the 80% frequency mentioned above was noted by White (1952).

Malformations were not always high in many earlier lists of conditions believed to underlie the persistently excessive perinatal death rate in diabetic pregnancy (Henley 1947; Pease et al. 1951), but even so their possible part in contributing to these deaths were matters of some dispute. For example Ronsheim (1933) held that deaths of "monstrosities" were part of the large number of mortalities, while Skipper (1933) equivocated, considering that though there seemed to be an "unusual tendency" for diabetics to have congenitally abnormal children, the facts were too scanty "to allow a definite conclusion to be drawn."

These mixed opinions continued into the next decades, as the following quotations illustrate. "The evidence does not suggest that congenital defects are responsible for the greatly increased mortality rate" (Henley 1947). "…not a single deformity was found" (Hall and Tillman 1951). "Congenital malformations…account for a very small proportion of neonatal deaths" (Pease et al. 1951). "There was no significant inc. Congenital malformations do not play a large part in fetal loss; their role is largely confined to late neonatal death" (Bachman 1952). "The evidence for the increased incidence of congenital abnormalities in infants of diabetic mothers is still unsatisfactory…. In none of these cases could the abnormality be considered to play any part in the death of the infant" (Cardell 1953). "Congenital anomaly was not responsible for an important segment of the fetal loss" (Jones 1958). Others, though they left no memorable quotations, found no malformations in the perinatal death occurring in their series, many of which were probably autopsied (Brandstrup and Okkels 1938; Herrick and Tillman 1938; Potter and Adair 1938; Mengert and Laughlin 1939).

Some bear looking into further. Hall and Tillman (1951) remarked they had not found a single deformity in 104 babies of diabetic women, but 19 perinatal mortalities were not autopsied. Or Palmer and Barnes (1945): "Although congenital defects were greater than normal in the group of living children they were not common...."

The negative impressions were no doubt the result of the high perinatal death rate then current, which obscured the level of malformations in the mortalities. This being the case it took the mortality rate falling in later years to allow this fact to be revealed. As will be seen below.

Stillbirth vs Neonatal Death

During the years when the perinatal death rate in diabetic pregnancy was extraordinarily high there was an intense search for its causes; whose close examination led to finding that the frequency of congenital malformations in stillbirths was about half that in neonatal deaths (partly due perhaps to the disproportionate spontaneous abortion of those with defects of the central nervous system—Kalter 1991).

Shifts occurred with time. From the 1930s to mid 1990s the malformation frequency recorded in stillbirths doubled, despite the substantial decrease in the perinatal death rate, while that in neonatal deaths almost trebled, the differential increasing continuously over the span in a fashion closely inversely related to the death rate. Despite the discrepancy however, the ratio between stillbirth and neonatal death rates remained fairly constant (Kalter 2000, Table 10.1, p. 104). These patterns no doubt reflected differences in the types of malformations usually predominating in stillbirth and neonatal death, those of the central nervous and cardiovascular systems respectively (Kalter 1991).

Diabetic vs Nondiabetic Mortality

The question remained whether the malformation frequency in deaths from diabetic pregnancies, many of which were autopsied and thus presumably closely examined, was greater than in those of pregnancies from nondiabetic women. Since control material was almost never collected, for comparison it was necessary to resort to data from hospital-based general population births in approximately the same stretch of time (Kalter 1991).

The data for the earliest decades showed that the impression of the clinicians of old that malformations in diabetic pregnancies, as reflected by those in mortalities, were not increased was correct. And for the most part the results for recent years continued to show no credible increase. Confirming this was ever more difficult, since perinatal death had so decreased that it was seldom mentioned in later reports.

Resorting thus to perinatal death, even with more complete and accurate account of major congenital malformations, yielded an almost uniformly negative answer to the question whether there was a significant elevation in the level of such phenomena in the children of diabetic women. Have pathology studies of perinatal mortalities from diabetic women confirmed this?

Pathology Studies

Since there was almost complete agreement that malformations played little if any part in the high diabetic perinatal death rate in older decades other explanations were sought for it. Pathology studies later joined clinical efforts, and though they revealed several unusual features they had no more success than the latter; perhaps justifying the skepticism of Baird et al. (1954), who said that numerous autopsies "showed no consistent pathologic change in any organ that could provide convincing explanation of death." Early studies often found pathology of one sort or another, e.g. hypertrophic and hyperplastic fetal pancreatic islet cells (Helwig 1940; Miller and Wilson 1943), thought to be the basis of the frequent transient neonatal hypoglycemia, but not to be directly related to it (Miller and Ross 1940).

The heart was noted to be markedly enlarged (Hurwitz and Irving 1937; Miller and Wilson 1943) in association with neonatal macrosomia, but disproportionately so relative to the increase in other organs (Naeye 1965). The enlargement proved to be transitory, serial x-ray examination showing progressive return of the heart to normality by two months of age or less (Miller and Wilson 1943; Given et al. 1950).

Later it was learned that cardiomegaly and cardiomyopathies were frequent in infants of diabetic women (Wolfe and Way 1977; Russell et al. 2008), and in recent decades received a good deal of attention. Advanced techniques identified the basis of fetal heart overgrowth as a transient hypertrophic subaortic stenosis (Gutgesell et al. 1976), and later more fundamentally as interventricular septal hypertrophy (Gutgesell et al. 1980), an exaggeration of the normally disproportionately thick fetal septum (Weber et al. 1991; Veille et al. 1992). Although the septal hypertrophy was found to be related to the 3rd trimester maternal glycosylated hemoglobin level, and good control of the maternal diabetes to reduce its incidence (Cooper et al. 1992); such management had not always insured its prevention (Rizzo et al. 1991; Weber et al. 1991), much as was true of macrosomia itself (Knight et al. 1983; McCance et al. 1989).

Two further points bear attention: first septal hypertrophy occurred equally in fetuses of women with insulin dependent, type 2, gestational, and class A diabetes (Cooper et al. 1992; Veille et al. 1992; Gandhi et al. 1995), indicating the condition to be a late gestational phenomenon unrelated to any possible consequence of the maternal condition during early gestation; and second septal hypertrophy was sometimes associated with septal defects (Cooper et al. 1992). A much smaller liability to ventricular hypertrophy was seen recently in gestational than type 1 and 2 diabetic pregnancy, altering none of the caveats above (Ullmo et al. 2007).

Considering the gravity in former years of the problem of diabetic perinatal death, it is remarkable that so few autopsy studies looking into its basis appear to have been conducted. A mere handful of reports comprising studies from 1931 to 1978 comprise the record. That they added little to understanding the problem hardly lessens the surprise. But even in what they might have been expected to accomplish—furnish an enlarged and more detailed picture of the morphological state of the dead children than clinical observations could do—they were a disappointment. Approximately the same malformation frequency was noted in the autopsied material as in clinical studies of perinatal mortalities, and as the latter had also shown, the difference from the admittedly sparse controls was not statistically significant.

One extraordinary matter should be pointed out: the malformation frequency in autopsied diabetic mortalities did not increase with time, remaining steady over the years at about 20%, contrary to its steady temporal increase in perinatal death generally; while in the sparse controls in that period it was about the same, at 17.4% (Kalter 2000, Table 10.3, p. 106). This fact may mean that autopsies were made on a selected sample of mortalities from diabetic births; as Farquhar (1965) commented, "the pathologist's population is not a fair sample of that seen at birth by the clinician."

The variety of malformations found was limited, predominantly cardiovascular and urogenital; the unusual one, a symmelia (Driscoll et al. 1960, originally reported by Gellis and Hsia 1959), obviously did not depend on autopsy for its revelation. Within organs, however, there was a wide spectrum of heart defects, a remarkable variety according to Rowland et al. (1973) as tabulated by Rowe et al. (1981, p. 677).

Only a minority of the autopsy studies reported stillbirths and neonatal deaths separately, and in these the proportion of the former was unrealistically small; part of the reason for which no doubt being that many stillbirths were autolyzed and thus poorly examinable; but also probably because neonatal deaths were the uppermost challenge.

A different slant came out of autopsies of nearly 3000 mortalities conducted by Mason Barr (personal communication, 1993). He noted a significantly increased frequency of several malformations in specimens from pregestational diabetic women than in those from nondiabetic women, including central nervous system and genitourinary, but not cardiovascular and skeletal malformations. The individual number of stillbirths and neonatal deaths was not stated however, making it difficult to accept the findings. Many of the specimens had been sent to Barr, presumably unselected for maternal diabetes; but this was made questionable by the greater than usual percentage of cases with pregestational diabetes and frequency of malformations—1.7% and 59.1% respectively.

Malformations in Surviving Infants

The final topic is the frequency of malformations in surviving infants, i.e. liveborn offspring not dying neonatally. The sources from which this information was gathered, in distinction to that from the specialized clinics caring for pregnant diabetic women discussed in the next chapter, were hospitals large and small, located in cities and communities of every size, extracted from over 100 publications. [They are listed individually in the Appendix in Kalter 2000.] Articles reporting survivors and perinatal death collectively were excluded.

The numerous articles that yielded the facts contained in that Appendix formed a relatively small proportion of the literature dealt with in the work in its entirety. These are the comparative few that explicitly reported the occurrence of major malformations in surviving offspring as defined above or from which this fact could be extracted.

The bottom line was that the frequency of major malformations in surviving infants of diabetic women in Europe and America rose from 1.6% in 1930–1949 to 2.2% in 1950–1969, and to 2.9% in 1970-mid '1990s (Kalter 2000, p. 109), comparable to that noted in hospital-based reports of surviving infants in overall populations. Although the comparison was hindered by the dearth of articles in which such information was given or could be ferreted out, and because the comparison required judgment as to which of the sometimes indiscriminately included defects was relevant, nevertheless the likely conclusion once more was that the frequency of congenital malformations is not significantly increased in diabetic pregnancy.

Minor Congenital Malformations

Differences of opinion about the definition, prevalence, and significance of minor congenital malformations and morphological variants continued. Some of these matters were touched on in pages above. The reader interested in fuller details is directed to articles and books especially concerned with these topics (e.g. Méhes 1983; Pinsky 1985; Hod et al. 1992; Merlob 1994). Such considerations impinge on considering whether these conditions occurred more often in the children of diabetic than nondiabetic women.

Aside from their intrinsic interest or importance, of greatest relevance here is a subsidiary role minor malformations have been assigned, that of being indicators or monitors of major prenatal maldevelopment. This possibility was bolstered by finding that unselected children with major defects had more minor ones than normal children (Ekelund et al. 1970; Leppig et al. 1987) and that children exposed in utero to known teratogenic anticonvulsant drugs had more minor defects than those not exposed (Janz 1982; Koch et al. 1992). According to these patterns, if insulin dependent pregestational diabetes is teratogenic infants of diabetic women should have a greater frequency of lesser defects than occurs generally (Pinsky 1985).

A primary obstacle to determining whether this inference follows was the practice of reporting congenital malformations in diabetic births without differentiating between those that are conventionally designated as major and those not so considered. In the section above in which the overall frequency of congenital malformations in diabetic pregnancy was dealt with, in the instances in which the abnormalities were actually named, by my judgment minor and other questionable ones were excluded. One rare example of an author drawing this distinction was Pengally's (1961) noting that patent ductus arteriosus "…can hardly be regarded as an abnormality…." Far more common, e.g. was Connor's (1967) practice of considering a minor deviation, in this instance a vestigial thyroglossal duct, an acceptable malformation and including it with the others found. Of course, only because the abnormalities were listed was it possible to discover this inclusion. In the following analysis, to avoid argument, only reports will be considered in which data for major and minor malformations were explicitly presented separately.

Twenty-seven articles published in the last 40 years of the previous century were identified in which such a separation was made. Only nine of them included a further vital ingredient, a control group, especially important for examining the frequency of minor defects because, compared to the fairly good agreement about what is a major congenital malformation, there is near chaos regarding what is reckoned a minor one. Hence only the inclusion of a comparably examined control with entities equally defined can permit a convincing judgment.

The 27 themselves typified the discord, by taking conditions as falling into this category that varied from narrowly delimited to widely inclusive. And as a result the frequency of whatever was called a minor defect, or any of its congeners, was found to range from 1.3 to 91.0%! The distribution of the percentages was very skewed, with 19 of the 27 finding levels of less than 10%, for a mean of 3.3%. The defects scored in these instances were probably the most obvious ones, those that might be adjudged a major minor.

But only the articles, nine in number, that included controls contributed to the inquiry here. In all but one the diabetic group did not have a statistically significantly larger frequency of minor conditions than the control. In the exception the defects scored (144 'minor physical features') were not individually named, and whether the cases and controls differed in type as well as in frequency was not noted and could not be determined.

In sum, the level of minor defects was not increased in the preponderance of studies of the offspring of diabetic women. So far as the theoretical inference noted above is concerned, with respect to insulin dependent diabetes this result may mean that minor defects do not "serve as reliable measures of intrauterine teratogenicity" (Pinsky 1985), but it was not explained why this might be the case for this category of environmental insult and not for others.

Chapter 12
Malformations and Diabetes

The clinical impression that offspring of women with diabetes have an increased occurrence of congenital malformations has a long history. As far back as 1933 Skipper considered that there was an "unusual tendency for the children of diabetics to show congenital abnormalities," though the evidence—various unrelated abnormalities reported in several publications—was too scanty "to allow definite conclusions to be drawn." Attention given to the subject during the ensuing 60 or more years largely dwelt on surveys of series of hospital-based births of diabetic women; but isolated instances of diabetic women having children with many types of malformations continued to be reported as well.

Of them certain malformations received special attention, namely, caudal dysplasia, caudal regression/sirenomelia, femoral dysplasia, and holoprosencephaly. Reports of the association of these malformations with diabetic pregnancy are considered in this chapter.

A Specific Diabetic Embryopathy

There have been two views regarding malformations in the offspring of diabetic women. One, that they formed no particular pattern but consisted of a cross-section of numerous types of defects, which continues to be the prevailing one (Driscoll 1965; Neave 1967, 1984; Pedersen 1977; Holmes 1992; Weintrob et al. 1996; Correa et al. 2008; Bánhidy et al. 2010).

Second, that as well as an increased frequency of an assortment of malformations the offspring of diabetic women have a disposition to particular syndrome of malformations, a specific diabetic embryopathy, as it was referred to by Lenz and Passarge (1965). [A similar term, embryopathia diabetica, was sometimes applied (Mayer 1952) which merely encompassed the long-recognized newborn features macrosomia, organomegaly, etc., though was later broadened to include congenital malformations generally (Mayer 1964) even as it continued to be used in the original sense (Majewski et al. 1979).]

H. Kalter, *A History of Diabetes in Pregnancy*,
DOI 10.1007/978-94-007-1557-8_12,

The name diabetic embryopathy syndrome was applied to a definite abnormality array, that of the lower limbs, which at first appeared primarily to consist of defects of the leg above the knee (Lenz and Maier 1964; Lenz and Passarge 1965).

This perspective changed when in orthopedic cases sacral defects were found about as frequently as femoral ones; which in turn made a change in the name of the syndrome necessary, from "caudal regression" to "caudal dysplasia," and a redescription, most commonly hypoplasia of the femur, absence of the sacrum and coccyx, or both (Passarge and Lenz 1966).

Then, and finally, a further modification ensued, which excluded femoral defects all together, with the entity considered to be composed only of lower vertebral abnormalities (Lenz and Kučera 1967).

[The prior emphasis on the femur may have stemmed from the deceptive appearance of the legs of individuals with sacral defects. In many of these instances, especially of more extreme examples, the legs were held in what was called the frog-leg position, being rigidly flexed at the hips and hyperextended at the knees. Despite the consequent bizarre appearance of the upper leg the femur was seldom shortened. The lower legs also usually appeared abnormal, but this was due not to their position but to hypoplasia or absence of muscles supplied by the affected spinal nerves, causing atrophy of the calves, giving them a withered look.]

In essence then, the malformations considered to be associated with maternal diabetes were those of the lower vertebral elements only, especially their absence. Inevitably though, what was meant to be a precise term designating a circumscribed anomaly-picture was soon loosened and the concept weakened by tampering and addition of an unrelated spectrum of defects of the caudal axis (e.g. Kaplan 1979; Ullrich 1979; Welch and Aterman 1984).

Frequency of the Proposed Embryopathy

Another matter to be considered is prevalence of the syndrome. It was estimated—guestimated perhaps, since how it was calculated was not stated—that this anomaly-picture occurred in "possibly about 1%" of infants of diabetic women; and further that according to the pooled data of several publications about 16% of all individuals with the picture were born to diabetic women (Passarge and Lenz 1966); figures that were uncritically cited in numerous publications (e.g. Jones 1988, p. 575; Buyse 1990, p. 297).

These conjectures had but a brief shelf life. The first figure was soon revised, in accordance with the analysis the authors made of reports of 48 series of diabetic pregnancies that extended over the previous 30 years, which yielded nine instances of "caudal regression" in 7101 births, i.e. a frequency of 1.27 per 1000 children of diabetic women (Lenz and Kučera 1967; Kučera 1971a). This was 227 times the frequency of the condition reported in all births in Czechoslovakia in 1961–1963 (Kučera and Lenz 1967), but only 4.5 times that in a multicountry control series (Kučera 1971a).

In addition to the many reasons noted by Kučera (1971a) himself to be skeptical of the validity of many of the series he cited, there was one he did not mention, namely the frequent misconception of what caudal regression or caudal dysplasia comprised, erroneous ideas that stemmed from the writings of Duhamel (1961), which will be returned to below.

To give but two examples of such misconceptions, anal atresia and other abnormalities, but not lower vertebral ones, were often labeled caudal regression (Miller 1972; Kubryk et al. 1981; Boutte et al. 1985; Lage et al. 1987; Shanberg and Rosenberg 1989); and even more ludicrously, miscellaneous skeletal abnormalities in a stillbirth and an abortus called the caudal regression syndrome for no more reason it seems than that they were the products of diabetic women (Perrot et al. 1987).

The 16% estimate of affected individuals born to diabetic women was also open to criticism. It was based on the information concerning 72 cases of congenital sacral abnormalities reported in three articles and a personal communication from one of the author (Blumel et al. 1959; Russell and Aitken 1963; Stern et al. 1965). Fifty of the cases had been reported by the first of these authors, but only eight were their own orthopedic patients, the others being learned of through a postal survey mainly of orthopedic surgeons—poorly replied to.

It is important in considering the frequency of these sacral abnormalities to know that most persons with them were first reported by neurosurgeons, urologists, radiologists, and orthopedic surgeons, and seen at ages beyond infancy, since these conditions were seldom diagnosed at birth (Pang and Hoffman 1980; Borrelli et al. 1985; Pang 1993; Van Dyke et al. 1995). For example, of the 56 persons whose ages were noted in the three papers cited in the previous paragraph, only two were neonates (Stern et al. 1965), the ages of the others when diagnosed or examined ranging from 2–41 years. Obviously this means that only the most severe examples of sacral abnormalities were recognized at birth, most instances in the general population of newborns being overlooked. Hence comparison of the prevalence of such defects in these individuals with that in the generally well-examined infants of diabetic women was hardly credible.

Case Reports of the Proposed Association

The association of maternal diabetes and a specific malformation complex was first proposed in the mid-1960s, hence the following overview refers to reports made following that time. In addition, since components of the complex are shared by various other entities, of known and unknown etiology (McKusick 1992, vol. 2, pp. 1028–1030), to lessen the possible heterogeneity of the material the condition in question was limited to sacral absence.

A search of the literature to the end of the last century identified 37 reports of 41 children with sacral absence born to 40 women with diabetes, many with other vertebral and nonskeletal malformations as well (Kalter 1993). Twenty-six of the 40 children whose ages were stated were diagnosed at less than 1 year of age, probably indicating that they were more severely affected than the majority of individuals with this abnormality. This surmise was supported by about 78% of them having total absence of at least the sacral elements of the vertebral column (in contrast with the smaller percentage in the examples reported in surveys of older patients noted below). In part early diagnosis may have been prompted as well by the growing awareness of the condition, which is attested by the increasing volume of such reports: six of the 37 were published in 1968–1969, nine in the 1970s, and 22 from 1980 to the end of the century. Finally, at least 27 of the 40 mothers of the children were insulin dependent diabetic; the status of most of the others was uncertain or not relevant.

Such case reports, even when valid, while possibly adding some details to the picture of the complex, did little to strengthen the connection between it and the disease, characterized as they were by their wholly biased ascertainment. The limitations of case reports for establishing etiology were well outlined by Leck (1993).

With respect to the frequency of the proposed association, the number of such occurrences reported during the final 30 years of the last century was but a minute fraction of those expected according to the estimate of 1.27 per 1000 offspring of diabetic women (Kučera and Lenz 1967). In the US alone, with approximately 113 million births from 1965 through 1995, and a frequency of insulin dependent pregestational diabetic pregnancy of about 5 per 1000 (Chung and Myrianthopoulos 1975a; Mills and Withiam 1986), over 700 such children should have been born to such women in this period. If far fewer were medically reported it may well be due to estimates of its frequency being exaggerated.

Retrospective Surveys of Caudal Dysplasia

The validity of the purported association of caudal dysplasia and maternal diabetes may be tested by determining the strength of the association in individuals brought to medical attention through these abnormalities. In a case-control study this would be attempted retrospectively by comparing the frequency of exposure to the imputed cause in affected persons with that in persons not so affected. Unfortunately it appears that no such comparisons were made, thus one must attempt to judge the question by the available information, namely from reports of individuals with the complex.

To my knowledge 26 reports of two or more instances of this abnormality complex were reported from 1965 to end of the last century, most of which dealt with the orthopedic and urologic problems of 342 patients that stemmed from their vertebral defects.

Most of them were older at examination or diagnosis than the subjects of the case studies noted above, not surprisingly since most of the reports were made by orthopedists, urologists, and radiologists. From which it should follow that more extensive defects were rarer among them, which was so, since less than half of the older patients had complete sacral or lumbosacral absence, compared to over three-quarters of the infants; and also that more of them should have lesser degrees of the defect, also true since about 14% of them had only unilateral absence of sacral elements, i.e. hemisacrum, versus perhaps as few as 3% of the younger cases.

About 15% of the patients for whom such information was presented had diabetic mothers, but for most the form of the diabetes and time of onset were not made clear. It must be recalled that it was only after 1965 that the supposed association of maternal diabetes and caudal abnormalities became known and accepted as fact. This cannot be discounted as a biasing factor in directing attention to this possible, and sometimes misunderstood, association; as when, e.g. gestational diabetes, so-called prediabetes, noninsulin dependent diabetes, or even a family history of diabetes was sometimes thought apropos (Banta and Nichols 1969; Sarnat et al. 1976; Mariani et al. 1979; Pang and Hoffman 1980). These data fell short of supporting the suggestion that caudal dysplasia and pregestational diabetes were associated.

A recent report it would seem supported a more positive view (Bruce et al. 2009). The subjects were nine prenatally diagnosed instances—abortuses and perinatal mortalities—of what was called the caudal dysplasia syndrome, discovered by searching surgical pathology and autopsy files in the Jackson Memorial Hospital, Miami, FL, from 1991 to 2006. Six of the nine had pregestational insulin-dependent diabetic mothers, a seventh a pregestational noninsulin dependent mother. Three of the six were abortuses (whether spontaneous was unstated), the other three perinatal mortalities. One of the three abortuses had an absent lower spine, as did two of the three perinatal mortalities. Two facts are obvious. The anomalies were lethal; also they were rare, the three reported instances of the syndrome occurring to diabetic women in the approximately half million births in the region in that period.

Other apparent instances of the syndrome were seen in infants of women with gestational and pregestational diabetes, whether insulin dependent not stated (Makhoul et al. 2001; Versiani et al. 2004), the former making the association suspect.

The Caudal Regression Syndrome

Now we return to consider the nature of the term "syndrome of caudal regression," as formulated by Duhamel (1959, 1961), and its evolution as it took on additional layers of meaning and came to be applied to the proposed diabetic embryopathy. Two issues are intertwined here. The first concerns the original concept, namely that there existed a complex of progressively more severe interrelated congenital malformations, the syndrome of caudal regression, and second that one of the features of this syndrome, lower vertebral absence, was increased in frequency in diabetic pregnancy.

Duhamel postulated the complex to consist of a graded series of malformations—limb, urogenital, anorectal, and lumbosacral—of increasing severity, extending from defects of the anal region at the mildest to symmelia (or sirenomelia) at the most extreme. The scheme was based on (a) clinical observations of the frequent association of such malformations in nonsymmelic individuals; and (b) experiments with chicken embryos that apparently supported the idea that the comprehensive syndrome stemmed from variably localized defects in the formation of the caudal region (Wolff 1948, pp. 165–170).

It was Duhamel's theory (formulated incidentally without reference to maternal diabetes) that formed the basis of Passarge and Lenz's (1966) suggestion that "minor malformations of the caudal region of the body [as seen in their cases]...were related to symmelia and sireniform monsters in a teratogenic spectrum which may include anorectal and urogenital anomalies," and hence that their cases possibly were examples of the caudal regression complex enunciated by Duhamel.

The suggestion that symmelia is sacral regression carried to its utmost degree (Passarge and Lenz 1966), later widely accepted (e.g. Källén and Winberg 1974; Kaplan 1979; Källén et al. 1992) and even equated with it (e.g. Schwartz et al. 1982), coupled with the supposition that sacral defects were associated with diabetic pregnancy, if taken to its logical conclusion led to the inference that symmelia too must be associated with maternal diabetes. This idea will be explored right after the symmelia complex itself is considered.

The Symmelia Syndrome

The existence of a sirenoid complex was accepted with little reservation. For example O'Rahilly and Müller (1989) wrote that "in less extreme forms, the caudal regression syndrome consists of sacral agenesis or merely imperforate anus." In their discussion of the developmental mechanisms of median anomalies these authors seconded an older theoretical scheme (Feller and Sternberg 1931), which ascribed the features of this complex to the extent of a median defect in the caudal region of the early embryo, narrower and shallower defects being associated mostly with vertebral abnormalities and broader and deeper ones with symmelia, etc.

In an extended critique of this theory (briefly summarized here) Gruenwald (1947) noted several difficulties with it. First, in Wolff's (1948) radiation experiments with chicken embryos the initiating cause of the symmelia was localized destruction of prospective axial organs, which was not the mechanism initially proposed for the origin of human symmelia (Kampmeier 1927), nor was it of any of the mechanisms since proposed (David and Fein 1974; Chappard et al. 1983; Stevenson et al. 1986). Second, the theory required that the defects (a) be determined in early stages (according to O'Rahilly and Müller 1989; by stage 11, i.e. about 24 days postovulatory); and (b) their extent and respective locations be unchanging in time—in other words that the parts concerned develop independently of one another. But such implied mosaicism, i.e. development without correlation of parts, is contrary to what was known about the interdependence of tissues and organ primordia in the early embryo (Hamburger 1988).

For these reasons it is doubtful that the several components of the symmelia complex can be due to variability in the extent of the putative initial caudal fault, and hence that any one or more of them by themselves represented intermediate degrees of the so-called symmelic syndrome.

Are Symmelia and Maternal Diabetes Associated?

In support of the claimed connection between caudal dysplasia and maternal diabetes, and the almost axiomatic contention that lower vertebral abnormalities and symmelia were lesser and greater forms respectively of one and the same syndrome of caudal regression, it was proposed that symmelia was also associated with maternal diabetes (Passarge and Lenz 1966). On the basis of the following facts this proposition cannot be accepted.

A search of sources from the mid-1960s to the beginning of the present century yielded 76 reports (plus personal communications) of 163 symmelic fetuses and infants (including a concordant twin and a sib pair). In 117 of the 120 accounts of pregnancies in which information regarding maternal health or the course of pregnancy was noted it was made clear or highly probable that none of the mothers had pregestational insulin dependent diabetes; and in the other three one mother had gestational and two had type 2 diabetes (Stocker and Heifetz 1987; Martin et al. 1990; Gürakan et al. 1996). [Most recently it was noted additionally that none of six instances of symmelia prenatally diagnosed in 1991–2006 occurred in infants of diabetic mothers (Bruce et al. 2009)]. Looking further back, of 28 symmelics reported in 1927–1964 (Stocker and Heifetz 1987) apparently only one had a known diabetic mother, who however was not clearly insulin dependent, and another a mother who had received insulin shock therapy for emotional illness.

Considering only the more recent cases with known maternal health status, and using the mean of several estimates of the prevalence of symmelia of 1.37 per 100,000 (Butler and Bonham 1963; Stevenson et al. 1966; Leck et al. 1968; Källén and Winberg 1974), the cases represent approximately 8.5 million births. Taking 5 per 1000 once again as the approximate frequency of pregestational diabetic pregnancy, among this number of total births over 42,000 should have occurred to diabetic women of this type. The apparent rarity of reports of symmelia in these diabetic births indicated that its relation to diabetes is minuscule or nonexistent. A nonrelatedness further indicated by the dissimilarity of the supposed pathogenesis of the two conditions (Jones 1988) as well as by various morphological considerations (Colwell et al. 1991).

Finally, in the innumerable articles published since the 1920s read by this author concerned with thousands of pregnancies of diabetic women, five instances of symmelia were reported, in three hospital-based and two population-based series (Gellis and Hsia 1959; Kučera 1971a; Steel et al. 1982; Vadheim 1983; Becerra et al. 1990), not all for certain occurring in offspring of indisputably pregestational insulin dependent diabetic women.

Femoral Dysplasia and Diabetes

Following the initial claim of the existence of a specific diabetic embryopathy (Lenz and Maier 1964) a large miscellany of isolated instances of congenital malformations and anomalies was alleged to be associated with maternal diabetes. Some of these defects, discussed here and below, were reported often enough to merit some attention.

In the light of hindsight it is ironic that the deformities of the very first infants considered to form a "special spectrum" (Lenz and Maier 1964; Passarge 1965) were not those that later came to represent the typical diabetic embryopathy. As was noted above, the first cases reported had femoral abnormalities, not the sacral ones that later came to be regarded as the hallmark of the anomaly-picture.

It is probable that Passarge's (1965) case was actually an example of a separate entity, one that has also been alleged to occur nonrandomly in infants of diabetic women. This infant, in addition to short femurs, had a pronounced cleft palate, micrognathia, and glossoptosis—i.e. the Pierre Robin syndrome (a photograph of this infant appears on p. 999 in Warkany's 1971 *vade mecum*), and hence is included among the cases with facial abnormalities considered below.

With respect to the femoral defect itself—known especially to orthopedists as proximal femoral focal deficiency (Ring 1961)—from 1965 to the end of the century, depending on definition, perhaps 18 alleged instances of the condition were reported. As with caudal dysplasia these cases were ascertained in various ways. They too will be discussed further below.

Facial and Femoral Abnormalitites

In another early report a child, described by Lenz and Maier (1964), with femoral and other long-bone abnormalities, was incidentally also noted to have "a remarkably long upper lip [and] a cleft palate…." (Kučera et al. 1965). A photograph showed that the child had an 'odd-appearing' face, not specifically alluded to. This child and its features were later recalled by Daentl et al. (1975), and together with further instances of this combination of femoral defects and unusual facial features (long philtrum, thin upper lip, short nose with a broad tip, etc.) were offered as representing a newly recognized entity, named the femoral hypoplasia-unusual facies syndrome. Up to the end of the century 42 instances or purported instances of this syndrome were reported. All were single cases of infants or young children, apparently ascertained through their malformations, by pediatricians and clinical geneticists. What makes this and the femoral dysplasia syndromes relevant here was the presence of diabetes in the mothers of some of the cases. This aspect will be considered below. [Incidentally, PubMed listed eight reports of single cases apparently of this syndrome since publication of the first edition of this book (Kalter 2000), in which various etiologies were postulated, but maternal diabetes in only one and that of uncertain form.]

Are These Different Syndromes?

The distinctiveness of the femoral dysplasia and femoral hypoplasia-unusual facies syndromes was also in doubt, many of their facial and other features overlapping, so that if they were different entities what demarcated them was unclear. Thereupon a tangled web was woven, and untangling it was hardly worth a try, but here goes.

What was perhaps the clue was the unusual facial features in the syndrome so named. These consisted of two different assortments of defects, one morphometric labeling a face as unusual, and the other of ordinary malformations—cleft palate and micrognathia. Both presented problems: the first because it was open to arbitrary judgment and because of its possible transience, and the second because the defects were frequently present in both syndromes.

There were differences of opinion about diagnosis. In the original delineation of the femoral hypoplasia-unusual facies syndrome all cases—not surprisingly—unequivocally shared the facial features (Daentl et al. 1975). But opinion was then divided, some felt that two of the original cases may not have had the syndrome; others questioned whether it had a separate identity, and even doubted that such an entity existed, on the contrary that the supposed unusual facial features were typical of the Pierre Robin syndrome (Eastman and Escobar 1978; Graviss et al. 1980; Maisels and Stilwell 1980; Lord and Beighton 1981; Johnson et al. 1983).

The orofacial malformations were also disagreed about. Those in the Pierre Robin syndrome, it was said, comprised a distinct entity, even when associated with femoral dysplasia, while also merely being considered additional components of the femoral hypoplasia-unusual facies syndrome. In any case cleft palate appeared of little use in differentiating the two syndromes (Walden et al. 1971; Holthusen 1972; Graviss et al. 1980; Maisels and Stilwell 1980; Hurst and Johnson 1980; Burck et al. 1981; Pitt et al. 1982; Johnson et al. 1983).

It seemed best therefore to consider these two supposedly distinct entities as one in getting to the nub of the question: their imputed association with maternal diabetes. Together, at the time, they amounted to 58 isolated cases of femoral dysplasia with or without facial anomalies. Eighteen had diabetic mothers: 12 insulin dependent (11 pregestational, one of uncertain onset time), two noninsulin dependent, three gestational, and one described merely as "diabetic." Thirty of the cases had cleft palate, but its conjunction with maternal insulin-dependent diabetes was not statistically significant. Ultimately however the question was clouded by biased ascertainment.

Some help was perhaps offered by the absence of diabetes in the mothers of 186 patients with the femoral defect, usually without the facial abnormalities, in three orthopedic surveys of affected individuals (Hamanishi 1980; Koman et al. 1982; Kalamchi et al. 1985). All in all, much detail and analysis, leading to little.

To return to reality a glance at PubMed found the subject, for better or worse, not yet expired, with 34 citations dated from 1986 to 2009, eight from 2001 and later; the latest still admitting that its "etiology…is unknown" (Figueroa et al. 2009).

Other Malformations

An assortment of congenital abnormalities not associated with vertebral defects was noted in infants of diabetic women in the later years of the twentieth century. Most were without merit and are ignored. One may be mentioned, neonatal small left colon syndrome, a transient functional intestinal obstruction, a report of which (Davis et al. 1974) led to further such discoveries (Davis et al. 1975; Berdon et al. 1977)—a suspect route of recognition, of course.

Similarly, notification of holoprosencephaly in two infants of diabetic women (Barr and Burdi 1978) led to recognizing five further instances of the association with one or another of the various forms of the defect. But were dubious, since one lacked the brain morphology typical of the condition and two others its usual facial features, in fact with various abnormalities unrelated to the supposed diagnosis. Further recognition of the association followed, namely, personal communication of nine other such occurrences. And last, three additional instances (including two of the seven noted above) identified through retrospective surveys of 189 diabetic deliveries at two medical centers, in sum suggesting a frequency of at least 1% for this condition in the infants of diabetic women.

As Barr et al. (1983) carefully pointed out, the evidence for the suggestion came solely from tertiary-level referral hospitals, and was thus open to the various biases residing in information from such sources. Therefore, the tacit assumption that their estimate of the frequency of the condition in diabetic pregnancy was greater than that in the general population presented problems from the start. Several variables affecting the prevalence of the condition at birth (Cohen 1989) further clouded this proposal.

Findings in genetic and abortion studies of holoprosencephaly may be noted. In 30 families of 32 patients two mothers were juvenile diabetics, and their children had less severe forms of the condition (Roach et al. 1975). Chromosomes were not examined, but neither case was considered of karyotypic origin. In a second study the mothers of 150 induced abortuses with holoprosencephaly had diseases of various sorts no more commonly than did matched controls (Matsunaga and Shiota 1977).

Population surveys of holoprosencephaly suddenly became popular in the mid-1990s, 381 occurrences with frequencies of 0.5–1.2 (mean 0.7) per 10,000 live- and stillbirths being reported. The most recent estimate, derived from a population-based register of congenital malformations in 1985–1998 in the north of England, found a prevalence including pregnancy terminations of 1.2 per 10,000 registered births (Bullen et al. 2001).

The available information regarding its associaton with insulin dependent diabetes indicated a frequency of 19 per 1000, much larger than the usual overall population level. But since holoprosencephaly has a heterogeneous etiology—chromosomal, syndromic, monogenic, nongenetic, etc.—without further information the purported association remained unresolved (Martínez-Frías et al. 1994; Croen et al. 1996; Rasmussen et al. 1996; Whiteford and Tolmie 1996; Olsen et al. 1997).

Bringing the record up to date, a search of PubMed from 2000 to mid-2010 dredged up the astonishing number of 701 citations in which the term holoprosencephaly was mentioned, of which possibly three noted unspecified diabetes as a risk factor (e.g. Croen et al. 2000).

To round out the discussion we note that the condition known as holoprosencephaly is in fact a general term for a series of progressively more severe median abnormalities of the face and fore- and midbrain (DeMyer et al. 1964). As the term cyclocephaly, originally proposed by Saint-Hilaire (1832–1837, vol. 2 pp. 423–24), intimated, the series of defects culminated in cyclopia, which displayed a single or partially divided median eye in one orbit and a large anterior cerebral cavity (see Kalter 1968 for an illustration of a cyclopic horse published by Orr 1888).

Which leads to this proposition: If cyclopia was the extreme expression of holoprosencephaly, as symmelia was said to be that of the caudal regression syndrome, and if holoprosencephaly, as claimed, was associated with maternal diabetes, it followed that cyclopia should also be so associated. Population surveys of the condition might be helpful with this question. Cyclopia, like symmelia, is rare. An overview of more than 10 million births in various countries since 1965 revealed perhaps 121 instances of cyclopia, for an estimate of about 1.2 per 100,000 (Källén et al. 1992). Later, more precise estimates reported a total of 28 cases in slightly over 4 million births, giving a mean frequency of 0.69 per 100,000 live- and stillbirths (Croen et al. 1996; Rasmussen et al. 1996; Whiteford and Tolmie 1996; Olsen et al. 1997). The condition of the mothers of these cases unfortunately was not stated. The earlier survey (Källén et al. 1992) found that in four of the occurrences maternal diabetes was recorded; but absence of information about the specific maternal disease made this number unhelpful. Skepticism is supported by the rarity of cyclopia in diabetic pregnancies in hospital-based reports; only four were discovered in articles published from the 1920s to the present: one in births at the King's College Hospital in London during 1951–1960 (Seligman 1963), one in 1950–1984 in the maternity hospitals of Dublin (Drury 1966), and two from India, whose mothers, said to be diabetic, turned out to be a gestational and a noninsulin dependent diabetic (Soni et al. 1989).

Conclusion

In evaluating the alleged association of malformations and diabetes, especially as made through case reports, it is obviously pertinent to recall that both congenital malformations and diabetes are common human afflictions. The relatively great frequency of the former has been mentioned often above (Kalter and Warkany 1983) and diabetes too is hardly less prevalent (Harris et al. 1987). Considering these facts, as well as the largely biased nature of the conduct of the majority of the case studies outlined above, it must be concluded, being extravagantly generous, that the evidence at most but barely suggested a causal relation between maternal diabetes and the various congenital malformations the condition has been alleged to be associated with.

Finally it must be said that association of specific congenital malformation patterns with maternal diabetes, as surely must be recognized intuitively, cannot be established by isolated reports of their concurrence. It is only by careful analysis of well-described surveys of unselected diabetic pregnancies, supported by meticulously conducted epidemiological efforts, that definitive conclusions regarding claims that they are causally related may perhaps be arrived at.

Chapter 13
Diabetes Center Studies

It will be useful in probing questions regarding diabetic pregnancy and its outcomes to review the activities of the most prominent of the US and European medical centers devoted to them, in order to look into the questions of interpretation and analysis.

The Joslin Diabetes Center

The first facility for the study and care of diabetic individuals, and still active today, was the Joslin Diabetes Center in Boston (originally named the Baker Clinic). By 1915, after 17 years, Dr. Elliott P. Joslin had treated about 650 severely affected female patients, of whom only 10 had become pregnant. This infertility greatly improved with the introduction of insulin. By the 1950s over 1000 viable diabetic pregnancies had been followed in the clinic, which by 1978 had reached 2307 (White 1978).

In an early summary of the outcome of the 125 consecutive completed diabetic pregnancies in 1936–1942, 115 of which occurred in women whose disease predated the index pregnancy, 20 infants were reported with "congenital anomalies" (White and Hunt 1943). This high frequency, of over 17%, as already noted, was clearly the result of including ineligible items, such as "cretinism, feeble mindedness, and Mongolian idiocy;" a figure later augmented to an unrealistic 80% by including every conceivable defective state found at various ages of childhood (White 1952), as confirmed in White's interview with Rubin and Murphy (1958) noted above.

In the publication introducing her convenient scheme for grading diabetic patients according to the prepregnancy state of the disease, White (1949) reported 439 pregnancies personally observed during the preceding 15 years. Since the clinic was a referral center it is not surprising that the great majority (95%) had insulin-requiring severe grades of diabetes. In this report however only the congenital defects found in the 78 perinatal mortalities (17.8% of those born) were reported, 2.9% in the stillbirths and 16.0% in the neonatal deaths.

H. Kalter, *A History of Diabetes in Pregnancy*,
DOI 10.1007/978-94-007-1557-8_13,

The next report of relevance was published 10 years later (Gellis and Hsia 1959), but mentioned only the congenital malformations associated with the neonatal deaths, 12.5% of 104, somewhat less than was found earlier. The deaths were autopsied and the malformations listed (Driscoll et al. 1960).

A later account provided some general data, but still had various gaps (Hubbell et al. 1965). It dealt with 504 pregnancies of diabetic patients of the clinic who delivered at the Boston Lying-in Hospital in 1959–1964, almost all of whom were insulin dependent. A control group of sorts consisted of consecutively delivered premature infants, i.e. of 2500 g birthweight or less, born in the same hospital to nondiabetic women in 1962–1964.

Both groups were part of the Collaborative Perinatal Study of the National Institute of Neurological Diseases and Stroke (as it was then named), and probably conformed to its protocols for examining newborns, stillborns, etc. (Niswander and Gordon 1972). But the malformations were not listed, which made it impossible to judge the acceptability of the assertion that "significant" malformations occurred in 13.5 and 6.5% of the test and control groups, and were the primary cause of neonatal death of 25.6 and 7.1% respectively. Findings obviously useless for judging the matter in question here.

The most ambitious investigation undertaken up to that time (and perhaps even to the present) to look into the possible teratogenic effects of maternal diabetes was made by Neave (1967), mentioned here because almost half of the subjects of the study were Joslin Center patients. It is considered below.

A rather different chapter in the story came with a prospective survey of neural tube defects in 18,155 live- and stillborn infants born in 1972–1975 in the Boston Lying-in Hospital (Holmes et al. 1976). Of them 283 were born to women said to be diabetic, i.e. 15.6 per 1000, a frequency far higher than usual (Kalter and Warkany 1983), partly due to many being Joslin Center referral patients, but possibly also to inclusion of other forms of diabetes. In the upshot there occurred one instance of a neural tube defect, 0.35%, compared with 0.14% in the presumably nondiabetic remainder, hardly of significance, especially in light of the various questionable matters in this investigation.

Carrying the Joslin Clinic series forward was a report of 175 diabetic pregnancies in 1975–1976, as usual, with no control group mentioned (Kitzmiller et al. 1978). Twelve percent aborted spontaneously, another 4% were electively aborted, about half after routine scanning revealed anencephalus. Malformations were found in 8.4% of the remaining offspring, including the abnormal induced abortuses. But since the condition of the others was not mentioned it was misleading to include any of them, which omitted gave a frequency of 6.8%. Two neonates had persistent ductus arteriosus, not ordinarily considered a serious abnormality since it frequently closes soon after birth. It was also left unconsidered that 16 of the women had gestational diabetes, and there being no major malformations in their infants, the malformation frequency in the pregestational diabetics (omitting anencephalics and the ductus) was therefore 5.3%.

Overlooked as possibly contributing to the high frequency of anencephalus—3/159 (i.e. minus the offspring of the gestational diabetics) or 18.9 per 1000—

is the fact that Boston had a considerable population of Irish ancestry, an ethnic group with a history of one of the highest newborn prevalences of neural tube defects in the world, in Boston as in Ireland (Naggan and MacMahon 1967; Coffey 1974). In this connection it is apropos to note that the clinic patients were predominantly white. Whether the increased anencephalus and overall malformation frequencies were related to the possibly biased ascertainment of the diabetic patients might have been answered by including a suitable control group.

Later studies dealt with the association of glycosylated hemoglobin level in early diabetic pregnancy and frequency of congenital malformation and spontaneous abortion, and sonographic diagnosis of malformations in diabetic pregnancy (Miller et al. 1981; Greene et al. 1989; Greene and Benacerraf 1991). These questions and related matters are addressed elsewhere in this work.

Malformations were next considered in patients who entered the glycemic level study in 1983–1987 (Greene et al. 1989). Omitting the spontaneous abortions, 17.2%—not an unexpectedly high rate—the frequency of congenital malformations in the remainder was 8.0%. All were called major but by no stretch of diagnostic imagination could six of the 19 different ones fit that designation (bifid thumb, undescended testicle, urethral cyst, etc.). As explained elsewhere in this work the malformation frequency in mortalities and survivors must be addressed separately. Doing so in this case was foreclosed because the total number of the former was not disclosed. Of those not fatal half were of minor varieties, whose omission left a malformation frequency of 2.4%, not unusual.

A search for later Joslin clinic reports on this subject came up empty handed.

Other American Studies

It is strange that aside from the Joslin Clinic in Boston few American clinics and hospitals have carried on long-term programs devoted to charting progress in the study and care of pregnant diabetic women, and most of these few entered the field fairly late.

An exception were studies from the University of Iowa Hospital at Iowa City, the first report from which appeared very early in this unfolding saga. It described the outcomes of pregnancies in 1926–1938 of 33 insulin requiring diabetic women. The seemingly high incidence of diabetes noted of 3.6 per 1000 hospital pregnancies was attributed to the patients' being a selected group. Apparently no congenital anomalies were seen, but not all the perinatal mortalities were autopsied (Mengert and Laughlin 1939), not a promising beginning.

Thirty-one years passed before the appearance of the next report, of 334 offspring born to diabetic women. A large number of the women apparently were referred, but no reason was given for any of the referrals. Congenital defects, undesignated except that no "particular defect predominated," affected 3.9%, again without further details, making for an unsatisfactory account (Delaney and Ptacek 1970).

The most recent report from this hospital, so far as can be determined, was primarily concerned with evaluating the postnatal development of 80 children of diabetic women, about 76% of whom were insulin dependent. Twenty of the children had abnormalities, mostly trivial or minor, supposedly found in the neonatal period, but several were probably diagnosed only postneonatally. The definition and means of detecting abnormalities were not spelled out. One abnormality, an L5–S1 fusion—thought possibly to represent a partial expression of the caudal regression syndrome—was no doubt found by x-ray examination, but what prompted that procedure and at what age it was done were not stated. Because of such considerations the frequency of major malformations in these children could not be calculated. Little, in fact, was certain other than that four of the nine neonatal deaths had major defects (Stehbens et al. 1977).

Reports from the Los Angeles Women's Hospital, the first only in the mid-1970s, had the shortcoming of naming only the malformations occurring in some of the mortalities, with the possible exception of one instance of sacral absence (Gabbe et al. 1977, 1978; Artal et al. 1983; Golde et al. 1984). No further reports from this center have been located. Fashions had changed.

Cincinnati Studies

A series of studies of pregnancies of insulin-dependent women made at the University of Cincinnati Medical Center extended into the 1990s. The reports began with a comparison of the effects of two treatment protocols instituted consecutively in 1956–1978 (Ballard et al. 1984). In all, 19 of the 176 infants had congenital abnormalities, mostly unnamed, but the admissibility of at least a third of them was dubious for different reasons; e.g. one was a chromosomal anomaly and another a persistent ductus arterious, whose fate beyond the age of examintion at 3 days was unknown. Focusing on three other defects, labeled caudal dysplasia, is instructive, one of which had sacral absence, another sacral vertebral abnormalities, and the third lower-limb defects, an example of the lumping of heterogeneous conditions under a single misleading rubric, as had been warned against (Benirschke 1987; Källén et al. 1992).

There was a puzzling difference between the earlier and later treatment periods. Before 1970, in the years when management consisted of the customary practice of the time, only one abnormality was noted in 69 offspring, a mere 1.4%, the ductus arteriosus already mentioned; while in the years after 1970, when "a more rigorous approach to diabetic control was undertaken," 16.8% of the offspring were malformed, with no explanation of the vast difference and no listing of the defects discovered beyond that mentioned above.

Succeeding studies from this ongoing program, covering different successive periods, also had conflicting results. The earliest reported a polydactyly (Lavin et al. 1983), a defect, though not further characterized, fairly common and usually negligible in blacks (e.g. Altemus and Ferguson 1965), a group that comprised a large proportion of the diabetic patients of this center (Neave 1967).

A lengthier series reported 205 infants of recruited insulin dependent diabetic women prospectively collected in 1978–1986, 13 (6.3%) with major malformations, predominantly cardiovascular, and three labeled caudal dysplasia, but apparently not including sacral absence, the supposed hallmark of the diabetic embryopathy (Miodovnik et al. 1986, 1988). Routine ultrasonography was performed in the 2nd trimester and thereafter to detect malformations, but whether any was discovered in this way was not mentioned.

The most recent reports of concern here, noting benefits to diabetic patients enrolled in a specialized prepregnancy program, included data regarding spontaneous abortion and malformation frequency (Rosenn et al. 1991, 1994; Miodovnik et al. 1998), are discussed elsewhere in this account.

London Studies

Another venerable center for the study of diabetes in pregnancy was the King's College Hospital in London, England. With the exception of an early publication, not until recently were its reports relevant to answering the questions of concern here. In 1942–1999 it surveyed 142 diabetic pregnancies and found nine, 6.3%, instances of "more serious" malformations (Peel and Oakley 1949). How many and which of these may have occurred in the considerable perinatal mortalities (25.5%) was not stated. The 6.3% was compared with the 0.9% in nondiabetic pregnancies in the same hospital during these years, and though it was implied that little trust could be placed in the latter figure it was felt that an increase could not be doubted. Exaggerated risk estimates based on such unrealistic background frequencies are not exceptional, as will be noted below.

A different opinion was expressed next. Reported were 201 pregnancies of 176 patients with preexistent diabetes in a series consecutive to the one just noted (Clayton 1956). Although the perinatal death rate continued to be high, a "disastrous" 27%, the possible role of congenital malformations in contributing to it was minimized because it was felt that "such abnormalities are seldom gross enough to cause intrauterine death, and the malformed foetus is usually born alive." [This judgment was partly right since the larger the perinatal death rate, in diabetic as in nondiabetic pregnancy, the smaller generally is the proportion due to congenital malformations, as was sagely noted by an author cited below.] The only malformations mentioned at all were those in five neonatal deaths, with the remark that their pattern varied greatly. This changed view was perhaps influenced by a pathology study in which congenital anomalies were not significantly more frequent in autopsied specimens from diabetic than nondiabetic pregnancies (Cardell 1953). A later report, of little helpfulness, stated that in 1958–1963 there were just four instances of significant (though unnamed) fetal abnormalities in 31 perinatal deaths (Oakley 1965).

The next communications were brief, but brevity was their least failing, since they reported results of examinations only of older children using a definition of anomaly that was unacceptably broad (Watson 1968, 1970).

Equally unhelpful was a report noting that in 1968–1972 seven infants from diabetic pregnancies were born with severe congenital abnormalities since the total number of such births during this period was not clearly stated (Essex et al. 1973). The report evaluating the significance of elevated glycosylated hemoglobin in diabetic pregnancy (Leslie et al. 1978) will be discussed below.

The most recent account, it seems, from this center, overlapping the previous one, reported 294 consecutive diabetic pregnancies in 1968–1976, including 34 gestational ones, all births presented together (Gamsu 1978). All told 20 infants, 6.8%, were said to have severe congenital abnormalities, seven in the 13 neonatal deaths, but the lumping of the diabetes types hindered the analysis.

Brief mention of congenital malformations (Essex 1976; Essex and Pyke 1979) noted that they were the commonest single cause of perinatal death in diabetic pregnancy in the hospital and that their overall 7% frequency in 230 such deliveries in 1971–1977 contrasted with the 2.5% found in a control group reported by Watson (1973) in an unpublished thesis, a comparison not to be taken seriously.

A note from another London hospital, Guy's Hospital, dealt with the familiar topic of sacral agenesis in older children (Wilmshurst et al. 1999). Remarked upon was the bimodal distribution of the ages of the affected children, one peak at less than 1 year and the other at 4–5 years; and that 12 of the 22 children had mothers with pregestational insulin dependent diabetes. It was stated in passing, without considering its outdatedness, that the association of the anomalies with maternal diabetes was "well recognized," citing estimates of its occurrence in infants of diabetic mothers that had long been repudiated (Passarge and Lenz 1966). Years later it was admitted that no cause of the condition had as yet been determined (Adra et al. 1994; Boulas 2009).

Edinburgh Studies

The first report from the Simpson Memorial Maternity Pavilion in Edinburgh mentioning malformations in diabetic pregnancy recorded only one such occurrence, an anencephalus in 16 perinatal mortalities in 1950–1953 (Rolland 1954). Years of studies followed, beginning with a general article whose predominant interest was the later development of children born to women "known to have diabetes mellitus" (Farquhar 1959); thus the physical abnormalities found (though unnamed) were those largely inferred to have been present at birth. In the first of these reports such conditions were found in 10 of 93 children when reexamined at older ages. This seemingly large frequency nevertheless furnished no comparson with the state of the children of 93 matched nondiabetic women, 13 of whom had abnormalities, especially since one of the index children had Down syndrome and two others "mental defect."

The upshot of the analysis of an enlarged series of babies of diabetic women born in 1948–1959 continued to be negative (Farquhar 1965). Those that died perinatally and a like number of randomly selected perinatal mortalities of nondiabetic women were compared and found to have similar frequencies of congenital malformations.

The next, apparently the final report, further enlarged the series (Farquhar 1969). The entire sample consisted of 329 children born in 1948–1966 to diabetic women 89% of whom were insulin dependent. Five of the 69 perinatal mortalities had malformations, none cardiovascular, as determined by the pediatric pathologists conducting the autopsies "with care," in whose opinion heart defects would not have escaped detection, even in the 28 macerated fetuses! These five plus the 10 malformations found in survivors, many examined at ages up to 18 years, that were likely to have been seen or diagnosed neonatally, gave a malformation frequency of 4.6%. The author concluded, based on the control data in his 1965 paper, that though "no difference in incidence was found, the nature of the defects in the diabetic group were more serious," an opinion commented on below.

The writer also recognized and called attention to the significant fact that the geographical variations that occurred in the frequency of certain congenital malformations in the general population may be reflected in the outcome of diabetic pregnancies, which despite being exaggerated maintained the regional variations. Thus in the sample the frequency of anencephalus was 4 in 329 or 12.2 per 1000 total births, while the population frequencies in Scotland in the years 1939–1958 and 1956–1966 were 2.6 and 2.8 per 1000 respectively (Record 1961; Elwood and Mackenzie 1971). This accords with the relation, e.g. in Copenhagen between the albeit lower anencephalus frequency in diabetic pregnancy of 4.7 per 1000 (Mølsted-Pedersen et al. 1964) and the overall one in that city in 1959–1961 of 1.6 per 1000 (Villumsen 1970). The question of the role of perinatal mortality in this apparent difference will be considered below. Increased occurrence of this malformation was not always the case however, as will be seen below in an account of neural tube defects in diabetic pregnancy.

Since Farquhar's articles (1959, 1965) focused on the follow up of children to older ages its results will be discussed in a chapter concerned with this aspect. Later studies from the Edinburgh center dealt mainly with the ameliorative effects on fetal maldevelopment of metabolic control of maternal diabetes begun very early in pregnancy or even before conception, again described below (Steel et al. 1982, 1984a, b, 1989, 1990).

Birmingham Studies

The earliest report of diabetic births in Birmingham was a brief note regarding 69 children of women with "frank" diabetes in 1960–1961 in the Maternity Hospital (Dunn 1964). The only malformation noted occurred in one of the 12 perinatal mortalities, a frequency apparently low compared with the 22.2% in perinatal mortalities of nondiabetic women born in the hospital during this period.

Not long afterward a further brief report noted a 5.8% frequency of unnamed congenital malformations in diabetic births in 1950–1964, but with details so sparse as making judgment difficult (Malins 1968). A fuller summary came 10 years later, of a succesively larger number of births in several intervals in 1950–1974, the total being 701, the congenital malformation frequency 8.1%, with 45.6% of the defects fatal, leaving according to my calculation 3.7% in survivors, all other things being equal; see below (Malins 1978). The most frequent were cardiovascular malformations, 2.3%, and neural tube defects, 1.2%, of all births, respectively; as well as three undescribed occurrences of the "caudal regression syndrome," said to be "about four times the expected incidence," the basis of which not stated. No other defects were named. A final comment had the consequence of leaving the number of insulin-dependent women vague: 1.7% of infants of women with "mild 'chemical' diabetes, i.e. White's class A, were deformed though none died."

An interim report confused the picture by reporting findings at overlapping times and also by muddying the composition of the diabetes types (Day and Insley 1976). Concerned were the outcomes of 205 babies born in 1969–1974, over half those of women of insulin dependent pregestational type, the others of type 2 and gestational diabetics. As a novelty malformations were defined: those causing death, needing surgical correction, or likely to lead to deformity or handicap classed as major, all others minor or posing insignificant problems.

This elaborate effort at categorization was for nought, since the malformations composing the supposedly increased frequency in the offspring of the insulin dependent women, 9.4%, were barely specified; but see below. However by dedging I found that 8.3% were perinatal mortalities, of which 41.2%, were malformed; thus 2.1% of the survivors were malformed, not different from the control. The minor malformations, not named, were relatively few.

A look at the malformations reinforced the conclusion, some whose admissibility as a serious abnormality being disputable: a microcephaly, which, as will be discussed below, is not often easy to diagnose; and two occurrences of patent ductus arteriosus, whose inclusion may be questioned since children only up to the age of 10 days were examined and anatomical closure of the ductus, which is frequent, may not occur until 2–3 weeks following birth (Taeusch et al. 1991). Omitting these, as noted, gave a malformation frequency not significantly increased. And the same was true of the malformation frequency in the offspring of type 2 women.

Now came a bit of a mystery, a publication by Soler et al. (1976) which preceded but repeated the findings given in Malins (1978), as well it seems as partly duplicating those reported by Day and Insley (1976). But because of the ways the malformations were listed, in the two jointly authored articles, it was impossible to establish exactly which were duplicated. For example, the malformations listed included some not eligible to be considered major, including two instances of patent ductus arteriosus and an isolated microcephalus. Others also probably misclassified were meconium ileus (apparently unaccompanied by other symptoms), congenital heart block, a condition frequently without obvious evidence of cardiac maldevelopment, and furthermore compatible with a long and active life (Warkany 1971, p. 583), and Hirschsprung disease, whose frequent familial occurrence suggested possible genetic involvemen. Discounting these malformations still further reduced the significance of the findings. A full description of this study is found below.

Moving forward, in 84 consecutive insulin dependent diabetic pregnancies in 1974–1997 there was again a supposed increased frequency of major malformations, over one-third of which occurred in perinatal mortalities (Soler et al. 1978). A flavor of the observations may be gotten by noting that two of the abnormal children had the Ellis-van Creveld syndrome (already reported by Soler et al. 1976; Day and Insley 1976), a relatively uncommon condition whose double occurrence and the high rate of consanguinity in parents of such cases strongly suggested recessive inheritance (Warkany 1971, p. 793); though Soler et al. (1978) seemed not to recognize this possibility and thus did not mention whether the two children were related.

A report summarizing some results of the Birmingham studies (Wright 1984) noted that malformations in fatalities were 4.5% of all diabetic births in 1974–1999, approximating that found in earlier years, a statistic less useful than the proportion malformed of all the perinatal mortalities would have been.

Later reports from Birmingam were few. Outcomes of pregnancy in insulin dependent diabetic women attending a university teaching hospital in 1990–1997 whose illness was complicated by nephropathy can be briefly summarized (Dunne et al. 1999a). In the 21 pregnancies there were no stillbirths, two neonatal deaths, and one presumably liveborn infant with skeletal malformations, all with frequencies said to be much greater than in births in the hospital population in this period, a mode of comparison irregular and unacceptable.

Also in a teaching hospital, outcomes were compared of pregnancies in pregestational and gestational diabetes in 1990–1988 in Indo-Asian and Caucasian women (Dunne et al. 2000). Congenital malformations occurred only in so-called established diabetes, by which was meant type 1 and type 2, but the confused manner of presenting the facts regarding their occurrence made estimating frequency a guesswork. It appeared that in whites with the established forms combined, if one may venture a stab at it, the frequency was 5.4%, with some unclear proportion occurring in the fatalities. In the others, Indians, Pakistanis, and Bangladeshis, again in the types combined, it was 8.1%. There were no stillbirths or neonatal deaths in these groups, so I would imagine that the few malformations were not of major kinds. Spontaneous abortion, not surprisingly, occurred only in the established pregnancies, 13.5% of the former and 9.1% of the latter, neither unusual; and of course none in the gestational diabetics. Nothing more on this subject from this region was forthcoming in recent years.

Northern Ireland Studies

The earliest studies of pregnancies of diabetic women in the Royal Maternity Hospital in Belfast, as in many described above, were principally concerned with maternal management and secondarily with the excessive offspring mortality. The findings were typical of many to come (Stevenson 1956). In the pregnancies in

1940–1955, of predominantly pregestational insulin dependent diabetic women, 3.3% spontaneously aborted (a surprisingly small and therefore suspicious number) and 25.8% ended in perinatal death. Congenital defects were seen in 5.8%, but none was named except for a meningocele in a neonatal death and an undescribed "foetal abnormality." Those in survivors were not mentioned.

The next report years later noted that despite good prenatal care the offspring mortality rate continued to be an increased (Harley and Montgomery 1965). It dealt with 115 offspring of mostly insulin dependent diabetic women delivering in 1956–1966, almost all referred from the diabetes clinic of the Royal Victoria Hospital, although without explicit indication of degree of illness. The 11.3% perinatal death rate, from a larger perspective was not unusual, but that of spontaneous abortions, 5.2%, on the contrary again seemed oddly low. Congenital malformations were found in 4.7% of infants (two cardiovascular malformations in survivors, one absent kidney in a neonatal death, two hydocephaluses, one with lethal defects, no others mentioned). The absence of controls made this figure unclear, but obviously the level was not impressive.

The high prevalence of diabetic pregnancies, about 6.6 per 1000 deliveries, the same as in earlier years, meant that the sample of women attending the hospital may not have been representative of diabetic women in Northern Ireland; as was perhaps true of many referral centers.

By the next report the situation had changed. The mortality rate had decreased and attention turned to the residual cause of death, prenatal maldevelopment, so much so that it was titled "Congenital malformations in infants of diabetic mothers;" these being defined as structural abnormalities present at birth and recognizable with the naked eye, by x-ray examination, or at necropsy, and divided into more severe, i.e. causing death or affecting a major organ system and resulting in serious incapacity, and less severe, not explicitly defined (Glasgow et al. 1979).

In 1963–1978 there were 195 consecutive pregnancies of referred diabetic women, none of class A, most treated with insulin. Of them 11 aborted (3 induced), and 19 of the remaining 184 had congenital malformations, 11 considered major, 7 in the 23 perinatal mortalities. Thus, of the 161 surviving newborn 2.5% were malformed, obviously not an excess; as was true also of the abortion rate. Four of the fatalities had cardiovascular defects and two anencephalus, the rate of the latter, 10.9 per 1000, apparently larger than the 3.95 per 1000 in the general Belfast population in that era (Elwood 1970, 1975), the excess owing perhaps to the women being a selected group.

Clouding the whole picture were the great regional variations within the city in the frequency of this defect and the high frequencies in women with abnormal reproductive history (Elwood and Elwood 1984). The authors felt it improbable that the anencephalies was related to the diabetes, rather that they reflected its high incidence in Northern Ireland as a whole. As for the cardiovascular defects there seemed to be no such doubt.

A further study (Traub et al. 1983) somewhat muddied things, since it surveyed diabetic births in years overlapping those examined by Glasgow et al. (1979), making it difficult to know whether the observations noted were additional or duplicating. It bears discussing nevertheless. In 1972–1981 there were 169 pregnancies of insulin-dependent diabetic women at the maternity hospital, 14% tranferred from elsewhere for various reasons, 7 ending as spontaneous abortions, the 4.1% still low, in the remaining 162, including twins, born after 28 weeks, 7, 4.3%, were perinatal deaths, 4 with cardiovascular defects, including 1 with multiple defects. as well an anencephalus in a terminated pregnancy; also 4 other heart defects and a sacral agenesis. At least half the total of 11 major defects were lethal, the frequency in the survivors thus being about 3.7%.

A further report, of diabetic births in 1979–1983, enlarged the purview by adding those from numerous other Northern Ireland obstetrical units (Traub et al. 1987). In the total of 221 pregnancies 15 conceptuses had major congenital malformations and four minor ones, but only the defects in the four prenatally diagnosed and therapeutically aborted were named. Omitting the 17 spontaneous abortions gave a major malformation rate of 7.4%. This was compared with the 2.5% malformation frequency in the overall population, a procedure that hardly satisfied the need for a well-matched control, especially since the most glaring residual problem, the overall diabetic perinatal death rate, approached the background level.

Despite a diligent attempt to trace all such patients, the prevalence of pregnancies in diabetic women was a low 1.6 per 1000 total deliveries, Agreeing, the authors commented, "It is disappointing that current record systems seem to be so inadequate…." Yet this may have been a true rate.

A later report, a brief summary, mentioned that major congenital malformations of about 11% occurred in offspring of insulin dependent diabetic women in 1979–1986, but aside from the cryptic remark that "half were potentially fatal" only the two anencephalies in induced abortions were named (Hadden et al. 1988). And yet the writers complained that another author's report was "incomplete."

Outcomes of pregnancies in numerous obstetrical units in 1985–1995 were reported separately for type 1 and gestational diabetic women (Hadden et al. 2001). In the former there were 17.4% spontaneous abortions and terminations combined, 3.8% perinatal mortalities, and 5.3% congenital malformations; the latter included those in the perinatal deaths, which were not named separately. It is a reasonable guess that a significant fraction of all the malformations occurred in the deaths. To reiterate, it is only by considering malformations in deaths and survivors individually that the fetal consequences of diabetic pregnancy can be truly evaluated.

For no discernable reason the outcomes of pregnancies in 2002–2003 of women with type 1 and type 2 diabetes in all maternity units in Northern Ireland, England, and Wales were incongruously admixed (Macintosh et al. 2006). There were a total of 2400 offspring, a prevalence of 3.8 per 1000 pregnancies. Despite the growing numbers of women diagnosed with type 2 almost three-quarters were type 1, the former more often borne by minority ethnic woman. Regardless of other differences between them, the two diabetic types did not differ in perinatal death rate, 3.2%, and little in congenital defects, 4.7% in type 1, 4.3% in type 2; though as the listing made explicit an appreciable number were not major ones. The frequencies of the two commonest and doubtlessly major defect types, comprising almost half of the entire array, neural tube and cardiovascular, were 4.2 per 1000 and 17.8 per 1000 respectively, all the former and over half of the latter diagnosed prenatally. About one-quarter of the perinatal deaths were malformed, but the fraction in the survivors so affected was not stated. I mention again the absence of any rationale for the combining of illnesses from the different geographical areas.

Nothing more seems to have been reported on this subject from this part of the world in later years.

Republic of Ireland Studies

The paper introducing the long-ongoing overview of the outcome of diabetic pregnancies in Dublin, the first Graves Lecture to the Royal College of Physicians in Ireland, began with the obligatory comprehensive historical review of the subject (Drury 1961). One of its main topics, offspring death in the National Maternity and the Combe Lying-in Hospitals was appreciable, 14.3% in the 178 pregnancies seen in about 1950–1960. Congenital malformations as one of its causes was not overlooked. Consistent with findings from other centers during those years malformations were seen in relatively few perinatal mortalities, as might have been expected of a time when the mortality rate was high and most deaths were not of developmental origin. Nine of the 12 stillbirths were macerated and probably unexaminable. Only five malformations were mentioned, three major ones in the deaths, and two of a minor variety, a talipes and a hypospadias. [Incidentally, the latter was also mentioned, as occurring in an adult, in an earlier work from a Dublin author Joyce 1922, reprinted 1986.]

Next, a fuller account considered 269 offspring born in 1950–1965, 14, 5.2%, of whom were malformed, four in the 26 perinatal mortalities, a cyclops being additional to the three with defects noted earlier (Drury 1966). An agreeable surprise—the abnormalities were named—thus making it possible to learn that five of them were inadmissible or questionable: a "Mongol," a laryngomalacia, two talipes, and a hypospadias. Ninety-eight percent of the women were said to be insulin dependent, though 9.5% were class A, a form not usually needing insulin. Again, many of the 16 stillbirths were probably not examinable. Nevertheless, balancing these facts it does not seem that an increased frequency of malformations occurred, but once again absence of a control left the question up in the air.

An intermediate study, of sorts, of 213 diabetic pregnancies, 12.2% of type A, in the National Maternity Hospital in 1962–1971 found a perinatal death rate of 12.7%, which was about three times that in nondiabetic pregnancies during the same years (Dundon et al. 1974). It is strange that no matter how hard one searches through this article one cannot find mentioned the total malformation frequency in the offfspring. "With regard," as it was stated, "to surviving infants, the incidence of major congenital malformations has been well documented…" but unrevealed except that…"the incidence of major and lethal congenital malformations is four times as high as amongst infants of non-diabetic mothers," leaving one in the dark. The only concrete figure given was that for lethal defects, occurring in eight of the

27 perinatal deaths, or 29.6%, which was almost identical to such deaths about that time in nondiabetic deaths, a rare revelation, again indicating the nonteratogenicity of maternal diabetes; which would have been fully recognized if another bit of evidence, the frequency of major malformations in survivors, had been stated. Regarding one other finding, that in the years reviewed there was not one case of anencephalus, is not surprising when judged against the mean background prevalence of the defect in that period of about 3.5 per 1000 births; not surprising therefore that there was no such occurrence in the small population of the 213 diabetic births. Another observation of wide significance was that over the brief period surveyed the overall frequency of anencephalus delined quite steeply, from a mean of 4.3 per 1000 in 1963–1967 to 2.5 per 1000 in 1967–1972; a remarkable decrease, of momentous significance discussed in full in my book on the story of neural tube defects (Kalter 2009).

Two publications over the next 10–15 years advanced the record. One gave a full account of the malformations in 616 offspring from 1951 to 1976 (Drury et al. 1977). In this sample 36 were malformed, including 11 with inadmissible defects, of the sorts enumerated above, leaving 25 with major malformations, 4.5%; the latter a major cause of perinatal death, leaving unclarified the matter of the malformation level in survivors.

Another more inclusive but not more illuminating report detailed the findings in 687 infants of consecutive diabetic pregnancies from early 1951 to mid-1979 (Drury 1979). Only the malformations in the 58 perinatal mortalities, 20.7%, were mentioned, and aside from two malformed stillbirths in 1975–1979, one anencephalus, the other iniencephaly, no other abnormality was specified.

One incidental fact may be helpful. Since the ordinarily rare malformation iniencephaly may have been more frequent in areas where anencephalus was common (Paterson 1944), the two instances of neural tube defects mentioned above may be considered together. These were apparently the only ones found in 1951–1979, giving a rate of 2.9 per 1000; not extraordinary in a population whose rate of anencephalus was among the highest then recorded, e.g. for the years 1953–1973 averaging 4.3 per 1000 (Coffey 1974), or as seen above 2.5 per 1000 in 1967–1972 (Dundon et al. 1974). A later summary brought the total of such defects to four, one iniencephaly and three anencephalies, in 941 viable infants, a rate of 4.2 per 1000 (Drury 1986), matching the population level, and thus different from the apparent increases in this malformation found elsewhere.

One further word. In the Banting Lecture given before his death Drury (1989) stated that 5.6% of major malformations had occurred in 1066 viable infants of diabetic women in 1951–1987. Drawing on evidence presented in earlier papers one can see that the 60 cases on which this frequency was based clearly included some number of minor abnormalities. Indeed Drury et al. (1983) remarked that nearly 40% of the malformations noted were minor ones, and an even larger proportion of minor defects was detailed by Sheridan-Pereira et al. (1983).

An ambitious though questionable procedure concerned births in 2006–2007 in prenatal facilities in a wide geographical area called the Atlantic seaboard; the doubtfulness consisting of combining the results in type 1 and type 2 pregnancies—

its rationale apparently being that both were pregestational—the former 77% of all (Dunne et al. 2009). [The preponderance of the former, though apparently not the usual pattern, was also the case in another study from this area; see Macintosh et al. 2006.] Nearly one-quarter of the pregnancies were aborted (but not examined), and despite this late date the perinatal death rate was still elevated, at 2.5%, whereas that of congenital malformations (not identified), despite the contrary assertion, was not.

In another recent study, outcomes of diabetic pregnancies in Dublin in 1995–2007 were compared (Carmody et al. 2010). In the very small number of the former the spontaneous abortion rate was 11% and in the latter 14%, both not unusual. Perinatal death was 0 and 3.5% respectively, and in the former there was one major malformation, a sacral agenesis, giving a frequency of 6.2% and in the latter an unnamed 3.1%, no doubt mostly in the perinatal mortalities. Awaited are further reports from Ireland.

Incidentally, the authors, citing the European Surveillance of Congenital Anomalies (www.eurocat.ulster.ac.uk), noted that the average yearly congenital malformation rate in 1997–2006 for all women delivering in Dublin was 1.8%, somewhat less than that usually reported.

Denmark Studies

An influential study of the outcome of births in 1926–1963 to women with diabetes was made in the Copenhagen University hospital, 80% after 1946 (Mølsted-Pedersen et al. 1964). All the women had pregestational diabetes, but only about 93% were insulin dependent. The case infants comprised 853 infants weighing 1000 g or more. In toto major congenital malformations occurred in 5.2% of the former and 1.2% of the controls, and in 12.2% of the diabetic perinatal mortalities and 4.1% of the control ones. All of which, having been of great importance in supporting the belief that maternal diabetes is associated with congenital maldevelopment, will be closely examined.

The Control Group

A word about the controls, which merit close examination. They consisted of births in the same maternity wards, but solely during a 6-month period in 1959–1960; part of a separate study of the possible teratogenicity of antihistaminic preparations (Zachau-Christiansen and Villumesen 1962). It goes without saying that controls must match the study group in all ways known to be relevant, but especially must also be contemporaneous to obviate changes in conditions and procedures that time may bring. Neither requirement was respected in this study. The majority of the diabetic births occurred only over the last 17 years of the study period, while the controls only in the 6 months toward its end. This is important, since conditions may change, but also because the frequency of particular congenital malformations may vary over time; instances of which were noted, e.g., during the years in question in a number of Czechoslovak maternity hospitals (Kučera 1971b).

Also important is the fact that both the diabetic and control mothers were in hospital for a variety of severe complications, and thus perhaps not representative of the diabetic or the general population as a whole; e.g. the maternity wards received women who were expected to have a pathological delivery, were unmarried, or were admitted during difficult delivery (Villumsen and Zachau-Christiansen 1963). Further making the appropriateness of the control doubtful was the large number of diabetic women among them, 15.8 per 1000, many times the prevalence noted in a part of Denmark in a series of insulin dependent pregestational diabetic pregnancies (Nielsen and Nielsen 1994).

A smaller matter perhaps, but infants of less than 1000 g were excluded from both groups, which may be relevant because Danish illegitimate infants at the time, as often elsewhere, had a increased rate of low birthweight (Matthiessen et al. 1967), and the frequency of malformations can differ in different weight groups (Goldenberg et al. 1983; Berry et al. 1987; Kalter 1991). Further, perinatal death rate, was not usefully detailed; nor, for neither group was the overall death rate noted, which made additional difficulties of comparison, since the rate in Denmark changed appreciably over the years surveyed (Matthiessen et al. 1967).

Finally, a question lingers whether the control infants were as well examined for congenital malformations as those of the diabetic women. An insight into this question was provided by a study of children born in the two Copenhagen maternity wards during 1959–1961 (Villumsen and Zachau-Christiansen 1963), which though focusing on the putative teratogenic effect of antihistaminics omitted many details that might have supported their validity as a control.

The Outcome

In the case group there were 55 malformed infants, 44 with major malformations, 5.2%, and 11 with minor ones, 1.3%. However, since the authors considered that the "classification of congenital malformations according to severity is largely subjective" their personal scheme was unclear, since the malformations were not listed in the publication.

Fortunately such a list, which included the designation of major and minor, was kindly made available to me at the time. Inspecting the list proved instructive. Four of the defects considered major for various reasons were clearly inadmissible: pseudohermaphroditism, male or female, can have a varied etiology (Warkany 1971, p. 1107 et seq.), and without details its status could not be judged; clubfoot is a fairly common malformation occurring more often in males than females, has a strong familial tendency (Wang et al. 1988)—strangely it was listed as a major malformation in one infant and a minor one in another, even though in the latter it was accompanied by a short femur; next, microcephaly not always easy to diagnose in newborns when occurring in the absence of other abnormalities, as was true in this instance, is frequently attributable to recessive inheritance; and last, Down syndrome, whose chromosomal origin was already established (Lejeune et al. 1959), of course could not be due to maternal diabetes. This was clarified much later, when an investigation from this same center found that insulin dependent diabetes did not increase the risk of chromosomal abnormalities (Henriques et al. 1991). Excluding these four abnormalities left 40 major congenitally malformed offspring in 853 births, or 4.7%.

The supplied list indicated that 17 of the malformed offspring died perinatally of their presumably lethal malformations. But the number of all perinatal mortalities was not specified, without knowledge of which the frequency of malformations in survivors could not be determined. A partial clue to this figure was derived from the information given for the 82 mortalities necropsied in the last nine and three-quarter years of the study, of which 16 had malformations (the only ones noted in a tsble in the article itself). Subtracting these deaths from the total born gave a malformation frequency in the survivors of 3.1%. From which it clearly appeared that an increased malformation frequency did not emerge from this study.

Incidentally, among the infants reported seven were of the cases cited by Kučera et al. (1965) in support of the theory that maternal diabetes was associated with a specific diabetic embryopathy. But the provided detailed list revealed that only one had a sacral abnormality.

The Aftermath

Important studies continued from this center. It was observed that the frequency of malformations in perinatal mortalities increased as improved maternal and neonatal care led to their overall frequency decrease (Mølsted-Pedersen 1967; Pedersen et al. 1974). The significance of this temporal variation in the overall malformation frequency was apparently not appreciated however. Malformation occurrence was reported spottily and uninformatively during the 1970s, only the total frequency given without specifying the defects found; this was true of the control as well, precluding close analysis (e.g. Pedersen 1975). Overall frequencies of major and minor ones were stated separately, which was helpful (Pedersen 1977, p. 192; Damm and Mølsted-Pedersen 1989). Autopsied infants from diabetic mothers, as noted above, continued to have a higher malformation frequency than controls, with cardiovascular and central nervous system abnormalities predominating.

During the mid-1970s a change was made in the manner of diagnosing congenital malformations. To the previous recognition at birth by external examination was added that by x-ray, upon clinically indicated need (Pedersen 1975); and then came a further addition: "some malformations were diagnosed only postmortem," both stipulations vague (Pedersen 1977).

Seeming to shift the earlier view that certain malformations (particularly short femur) were characteristic in offspring of diabetic women (Pedersen 1977, p. 105), it was later stated that "the correlation between maternal diabetes and congenital malformations in the progeny is of an unspecific nature," and that the apparently increased frequency of certain malformations in such children was due to an "increase in incidence and severity of the usual types of malformations," a statement that is nothing if not ambiguous (Pedersen 1977, p. 194).

By the mid-1970s the Copenhagen series included four cases of "total caudal regression" (Pedersen 1977, p. 194), a term supposedly meaning sacral absence, which constituted a 600-fold increase than in the general population rate (Kučera 1971a). As noted, the provided list of malformations mentioned above included only one sacral abnormality, though Kučera et al. (1965) considered that there were seven such cases in this material. What accounted for the discrepancies? Was it partly caused by change of definition of the entity in midstream? Or was it as well, as the pathologist Benirschke (1987) suggested, that the term "embraces…a host of malformations that are very dissimilar," or as a team of epidemiologists put it, that its prevalence "depends on which forms are included…" (Källén et al. 1992).

Later reports were mainly concerned with prenatal evaluation of fetal growth and development in diabetic pregnancy, etc; they will be discussed elewhere in this work. Others summarized findings in series during different time periods. One, comparing diabetic pregnancies cared for in 1966–1977 at the two hospitals in Copenhagen with those outside the area (a comparison discussed below), introduced further changes in the definition of malformations and further increased the difficulties of analysis (Pedersen and Mølsted-Pedersen 1978). A distinction was made between major malformations and a subset, 'severe' ones, the latter causing death or necessitating major surgery in the first 6 months of life. The total rate rate was 8.2%, but since none of the defects was named scrutiny was again defeated. The mention in a contemporary paper (Pedersen 1979) of five occurrences of "caudal regression" did nothing to lessen the difficulty. A later appearing publication (Damm and Mølsted-Pedersen 1989) presented data for a series of patients considerably overlapping the one just mentioned, yet only one case of sacral absence was reported in this larger group of infants.

Other findings of Pedersen and Mølsted-Pedersen (1978) were of great interest; including the claim that the congenital malformation rate was "normalized" in insulin dependent diabetic women whose pregnancies were planned and hence in which strict metabolic control at conception and during the early weeks of gestation was enabled.

A later study, considering the years 1979–1987, was mainly concerned with alphafetoprotein levels in amniotic fluid and maternal serum in a selected group of diabetic pregnancies (Henriques et al. 1993). The malformations found, major and minor, were listed, and they and various other matters are analyzed in the section dealing with maternal factors associated with diabetic pregnancy.

Studies in the most recent years were concerned with diabetic pregnancy in women with certain problems such as microalbuminuria and nephropathy, but without finding an increased frequency of perinatal death or congenital malformation (Ekbom et al. 2001; Nielsen et al. 2006b, 2009).

Finland Studies

The study of diabetes in pregnancy in Finland has a long history perhaps due to the relatively high prevalence of type 1 diabetes in that part of the world (Saxén 1983; Tuomilehto et al. 1991a). All of the several hospitals in Helsinki that were engaged in this work will be considered. The earliest identified report, from the First Women's Clinic of the University of Helsinki, noted two abnormal infants in 81 births in 1949–1955, one with "frog position of the limbs," often a sign of caudal dysgenesis, the other not named (Jokipii 1955). Congenital malformations were not mentioned among the causes of the neonatal deaths, their number not clearly specified.

The next report, just as unsatisfactory, noted abnormalities in seven of 162 infants born in 1951–1960 in the Central University Hospital (perhaps partly duplicating the cases presented by Jokipii 1955), three in the 16 neonatal deaths, one perhaps with major defects, others undescribed (Österlund and Rantakallio 1964). There were the usual uncertainties: the diabetic women were a selected group, having "complications" of pregnancy, referred from all parts of the country; over 20% gestational diabetic; stillbirths were frequent but their condition not mentioned, most were macerated, etc.

Congenital abnormalities called major were seen in six of 76 births of insulin dependent diabetic women in the Institute of Midwifery in 1961–1966, though only one was described, a "defect of sacrum"; six others in 47 children of class A mothers had minor defects, including a Down syndrome, all in all hardly worth mention (Tiisala et al. 1967).

A report from the Department of Obstetrics and Gynecology of the University Central Hospital compared the outcome of pregnancies in 1970–1971, in which the diabetic management was the conventional one of the day, with those in 1975–1977, given intensive metabolic control (Teramo et al. 1979). In the first period malformations occurred in four of 54 infants and in the later period in four of 136, in neither were the defects named. Nor considered was whether the apparent improvement was connected to the difference in management.

All the Finnish studies mentioned above contributed nothing to the tale unfolding here, and were included for the historical record only.

A study from this hospital some years later, hardly more contributive, summarized the outcomes of pregnancies in 1978–1982 of women with insulin dependent diabetes (Ylinen et al. 1984). There were 146 fetuses including twins and abortuses, 11 classed as having major malformations. Only mentioned were two perinatal deaths and three induced abortuses, two with anencephalus diagnosed by ultrasound (a topic expanded upon below), and one with caudal regression syndrome (called "typical" raising the questions of what that meant, and whether the second was not typical). The total number of deaths and abortions was not noted, nor were other matters, the focus of the study being maternal glycosylated hemoglobin values in early pregnancy, a topic discussed elsewhere. Thus, again an unsatisfactory account.

After a gap of years a report appeared from an area of southern Finland of births in 1988–1997 of type 1 diabetic women whose main purpose, glycemic control, will be turned to below (Suhonen et al. 2000). Considered here are the findings regarding pregnancy outcome. The frequency of malformations, diagnosed by prenatal ultrasonography and at birth, was 4.2%; while in controls, offspring of nondiabetic women born in the area in 1993–1994, it was 1.4%. The former is an exaggeration, since it included defects, about half the total, whose classification as major is in doubt, e.g. patent ductus arteriosus, pulmonary stenosis, club foot, hypospadias, etc., etc. Omitting them left a frequency of 2.3 per 1000. The control figure, on the contrary, may be an underestimate.

Another recent study concerned 296 births to insulin-dependent diabetic women in 1986–1995 in hospitals in two northernmost provinces of Finland (Vääräsmäki et al. 2000). Boiled down to essentials, the perinatal death rate was 3.0% and that of congenital malformations called major 3.7%, almost two-thirds cardiovascular and one other a caudal regression syndrome, the latter and a heart defect one of the nine perinatal deaths. The glycemic control aspects of the study will be discussed below.

A later study using data from four national health registers from 1991 to 1995 found a rate of major congenital malformations in offspring of type 1 diabetics from midpregnancy to 1 year of age of 6.3%, a meaningless figure (Vääräsmäki et al. 2002). The rate of perinatal death was 1.4 per 1000, almost one-quarter of them malformed. With this unsatisfactory note such communications from Finland seemed to have come to an end.

It is of much interest that a study of the freqency of newly diagnosed type 1 diabetes in Finish children found that they possess the highest rate worldwide, rising from of 31.4 per 100,000 in 1980 to 64.2 per 100,000 in 2005 (Harjutsalo et al. 2008). Nor has this increase been confined to Finland (Patterson et al. 2009, etc.)

Birmingham Hospital Study

In conspicuous contrast with the Finnish reports are the detailed accounts from Birmingham. Since they were influential in engendering the belief in the teratogenicity of diabetes it will be useful to scrutinize them closely.

It began with the report, as mentioned briefly above, of the 701 births to diabetic women in the Birmingham Maternity Hospital in 1950–1974 (Soler et al. 1976). About 16.5% of the women were of the White class A variety, i.e. not insulin dependent, and 1.7% of their children were malformed, none fatally. Of the 585 others 9.4% were malformed, a rate claimed to be "three to four times higher" than the frequency in the contemporary population of Birmingham. It is this claim that will be examined, together with other details regarding the insulin dependent women and their pregnancies.

The women were probably not a random sample of the diabetic women in the Birmingham of the day, especially during the last years of the study, when the hospital became a referral center for the more severely affected. While the malformation frequency fluctuated somewhat from year to year, in the last 5 years of the study that of malformations generally and of lethal malformations especially greatly increased with no attempted explanation.

Important considerations are the perinatal death and autopsy rates, since as pointed out, "…infants of diabetics are likely to have been examined in greater detail; more *post mortem* examinations were carried out amongst infants of diabetics because of their higher perinatal death and the rate of recognition of congenital abnormalities at autopsy is higher than in living infants." These were 16.9 and 90% respectively, the latter far greater than the usual contemporary 60% (Leck et al. 1968). Though the malformation frequency was greater in the later period the mortality rates in the two intervals were almost identical.

Congenital malformations, as noted, were seen in 9.4% of all offspring (55/585), 26.3% (26/99) in perinatal mortalities (stillbirths 17.5%, neonatal deaths 38.1%). Thus 47.3% of the malformed offspring (26/55) were mortalities; the high frequencies no doubt owing in part to the high autopsy rate and the special interest of the pathologists. The complete list indicated which were considered major and which fatal. [Unmentioned was the frequency of spontaneous abortion, which a later study found to be 25.9% (Wright et al. 1983).]

Of the 99 perinatal mortalities 26.3% were malformed, all called major but several erroneously so labeled, e.g. an apparently isolated meconium ileus, an Ellis-van Creveld syndrome, probably an autosomal recessive trait, etc. Of the 486 survivors 31 had what was called a congenital malformation, many labeled major; a designation that could be challenged in many, especially those categorized skeletal, but others as well. The upshot being that the frequency of indubitable major congenital malformations in the survivors was 2.3%, approximating the 1.9% in all births in Birmingham at that period (Leck et al. 1968).

The outstanding difficulty was the absence of a contemporaneously collected group of matched pregnant nondiabetic women whose offspring were as carefully examined for malformations as were those of the diabetic women. The authors recognized that a control was necessary and resorted for comparison to the findings of a study of births in Birmingham in the 1950s (McKeown and Record 1960), but acknowledged this to be a poor choice. [A control group included in a smaller study, described in detail elsewhere in this work, collected at the hospital during the later years of the study under consideration, when compared with the malformation frequency in the diabetic births, revealed the increase not to be statistically significant (Day and Insley 1976).]

The most frequent were cardiovascular malformations, 2.3%, not all lethal, and anencephalus and spina bifida, 1.2%, of all births, the latter greater than the 3.6 per 1000 noted in all births in Birmingham in 1950–1999 (Leck et al. 1968). At the same time it should be recalled that a similar or even greater overall propensity to neural tube defects existed in Ireland, yet, as the authors noted, no such diabetes related increase was discovered in that region. There occurred as well three instances of the "caudal regression syndrome," not described, said to be "about four times the expected incidence," the basis of which was not stated. Other defects were not named.

Thus four tendentious matters—biased ascertainment of diabetic women, intensive examination of children, inclusion of ineligible malformations, and frequent absence of controls—were present here—as in study after study of the outcome of pregnancy of diabetic women reported by specialized clinics.

Johns Hopkins Study

All presumedly diabetic women delivering at the Johns Hopkins Hospital in 1946–1970 were identified and a random sample of the births of about 600 of them and an approximately equal number of nondiabetic births selected for study (McCarter et al. 1987). The former were divided into definite, probable, and suspect diabetics, with nearly twice as many of the definites diagnosed before age 20 and insulin treated, as were the probables. It is not surprising that this unclear means of classification, and other opaque features of the investigation, compromised the analysis of the malformation picture, and yielded the ambiguous conclusion that the malformation risk was not increased in diabetic women, made even more imponderable by some caveats. It cannot possibly be irrelevant that three-quarters of the definite and probable diabetic women were black.

Critique

The preceding pages described studies of the outcome of pregnancies of diabetic women made over many years. As medical and social progress brought improvement in the perinatal death picture of these pregnancies and pregnancies generally a continually increasing fraction of the deaths seemed to be associated with the most refractory of the causes of offspring mortality—congenital malformations. Much interest then turned to documenting these conditions and later to attempts at reducing their prevalence.

Outlined above were not only the findings of centers examining the spectrum and frequency of malformations, to the extent possible, but as well the difficulties impeding efforts to establish beyond doubt that they were extraordinary in type or degree. For the reviewer the virtual absence of any consideration of these many important aspects by the various authors made the task perilous. It is tedious to repeat, but these vital ingredients must be emphasized. Doubts largely remain about: how the diabetic women cared for at specialized centers were selected or otherwise identified; how representative they were of the entire population of diabetic women of reproductive age in the regions served by these centers; the definition and means of diagnosing the phenomena considered malformations; the assiduity and competence of personnel examining dead and surviving infants for malformations; the validity of the composition of control pregnant women and the diligence of the examination of their children for malformations, in the infrequent instances where controls were recognized as necessary at all; and last the many almost uniformly neglected subsidiary relevant elements in the scheme, familial, socioeconomic, demographic, etc. (Little and Carr-Hill 1984).

But perhaps greatest among these prejudicing aspects was the practice of specialized centers of typifying the situation by generalizing from individuals who in one way or another were apparently unrepresentative of diabetic women generally. The patients in these clinics were usually a selected group, referred e.g. because of their poor previous reproductive history or the unusually severe nature of their illness, and observations made upon them are not to be considered typical without good evidence. As Williams (1930, p. 602) said years ago of maternal and fetal death in diabetes, so it also may be true of other pregnancy outcomes of diabetes "...such statistics give too gloomy a picture, as they are based mostly upon severe cases, and do not take into account the milder ones which are usually not reported."

Sometimes even what is meant by 'selected' or its opposite 'random' may be misunderstood. For example, Pedersen (1954b) called his patients "unselected" because they came to the clinic at all stages of pregnancy, but at the same time noted that they were referred by various private and provincial hospitals and general practitioners. And Froehlich and Fujikura (1969), on the contrary, thought that since "the Collaborative Study is a prospective one and the mothers randomly selected, the proportion of 'high-risk' cases such as maternal diabetes would be relatively low;" but Mitchell et al. (1971) reported a prevalence of 'diabetes' among these women of 14 per 1000, some three times that usually found of type 1 diabetes, indicating that the condition had been defined very broadly.

An explicit admission of the occurrence and perils of nonrandom selectivity was made by Takeuchi and Benirschke (1961) when, in studying autopsied offspring of diabetic mothers, they stated that it was possible their material was "biased because of the higher incidence of maternal diabetes at the Boston Lying-in Hospital due to its affiliation with the Joslin Clinic," and then, calling attention to another biasing element, noted that "a high percentage of autopsies is obtained in this group because of the interest by the physicians taking care of this group of patients."

Ultimately problems arose because in the aggregate and for many kinds individually congenital malformations were relatively common. Thus a comparatively small increase in their frequency, such as was claimed diabetes caused, because of the numerous variables confounding the picture, made recognizing possible augmentation problematic. The relevance of these facts here can be illustrated by the following. If for purposes of analogy one considers pregnancy in diabetes a pandemic, then the problems entailed in determining whether this state was associated with an excessive level of malformations can be compared with the task undertaken in the early 1960s by those trying to identify the cause of the rash of unusual limb malformations that had suddenly appeared in Germany and elsewhere (McBride 1961; Lenz 1961). It proved incredibly complicated to do so, and only upon profound epidemiological analysis, greatly facilitated by the fact that among the most frequent malformations induced were the conspicuous and ordinarily quite rare phocomelia and amelia, was it nailed down that the culprit was the recently introduced sedative thalidomide (Lenz and Knapp 1962; Sievers 1969; Weicker 1969).

In the case of diabetes the situation is reversed. The supposed cause is known and common, and the effects have to be proved. Would it help to do this if the frequency of ordinarily rare and conspicuous malformations were increased? Does sacral absence or holoprosencephaly, both said to be increased in diabetic births (Kučera 1971a; Barr et al. 1983), fit this bill? Several difficulties attend this proposition.

Sacral absence is apparently seldom diagnosed in newborn infants; a worldwide review of hospital births noted a frequency of 4.8 per million (Kučera 1971a). But such a scarcity is not true in older individuals, as was shown by a survey of a relatively small number of American orthopedic surgeons, which had no trouble identifying at least 50 cases of partial or complete absence of the sacrum (Blumel et al. 1959). This discrepancy appeared to indicate that the condition mostly went unrecognized at birth, and that the alleged increase in diabetic pregnancies was owing to diligent examination, more severe defectiveness, or both.

Holoprosencephaly, the general term for a set of related conspicuous craniofacial abnormalities, can hardly be overlooked (DeMyer and Zeman 1963). Though etiologically heterogeneous (Roach et al. 1975; Corsello et al. 1990), it is uncommon, with a mean frequency recently determined to be about about 0.75 per 10,000 total births (Martínez-Frias et al. 1994; Croen et al. 1996; Rasmussen et al. 1996; Whiteford and Tolmie 1996; Olsen et al. 1997). There was evidence that many embryos with these severe malformations were spontaneously aborted, since the frequency in induced abortuses in Japan in 1962–1974 was many times greater than that found at term (Matsunaga and Shiota 1977). The condition should thus be overrepresented in abortuses of diabetic pregnancies, but pathology studies of perinatal mortalities described above supplied no support for this conjecture.

Chapter 14
Broad-scale Studies

Various comprehensive approaches have been taken over the course of time in studying the outcomes of diabetic pregnancy, including broad-scale, multicenter, and population-based surveys, discussed in this and the next chapter.

Reviews and analyses of congenital malformations in diabetic pregnancy, of information gathered from multiple sources, were used to survey the broad landscape. The purpose was to overcome the limitations imposed by the sparse numbers of diabetic pregnancies any one clinic or hospital could supply, by collectively examining and interpreting the findings of many isolated and more limited reports. The conduct and findings of extensive reviews first and then multicenter ones will be examined.

The Kučera Analysis

Not long after the publication of the report by Mølsted-Pedersen et al. (1964) a broad review appeared that supported its finding of an increased occurrence of malformations in diabetic pregnancies (Kučera 1971a). It presented an analysis of a compilation of 7101 births to diabetic women drawn from nearly 50 case-series originating from many European countries and the US in about the previous 30 years. Noting that 4.8% of the offspring "showed anomalies," compared with 1.6% in a control series (the article's summary erroneously gave this figure as 0.6%) derived from a World Health Organization study (Stevenson et al. 1966) and his "own series of anomalous cases," the author suggested that there was an increased incidence of anomalies in the offspring of diabetic women.

The conclusion, as was conceded, was based on data flawed in a number of ways, methodological and conceptual. One matter not mentioned was the noncomparability of the test and the control groups with regard to national origin; e.g. about three times as many controls were German or Czech as the diabetic group; some controls were Australian and South African, nationalities not represented in the diabetic births; and many countries present in the latter were not present in the controls.

H. Kalter, *A History of Diabetes in Pregnancy*,
DOI 10.1007/978-94-007-1557-8_14, © Springer Science+Business Media B.V. 2012

The source of a considerable fraction of the control series appeared to be a study sponsored by the World Health Organization, and some clues as to its formulation and characteristics could be gleaned from the report of it (Stevenson et al. 1966). It seems that only the largest hospitals were recruited for the study, and that such hospitals, as was noted, "with so many births each year are inevitably very busy places and understaffed, so that it would have been unrealistic to expect recording of elaborate information about births." Hence, all other matters apart, the Kučera findings are challenged by the familiar objection that relatively competently and conscientiously examined infants of diabetic women were compared with superficially and casually examined controls.

The Kučera publication noted that certain malformations occurred in great excess in the children of the diabetic women, especially "spinal anomalies including the syndrome of caudal regression." What was meant by the latter was not entirely clear, but if "caudal regression"was synonymous with absence of the sacrum, as the introduction in this publication held it to be, and the latter was considered a "specific malformation of fetuses of diabetic women," then this malformation as it occurred in the case-series, is to be looked at closely.

There were nine instances of "caudal regression," two from the US, one from the United Kingdom, two from Germany, one from Bohemia, and three from Denmark. Reading the sources from which this information was gleaned I found the following: In none of the US articles was sacral absence mentioned; in one a "spinal defect" was recorded (Thosteson 1953) and in another a "sireniform monster" (Driscoll et al 1960; the last was a report of a pathology study of malformations in neonatally dying children of diabetic mothers first reported by Gellis and Hsia 1959 discussed above). Although sirens often have sacral abnormalities the sacrum is seldom missing. Four of the other seven cases were reported to have sacral absence (Farquhar 1959; Herre and Horky 1964; Mølsted-Pedersen et al. 1964; Kučera et al. 1965); another was a siren (personal communication from Mølsted-Pedersen to Kučera et al. 1965), and two others had unspecified vertebral-column abnormalities (see Kučera et al. 1965).

Since sacral absence in neonates seldom comes to medical attention, only a well-examined matched series of nondiabetic births gathered concurrently with a series of diabetic ones could have decided whether the four clear occurrences of the defect in the 7101 infants of diabetic mothers collected by this review was truly an excess frequency. Questions regarding the frequency of this defect in diabetic and nondiabetic pregnancies are discussed below in the section on particular malformations. Little else in this report was of significance.

The Neave Analysis

Almost contemporaneous with the articles by Mølsted-Pedersen et al. (1964) and Kučera (1971a) a doctorate thesis was submitted to the Harvard School of Public Health on the subject of congenital malformations in the offspring of diabetic women (Neave 1967). Excellent in conception and execution, it has been relatively little known, perhaps because it was not otherwise published, except for a relatively brief summary appearing 17 years later (Neave 1984), it presented a substantial and meticulously analyzed body of data that made a case for malformations being much increased in diabetic pregnancy.

The data came from the records of births in 10 university-affiliated hospitals in the US and Canada, located from Cincinnati to Montreal, and covered different lengths of time from hospital to hospital in the years 1928–1966, but mainly the 1950s and 1960s. Very different proportions of the births came from the various hospitals, ranging from 2.1 to nearly 47%, the latter from the Boston Lying-in Hospital; the same was true of the number of diabetic women delivering, an indication of hospital size or referral status, which ranged from about 5 to 35 per year.

The records, abstracted by trained personnel, concerned births to women known to have been diabetic during pregnancy; hence may have included women not insulin dependent and not diabetic before conception of the index pregnancy, in both cases with and without clinical symptoms. Controls consisted of nondiabetic women delivering next at the same hospital matched for age, parity, and race. This then was a thorough investigation of historical records, albeit unavoidably containing much heterogeneity.

The Malformations

The infants were observed from birth to the time of discharge, but the malformations were mostly discovered in the first 2–3 days of life. Thus, abortion, spontaneous or induced, was not included. About 65% of stillbirths and 80% of neonatal deaths, index and control, were autopsied. Records of the births of 2592 index and a like number of control infants were available. The malformations were coded according to a modification of the framework presented by Edwards et al. (1964); and the abnormalities of each infant were encoded and listed in an appendix of the thesis.

In the index group 13.1% were stated to be congenitally malformed compared with 5.3% of the controls, the large frequencies due to inclusion of questionable entities. The most frequent of which were various morphological abnormalities of the placenta and umbilical cord, recorded in the absence of any serious congenital abnormality in 75 diabetic and 34 control pregnancies, phenomena that by no stretch of the imagination can be considered malformations of the infant. [Such conditions, incidentally, were not mentioned in reports of a number of pathological studies of the placentas of diabetic pregnancies (Warren and LeCompte 1952; Driscoll 1965; Singer 1984; Labarrere and Faulk 1991)]. In addition, numerous other isolated abnormalities (i.e. occurring in the absence of any others) were included that in themselves are usually trivial or have doubtful health implications (see entire list in Kalter 2000, p. 136).

The large number of one of these isolated defects, single umbilical artery, all but one of which were diagnosed at the Boston Lying-in Hospital, was explained by the special interest in this anomaly by the pathologists at that facility. That this was exaggerated was made obvious by the fact that in a pathology study from the same hospital this defect was found only once in 95 autopsies, and that without associated abnormalities (Driscoll et al. 1960).

The inadmissible defects included isolated microcephalus, which as was conceded is not ordinarily a clear-cut deformity; hypospadias, a relatively common and usually trivial defect with an important hereditary component (Harris 1990), seldom associated with unrelated defects (Calzolari et al. 1986); undescended testis, even commoner than hypospadias, in most cases of which the offending organs have descended by 3 months of age (Berkowitz et al. 1993); and Down syndrome, of which there were six instances, being due to a chromosomal aberration (Lejeune et al. 1959; Gardner et al. 1973) obviously cannot be the responsibility of maternal diabetes.

When these and the other disqualified conditions were omitted the malformation frequency became 5.8% in the index infants and 1.4% in the controls, a more realistic but still appreciable difference (perhaps indicating intense examination of the former and inadequate examination of the latter).

Perinatal Death Questions

These were total frequencies, in survivors and nonsurvivors combined. Not given special attention, but of obvious importance, was the frequency in each individually. These were 3.5 and 17.2% respectively in the diabetic and 0.9 and 14.7% in the controls; thus being about the same in the diabetic and control perinatal mortalities; but larger in the diabetic than the control survivors.

Setting aside the roughly similar frequencies in the deaths, there is left the differential in the survivors, which can perhaps be looked upon as meaning that maternal diabetes caused an increase only of less serious abnormalities, of the sorts that may present ambiguities in diagnosing; not ignoring the even greater likelihood that the controls were not as well examined as the index infants.

Race Considerations

Race may have had some relevance. Overall 12.7% of the diabetic women were nonwhite, predominantly black, although the proportions in the different hospitals varied, ranging from 1.2% in the Boston Lying-in Hospital to 75.6% in the Cincinnati General Hospital. Since race is markedly related to the frequency of several different congenital malformations, serious and trivial (Altemus and Ferguson 1965; Ivy 1968; Erickson 1976; Christianson et al. 1981; Polednak 1986; Chávez et al. 1988), pregnancy outcome may have been related to this factor. This matter divided the hospitals into two almost discrete sorts: five with a large mean percentage of nonwhite diabetic pregnancies, 41.2%, and five, with 2.3% nonwhite, a huge difference.

In hospitals with a large percentage of nonwhite patients twice as many nonwhite infants were malformed as white ones (7.0 vs 3.4%), while in hospitals with a small percentage of nonwhite patients, the frequencies were about equal (6.1 vs 6.8%). Unfortunately the malformations were not listed by hospital, so the analysis cannot go further. But it cannot be ignored, constituting as it did a further source of heterogeneity.

Research Biases

Neave encountered several difficulties in the course of his study. A particularly important one, called "observer bias," was characterized as follows: "Offspring of diabetic mothers often present formidable clinical problems.... There is no question that these infants are preferentially treated and that the chances of observing and recording malformations are greater [in them] than in the offspring of nondiabetic mothers." He attempted to allow for this by determining the frequency of malformations likely to be easily recognized because of being "grossly evident," and hence not subject to this bias. These defects too he found occurred almost twice as often in index as in control infants; and thus felt that this bias, and other possible ones that he enumerated, had not influenced the recorded data. But this reasoning was contradicted by another fact not emphasized by him, namely that the frequency of these conspicuous types of malformations was not greatly different in the index perinatal mortalities than in the control perinatal mortalities.

One malformation of special importance, sacral absence, because it has been thought to be part of a specific diabetic embryopathy, must again be given particular attention, though it was not included in the list of defects considered exempt from observer bias. Two infants with total sacral absence occurred in the index births in the Boston Lying-in Hospital, and one with absence only of the coccyx in the Johns Hopkins Hospital, all three being perinatal mortalities.

Indirectly, through the former two cases, a question arose about the adequacy of the search of the hospital records made by the abstracters hired to perform this task. Though Rusnak and Driscoll (1965) recorded three children with this condition as born to diabetic women at the Boston Lying-in Hospital between 1952 and 1964, only one was among the cases included by Neave; and Neave's second Boston case, born in 1956, was not one of those described by Rusnak and Driscoll. Apparently also absent from the records of index births made available to Neave was the symmelic infant noted by Gellis and Hsia (1959) and Driscoll et al. (1960). One is left therefore with the suspicion that, since relevant records were possibly overlooked or erroneously included, others pertaining to children malformed and not malformed may have been similarly mishandled.

It can thus be concluded that, being pervaded by so many loose ends, and especially in the face of a malformation frequency not excessive, an association between diabetes and malformations was not unequivically proven.

Multicenter Studies

Until the 1980s multicenter studies were relatively modest in size and made no pretense of surveying the entire population of a region. In time, however, as the number of units cooperating in these studies increased they began to overlap and were sometimes indistinguishable from those that intended to cover the entire populations of their respective geographical areas. The latter, the strictly population-based studies, will be discussed further on.

To begin at the beginning, the perspective of the earliest multicenter studies reflected their time by paying little or no attention to congenital malformations (Miller et al. 1944; Peel and Oakley 1949; Medical Research Council 1955). The first of these obtained data from the records of three hospitals in New York City, New Haven, and Boston, the second, by questionnaire from 26 hospitals and hospital-based centers in Great Britain and Ireland, and the third, from nine British diabetes centers. They all dealt almost exclusively with the relation of several maternal and treatment variables to the predominant concern of the day, the high level of perinatal death, and showed by their almost total neglect of malformations how little influence they considered such conditions to have on this problem. This was redressed by the next study of this sort.

Sweden Studies

An early such study consisted of a comprehensive analysis of records of diabetic pregnancies delivered in 1948–1954, mostly of patients insulin treated for several years, obtained from the obstetric departments of 21 general hospitals located in many parts of Sweden (Hagbard 1956, 1961). Information on a total of 472 children weighing at least 1000 g at birth or from pregnancies proceeding beyond 28 weeks were collected. As was usual for the time a large number, 36.3%, were stillborn or died in the first postnatal week.

The impact of congenital malformations on this outcome, it is obvious from the space allotted to these conditions—a bit more than one of the 180 pages in the entire 1956 monograph—was not thought of much importance. Yet sufficient information was given to reveal that such abnormalities were found in 6.4% of the offspring; and the list of the defects provided revealed that for the most part they consisted of the major varieties and represented various systems and parts. But which of them occurred in the mortalities was not designated. And this is of significance since a large proportion of the defective offspring, 63.3%, were found among the perinatal mortalities, leaving the remaining defects, for the most part probably of the less serious sorts, in 4.1% of the survivors.

Almost nothing was said of the way these abnormalities were detected, aside from the children usually being thought of as premature and therefore carefully watched for the first 5 days of life, with most perinatal mortalities, except for a few macerated stillbirths, being autopsied. The protocol from hospital to hospital apparently varied, as did the patient representativeness, but this was not detailed. The need for a control apparently was never entertained. Later studies in Sweden are considered elsewhere in this monograph.

Large Studies

The purpose of multicenter studies of reproductive outcomes of diabetic pregnancy should not merely be collecting the large number of subjects that may be needed to come to grips with difficult questions and their statistical analysis. The prime purpose, rather, is to reach for greater representativeness of pregnant diabetic women overall, something not to be expected of patients referred to specialized clinics and large hospitals, who usually constituted a biased sample of this population. To the extent that investigators were alert to the dangers of misinterpretation presented by selection factors, and their success in minimizing them, the findings of multicenter studies are credible. It might be argued of course that population-based studies would have an even greater advantage in this respect, a proposition examined below. Many multicenter studies have been conducted in recent years. Some of the more important ones are described here.

The Collaborative Perinatal Study

The mother of all multicenter studies was the Collaborative Perinatal Study sponsored by the then National Institute of Neurological Diseases and Blindness of the US National Institutes of Health (Berendes and Weiss 1970; Niswander and Gordon 1972). It was a grand scheme whose purpose was to examine the relation between pre- and perinatal factors and later aberrant neurological development. To achieve this goal 14 university-affiliated medical centers were recruited to collect the required obstetric and pediatric information. The study continued for 7 years, ending in December 1965, with the final registration of 55,908 women and their pregnancies.

The first report of the study concerned 39,175 women, about half of whom were white, half black, and dealt with perinatal death and neurological state at 1 year of age (Niswander and Gordon 1972, pp. 239–245). Relatively few of the women had diabetes, by which was probably meant pregestational diabetes, all together 254, giving the perhaps exaggerated prevalence of 6.5 per 1000 pregnancies, again about the same in whites and blacks. The only outcome of interest here, the so-called perinatal death rate, 14.2%, was excessive because it included deaths from the 20th week of gestation to the 28th day postnatal. White and black pregnancies were not different in this respect, perhaps because the black women included in the study were of urban origin and probably relatively well off socioeconomically (Berendes and Weiss 1970). Congenital malformations were not mentioned at all, not too surprising since the thrust of the study were neurologically handicapping conditions. All in all a big disappointing report.

More complete analyses of the voluminous data that dealt with aspects relevant here appeared in later years, but were not always useful. For example, from Boston came a report about newborns of diabetic women, providing data regarding over 500 diabetic pregnancies, but whose incompleteness prevented their clear analysis (Hubbell et al. 1965).

A general inquiry into the etiological bases of cardiovascular malformations in the offspring of diabetic women found a frequency of 2.5% up to 1 year up of age, which was about three times that in children of nondiabetic women (Mitchell et al. 1971a). This large figure was based on examinations "undoubtedly…more complete in some centers than in others," by pediatric cardiologists and other interested physicians, of children with definite or suspected congenital heart disease (Mitchell et al. 1971b). Although it cannot be compared with the frequency discovered in the perinatal period it is relevant because it is the result of augmentation by the emergence or recognition of such abnormalities during postnatal months and years (e.g. Neel 1958; McKeown and Record 1960; Mellin 1963; Hakosalo 1973; Klemetti 1978; Hoffman and Christianson 1978; Christianson et al. 1981), even taking into consideration the deaths of some malformed children at various postnatal ages (McDonald 1961; Hardy et al. 1979; Myrianthopoulos 1985). This matter will be adverted to again below, when it will be seen to have made for imponderabilities in analyzing an even wider range of observations (Chung and Myrianthopoulos 1975b).

Another matter of confusion in the Mitchell et al. (1971b) report is that it included 786 women as diabetic, a far greater number than the 254 so reported by Niswander and Gordon (1972). This gave the unusual prevalence of about 14 per 1000, which undoubtedly means that as well as pregestational diabetic pregnancies women with gestational diabetes and abnormal glucose tolerance were included, a conjecture supported by Naeye (1978) and notations seen elsewhere in this work.

A vast effort using the data of the Collaborative Study to examine the teratogenic potential of drugs found that 13 of 333 (3.9%) children of diabetic mothers had malformations, a frequency believed to indicate an increased relative risk; but again this figure was inflated by the children being periodically examined during their first 4 years of life (Heinonen et al. 1977, pp. 31, 430), as well no doubt as being based on inadequately examined controls. Mention of the outcome of diabetic pregnancies elsewhere in this publication was unclear.

The sparse details in the papers cited above were added to by several reports of the Collaborative Study which pertained to congenital malformations generally and to those in offspring of diabetic mothers in particular. It is not amiss to recall that the Collaborative Perinatal Study (which later was also sometimes called the Collaborative Perinatal Project) was a prospective investigation of the etiology of neurological and sensory disorders of children detected during the first 7–8 years of life.

Very complete accounts of the great variety of congenital malformations encountered in the entire number of children appeared in time (Myrianthopoulos and

Chung 1974; Chung and Myrianthopoulos 1975a; Myrianthopoulos 1975; Hardy et al. 1979). The account in Hardy et al. (1979, pp. 292–293) is especially revealing, since it presented the number of children with each listed abnormality diagnosed in the nursery and at 1 year of age, and thus revealed the greatly increased frequency that results from the protracted period of examination.

A full report of the malformations in the offspring of diabetic mothers enrolled in the study was made by Chung and Myrianthopoulos (1975b). But its design and intent defeated any great usefulness the findings may have had for the present monograph. In one respect it was an advance, since it differentiated between the several forms of diabetes, but continued the hindrance that the numbers and types of abnormalities noted were those diagnosed throughout the first year of life. It had other problems as well. Though one can agree with the authors (Myrianthopoulos and Chung 1974) that the division of malformations into major and minor is sometimes arbitrary, still there is much agreement as to what is one or the other, and in this paper this was often disregarded—over half of the cases with abnormalities that were listed as major are generally considered minor or dubious. (The extent to which this practice can influence outcomes was articulated when Klemetti 1978 found "a trebling of…frequency if the definition is made wider than strictly structural malformations to include minor deviations and functional disturbances.")

Another bias was introduced by including a large number of diabetic pregnancies from the Joslin Clinic. Since it was impossible to learn which defects were found neonatally and which discovered later the roughly doubled frequency of purported major malformations recorded in the children of the diabetic women was of no help in assessing the question of the teratogenicity of pregestational diabetes.

The Collaborative Study was also weakened by the number of women contributed by the participating centers being very uneven. Almost 42% came from just two of them—the Boston Lying-in Hospital and the Pennsylvania Hospital in Philadelphia (Niswander and Gordon 1972). Which probably led to a serious bias as far as the ascertainment of congenital malformations was concerned—variable racial composition, which ranged from 0% white in New Orleans to 97.6% white in Buffalo (Myrianthopoulos and Chung 1974)—though the overall sample that was analyzed for the relation between maternal diabetes and congenital malformations was fairly evenly divided in this respect (Chung and Myrianthopoulos 1975b). Nevertheless, this wide disparity and the undoubted difference in patient selection and malformation diagnosis further diminished the value of the data so laboriously collected and analyzed.

United Kingdom Study

A questionnaire survey of many hospitals throughout the United Kingdom identified 773 women with pregestational diabetes giving birth in 1979–1980, almost 90% insulin treated (Lowy et al. 1986b).

Major congenital malformations were noted in 4.0% of births, which included some ineligible conditions such as Down syndrome, uncomplicated talipes, patent ductus arteriosus, and ventricular septal defect. The perinatal death rate, 5.6%, though less than in former years was still nearly four times that for all babies in the United Kingdom at that time. Nearly half of the malformations occurred in perinatal mortalities, which was probably an underestimate, as indicated by the malformation frequency in stillborns being 12.0%, far less than the 55.6% in neonatal deaths, which probably meant that many of the former were not or could not be autopsied.

The malformations were of many parts, some of them considered "relatively specific," especially those of the heart and great vessels (which included, as noted, an unspecified number of offspring with patent ductus arteriosus and ventricular septal defect) and certain central nervous system defects. But no instance of anencephalus and only one of spina bifida was mentioned, which is strange since these defects had a relatively high frequency in many regions of the United Kingdom. Of interest, because of their notoriety, but given no special attention by the authors, was the occurrence of three cases of sacral absence (the manner of whose diagnosis was unmentioned) and two of holoprosencephaly. In addition, minor malformations (defined as those "unlikely to interfere with the baby's life") were noted but whether associated with the major ones was not mentioned. Also an attempted analysis of the relation between 1st trimester blood glucose level and malformation incidence had no useful outcome, mainly because major and minor malformations were not considered separately.

Whether the surveyed women were representative of the overall pregnant diabetic population was uncertain, since only 38% of the 474 hospitals from which information was requested participated in the study, and on average less than one pregnant diabetic woman was reported for every 1000 pregnancies, though this varied geographically from 0.3 per 1000 to 1.9 per 1000. [Such variations may be common; they were also noted in the many hospitals of an American metropolitan area (Miller 1965)]; whereas pregestational diabetes usually occurred in about 5–6 per 1000 pregnancies [(Niswander and Gordon 1972; Kalter and Warkany 1983)]. Finally, the outcomes of the pregnancies comprised only those that were "fully analysed," which was not explained.

National Institute of Child Health Study

The National Institute of Child Health and Human Development engaged with five US medical centers in a collaborative study of malformation and fetal loss in diabetic pregnancy in 1980–1985 (Mills et al. 1982, 1983, 1988a, b). Of the 626 insulin dependent diabetic women ascertained, 86% entered the study before or within 3 weeks of pregnancy and 14% later than this time. Controls were obtained only for the early-entry group. Malformations were usually diagnosed only on the 3rd day after birth by trained examiners guided by a checklist of defects.

The frequency of major congenital malformations in the early-entry group was 3.7% (or 2.3% if the isolated ventricular septal defects are omitted; the argument for doing so is presented below in the chapter dealing with specific malformations in offspring of diabetic women), and in the late-entry group 7.2% (or 6.1% if again the venricular septal defects are omitted). The controls had a 1.0% frequency of major congenital malformations with no explanation offered for this unrealistically low level.

The apparently increased frequency in the early-entry group was not thought to be related to mean blood glucose and glycosylated hemoglobin levels during early pregnancy, a conclusion departing from conventional ideas about glycemic control and maldevelopment, and criticized, as will be seen in pages below where these topics are dealt with.

Matters regarding the design of the study must be considered. Both the diabetic and control subjects were highly selected. The former, recruited "by means of public appeals as well as through the medical system," were without hereditary teratogenic tendencies themselves or in first-degree relatives, and diabetes in the latter was excluded; as were those being treated with potentially teratogenic pharmaceutical drugs for various diseases or disorders. The controls, employees of business corporations, medical centers, and prepaid health plans, were highly motivated volunteers whose pregnancies were planned.

The discrepancy between the number of diabetic women entering the study early who spontaneously aborted (as reported by Mills et al. 1988a; discussed above) and the number continuing their pregnancies was not explained. Last, the number of perinatal mortalities and the malformations occurring in them were not specified. The aspects of the study concerned with the relation between abnormal prenatal development and glycemic control in early diabetic pregnancy (Mills et al. 1988b) and with fetal growth delay (Brown et al. 1992) will be addressed below. All in all, an unsatisfactory study and report.

Recent Studies

A California program encompassing 19 clinical units in eight perinatal centers during 1986–1988 registered 572 pregestationally diabetic women (Cousins 1991c). The fraction this number comprised of the total of such pregnancies in the areas of the state surveyed during this time was not mentioned. The report of this apparently ambitious program was especially disappointing because its many numerical discrepancies and other inadequacies made its congenital malformation and perinatal death data difficult to interpret.

Diabetes Control and Complications Trial

In a US nationwide multicenter study in 1983–1993 half of the 270 pregnancies of insulin-dependent diabetic women were managed intensively and half conventionally (Anon. 1996). But because the project ended unproductively, so to speak, there being no significant difference in outcome between them, the pregnancies will be considered together. The rate of spontaneous abortion was 11.8%, i.e. within expected limits; another 2.2% were induced abortions, half with congenital malformations. Finally, the perinatal death rate was 15.2%. This left 191 live births, nine, 4.7%, with congenital malformations called major, but omitting three of the improbable ones left 3.1%, close to the usual level. The conclusion was that intensive therapy begun early had no effect on pregnancy outcome.

Denmark Studies

The earlier series of studies in Denmark, described above, of the detrimental effects on offspring of maternal type 1 diabetes, continued with a study noting a significant discovery regarding such births in the Rigshospital in Copenhagen in 1967–1986 (Damm and Mølsted-Pedersen 1989). Namely, major malformations whose frequency in 1967–1981 had been constant at 7.4% declined thereafter to 2.7%. And while this was greater than the 1.7% in nondiabetic controls it no longer seemed to be related to severity of the maternal disease. The feeble explanation of the decline was that the later pregnancies had been planned. More likely ones, such as modified malformation definition and mortality trends (prenatal and perinatal death were unmentioned), were neglected. Other aspects of this report are discussed below.

The series, overlapping somewhat, continued with a multicenter study of consecutive pregnancies of type 1 diabetic women in 1976–1990 in 11 hospitals in Northern Jutland, the majority in the main obstetric hospital at Aalborg (Nielsen and Nielsen 1993). Early spontaneous abortions occurred in 11.1% of uninterrupted pregnancies, not an unusual level; while in the remaining ones 4.3% died neonatally; all were autopsied and one found multiply malformed, giving a rate of major malformations of 3.1%, and an additional 2.4% minor; the number of the former in mortalities was left unstated however, clouding the full analysis.

A prospective large scale study of consecutive type 1 diabetic pregnancies was conducted in eight nationwide centers in 1993–1999 (Jensen et al. 2004). Admission to hospital was later than the first trimester, spontaneous abortion thus was not noted. The perinatal death rate was 5.3%, significantly greater than the population one of 1.2%; as was the 5.0% of congenital malformations (comprising many systems, predominantly cardiovascular) greater than the background of 2.8%. However, only half of the malformations were major and the proportion that occurred in the perinatal mortalities was not stated. Thus the important fact of the individual frequency of major malformations in perinatal mortalities and in survivors was again left unstated.

A recent report contained a startling number (Nielsen et al. 2006a). In a study, whose focus was the association of adverse pregnancy and glycemic level, insulin dependent pregnancies in North Jutland County during the wide interval of 1985–2003 had a spontanous abortion frequency, unless I am seriously misreading the article, sharply increased to 21.6%—unremarked upon—from the earlier reported

11.1%. Unnamed major and minor congenital malformations were seen in 4.3 and 4.5% respectively of uninterrupted pregnancies; which is an exaggeration, since once more it included those in perinatal mortalities.

The latest identified report concerned type 1 diabetic pregnancies from eight centers notified to a central regisry in 1993–1999 whose purpose again was examining the association of adverse pregnancy outcome and glycemic status (Jensen et al. 2009). The overall frequency of major congenital malformations was 2.5%, just less than the 2.8% in perinatal mortalities. Overall the malformation frequency appeared to be related to the degree of periconceptional glycemic control, ranging from 10.9% at levels greater than 10.4% HbA_{1c} to 3.9% at less than 6.9%, but without a significant relation.

France Studies

A survey evaluating outcomes of pregnancies of pregestational diabetic women was conducted in numerous perinatal centers in 2000–2001 (Boulot et al. 2003). The outcomes in type 2 women were summarized above. Those in the type 1 women were similar, perinatal death, 6.6%, and congenital malformations, 4.5%, unnamed, but occurring largely in the mortalities, again despite preconception control efforts.

A report of type 1 diabetic pregnancies in Nice in 1999–2002, mentioned above with respect to type 2 pregnancies (Hiéronimus et al. 2004). Again it was not possible to analyze because the malformations were not named and the proportion of malformed offspring that died perinatally was not stated.

In a retrospective multicentric study women with type 1 diabetes were treated during pregnancy with insulin glargine, a long-acting insulin analogue (Lepercq et al. 2010). In the 102 pregnancies the low frequency of one stillbirth and two major congenital malformations was, of course, attributed to the treatment.

Chapter 15
Population-Based Studies

Most of the studies this monograph is concerned with—hospital-based studies of pregnant diabetic women—were conducted in special medical facilities, including diabetes clinics, i.e. facilities whose patients may have needed special care, and who therefore may not have been a true cross-section of all pregnant diabetic women in that time and place.

The consequences of the diabetes in these women may therefore not truly represent the consequences in all its sufferers. This uncertainty may have been added to by the limited number of subjects that such studies included, regardless of the size of the facility and the number of years of the study; in fact the longer it continued, owing to changes over time, the less typical the study group may have been, making generalization more hazardous.

Two types of study were made—multicenter and population-based—to reduce unreliability and yield more valid interpretation. The main purpose of the former was to enlarge the sample and allow more acceptable conclusions. What it could not do was minimize unrepresentativeness; although the aggregate number of subjects may have been much greater than most centers could each provide, they were still usually composed of diverse and nonrandomly selected women.

The goal of the latter was to survey the entire population of subjects in a geographical area during a prescribed interval. But such studies had their own brand of problems, since they relied on sources of information—public-health and vital statistics certificates, alone or sometimes supplemented by various hospital records—that often proved to be deficient in important details regarding both mother and child; exemplified by the difficulties encountered in various studies of congenital malformations (Knox et al. 1984; Greb et al. 1987; Calle and Khoury 1991; Snell et al. 1992; Stone 1992).

Population-based studies nevertheless can provide insights not obtained otherwise. Such efforts proceed along two paths, from alleged cause to supposed effect or vice versa. Thus in the examples examined below the studies started either with diabetic pregnancies to learn whether they resulted in congenitally malformed offspring more often than did nondiabetic pregnancies; or with malformed offspring to learn whether more of their mothers were diabetic than those of nonmalformed offspring. The first type is called a cohort study and the second a case-control study.

H. Kalter, *A History of Diabetes in Pregnancy*,
DOI 10.1007/978-94-007-1557-8_15,

In both the key ingredient is unbiased ascertainment of the subjects and suitability of the controls.

Cohort studies of the outcome of pregnancy in diabetic women have sometimes relied on information obtained from vital statistics documents, supplemented by cross reference to hospital records of births and deaths and other sources of data; and sometimes, when the study was confined to a limited region, on information obtained from all or most of the hospitals in a region. The latter thus became magnimulticenter studies, and were often beset by some of the difficulties inherent in more conventional multicenter studies.

Cohort Studies

The ultimate cohort study relied on congenital malformations recorded on birth certificates—which it may be noted are seldom to be relied on for completeness or accuracy (e.g. Hexter and Harris 1991; Cooper et al. 2008). Nevertheless—

Birth Certificate Studies

Certificates of live birth and fetal and infant death in 1958–1959 from the New York City Department of Health disclosed that the frequency of congenital malformations in offspring of diabetic women, as noted within 48 hours of delivery, was 8.3%, versus 1.5% in the entire sample of births, the rate in fetal deaths being about five times that in live births (Erhardt and Nelson 1964). These figures are based on abnormalities many of which were not major malformations, e.g. clubfoot, hernias, hemangiomas, neoplasms, etc. (some whose admissability the authors themselves were skeptical of), or ineligible, "Mongolism," or unspecified, digestive system, bone and joint, etc. Some clearly major ones, such as anencephalus and spina bifida, however, were ascertainable, at 1.71 per 1000 births, and showed their usually ethnic proclivities. The type of the diabetes was not specified, but its apparently low prevalence, 2.1 per 1000, perhaps indicated failure to identify all diabetic women. These uncertainties, plus unreliable control data, make any overall conclusions regarding outcome of diabetic pregnancy from such sources precarious.

A similar survey of birth certificates, but of live births only, in Hawaii in 1956–1966, revealed far smaller frequencies of malformations, still larger however in diabetic than nondiabetic pregnancies, 1.8% vs 0.9% (Goodman 1976). The low frequency in the former may have been due to the dilution of the outcome by the inclusion of gestational diabetic and glucose intolerant pregnancies; but was not likely to have been significantly affected by only live births having been surveyed. However, even this low rate was magnified by including defects that could not be attributed to maternal diabetes: a Down and rubella syndrome, as well as several other inadmissible defects, omitting which reduced the frequency to 0.9%, almost identical with that (the unrealistically small one) in the nondiabetic pregnancies.

Swedish Birth Registers

Motivated by the thalidomide catastrophe (Lenz 1961; McBride 1961) Swedish medical authorities in 1964 set up a national system of surveillance of congenital malformations, accounting for more than 99% of the births in the 50 hospitals in the country, for the purpose of prompt warning of the presence of new environmental teratogens (Källén and Winberg 1968). Fortunately, little evidence of such a presence was detected (Källén 1987a, 1989). But another use to which the registry was put—examining the possible effects on offspring of maternal diabetes, among other selected maternal diseases and various problems—furnished some positive results, which however were only sparsely published (Källén 1987a, b, 1989).

Dr. Bengt Källén (1985, Analysis of deliveries among diabetic women in Sweden: 1978–1981. Personal communication) was kind enough to send me a detailed list of the malformations in offspring of women with diabetes "during pregnancy" in 1978–1981. The Medical Birth Register noted 1,512 such pregnancies, being a prevalence of 4 per 1000 births (close to that found somewhat later in Sweden—Pradat 1992a). This was considered to be higher than usual, an excess believed to be due to "25% of cases which do not fulfill the criteria of what is usually called diabetes…." From this it was further reasoned that the pregnancy outcome risks discovered probably were underestimates in the same proportion.

As defined by the then current ICD (WHO Classification of Diseases) 7.5% of the offspring were congenitally malformed, whereas the Swedish Register of Congenital Malformations noted 2.3%, the difference accounted for by exclusion of numerous minor or doubtful defects (Källén and Winberg 1968). The rate of perinatal death was 2.7%, of which 24.4% had "significant malformations" (4.2% of stillbirths and 52.9% of neonatal deaths—a difference of a sort found elsewhere noted in the present writing; the reason for the low frequency in the former thought to be that malformations were a lesser cause of such deaths. The frequency of undoubted major malformations in the survivors was 2.7%; while the 24.2% malformation frequency in the perinatal mortalities of the diabetic women was not statistically significantly different from the 20.0% in the entire population surveyed (Källén 1989).

A wider-ranging survey, in 1960–1980, of death of offspring of diabetic women noted a continuously and rapidly declining perinatal death rate, from 24.3% in 1960–1966 to 1.1% in 1974–1980, till the difference between it and that in nondiabetic births became almost negligible; while the infant death rate remained twice that in the nondiabetic population, due to the high level of lethal malformations (Olofsson et al. 1984b).

A prospective nationwide study of 80% of the pregnancies with type 1 diabetes in 1982–1985 was conducted at 36 regional and county hospitals (Hanson et al. 1990; Hanson and Persson 1993). The pregnancies were followed from the time the women were enrolled in the study, which was at about 9 weeks of gestation, which may have been the reason for the low spontaneous abortion frequency, 7.7%. Still this was very close to the 7.2% in the randomly chosen nondiabetic control pregnancies. Despite the women receiving the best medical care of the day the perinatal death rate continued to be over four times that occurring in the general population. A total of 4.2% congenital malformations was found at examination on the day of birth, over half of minor varieties, leaving 2.0% major, compared with a low 1.0% in the controls (none of which were specified in either group).

Little further has thus far appeared regarding the total population, most recent studies being limited to certain regions of the country or to certain malformations. One compared the effects of metabolic control during different periods in 1982–1993 in a county hospital in rural Ostersund, in a diabetic care program said to be efficacious, as judged by the perinatal death of 4.2% and a similar somewhat elevated congenital malformation 4.2%, while the miscarriage rate, 14.3%, continued along the usual line (Nordström et al. 1998).

Records in several health registries in 1987–1997 indicated that births to women with preexisting and gestational diabetes had total congenital malformation rates of 9.5 and 5.7% respectively, the latter similar to the population rate, while the excessive one in the former was due to including minor and otherwise ineligible defects such as hypospadias and polydactyly (Aberg et al. 2001).

A national study focusing on the fertility of type 1 diabetic women was limited to live births, and only secondarily noted congenital malformation frequency; which was said to have continuously declined, from 11.7% in 1973–1984 to 6.9% in 1995–2004, the overall frequency in the whole period being 7.4%, and 4.2% in the general population (Jonasson et al. 2007). Details allowing judgment of these figures, said to be noted in an Appendix, was inaccessible however.

The most recent report of the subject available to me was a population-based study of type 1 diabetic pregnancies in 1991–2003, encompassing almost all such pregnancies (Persson et al. 2009). Even at this late date unfavorable outcomes continued to be significantly more frequent than in the control group, i.e. the general population, namely, perinatal death 20.0% vs 4.8%, early neonatal mortality 5.1% vs 1.8%, major malformations 4.7% vs 1.8%. Although the malformations were not named a significant proportion were lethal. Here and in the Jonasson article, how the general population data were derived was not noted.

All in all, reports from this part of the world in the last 50 or so years seem not to have recorded any remarkable improvement in the fate of conceptions of diabetic women.

Washington State Birth Register

A review of diabetic pregnancies in Washington in 1979–1980, as identified through birth and fetal death certificates supplemented by records from hospitals and birthing centers, aspired to include about 95% of births in the state (Vadheim 1983; Connell et al. 1985). This ambitious attempt fell far short however, fewer than half the diabetic pregnancies being recorded on vital statistics certificates; yielding a prevalence of 2.1 per 1000 live births and fetal deaths, significantly less than often found elsewhere. The control consisted of pregnancies of nondiabetic women randomly accessed from birth and death certificate files.

About a quarter of the pregestational diabetics did not require insulin, making it likely that some of them were mislabeled, and the prevalence even less than 2.1. Also separately ascertained were women with gestational diabetes, with a prevalence of 2.9 per 1000, lower than often noted, suggesting underdiagnosis or underreporting.

Numerous inconsistencies and inadequacies regarding congenital malformations found their way into the findings, probably because the study depended on sources of data of variable quality. The inquiry having essentially an epidemiological thrust, the authors gave much attention to its design and to the classification of diabetes in pregnancy and less to considering the possible incompleteness and unreliability of the civil and hospital records the survey was based on.

The data, as presented in two discrepant tables, showed that the frequency of major congenital malformations in the offspring of pregestational diabetic women was about 13.0%, significantly greater than the 1.8% in the nondiabetic controls. The likelihood that the former was inflated and that the latter underreported were not considered. Nor was it mentioned that findings at postnatal ages were included in the figures.

The detailed list of congenital malformations in the case infants, appended to the thesis, revealed as supposed that many of them were not major. One set of the listed malformations is worth describing. It consisted of five instances of the caudal regression syndrome and two of sacral absence, three of the seven in gestational and four in pregestational births, an unusually large number of these rare abnormalities to exist in a relatively small sample. Descriptions of the defects offer a clue to this abundance. One of the sacral ageneses was described as follows—presumably copied from the original record: "Hypoplastic lower extremities, with flexion contractures of ankles (sacral absence)," which probably means that the person originally diagnosing the abnormalities, following the misconception of the day, interpreted the lower-limb defects as being equivalent to sacral absence. The second was described as consisting of "sacral agenesis and caudal regression," together with facial asymmetry, etc., leaving an unclear picture. One of the five instances of the caudal regression syndrome was accompanied by urogenital and other defects, including polysplenia, and another by imperforate anus. Those remaining were called "classical," a designation not without ambiguity. Since no definition or description was given of what caudal regression syndrome was considered to consist of, doubt must remain that the defect in these cases was that thought to be specific for diabetic embryopathy—especially since three of the seven instances occurred in infants of gestational diabetic women, in whom the frequency of congenital malformations was not increased (Kalter 1998).

Such indefiniteness was rife [but shared by many authors who were equally vague about such matters; e.g. Ramos-Arroyo et al. (1992), in a table listing malformations included "caudal dysgenesis," by which was meant "agenesis or hypoplasia of the femur, sacrum and/or lower vertebrae," a truly mixed bag, and truly and hopelessly confusing any attempt to relate a specific embryopathy with the maternal disease].

A bit helpful in compensating for the overall inadequacies of the study were the perinatal death data. Regarding its rate there was little difference between the pregestational diabetic and control pregnancies, 11.6% vs 8.4%. Malformations overall suffered from inadequate information, but its frequency in the diabetic mortalities was significantly larger than in the controls, 43% in perinatal mortalities and 21% in late fetal losses, probably owing to toutomehe special attention given the former.

Finally, the validity of the composition of the control was questionable. The births of the diabetic women took place in 38 of the nearly 90 hospitals in the state (Connell et al. 1985), while those of the control women, being a random selection from the vital statistics documents, had apparently occurred in all or nearly all the state hospitals. Further biasing the outcome, 79% of the diabetic women gave birth in just 16 of the 38, the largest and best equipped hospitals, those in which it can be safely assumed the offspring of women referred for special treatment received close attention. For all the reasons mentioned no great trust can be put in the supposedly increased congenital malformation frequency in diabetic pregnancies found by this population-based study.

Norwegian Birth Register

A population-based study in Norway made use of the national legal requirement that all offspring of at least 16 weeks' gestation be registered 7 days after delivery (Jervell et al. 1980). Such records revealed a prevalence of diabetic pregnancy in 1967–1976 of 1.6 per 1000, low according to some type 1 population estimates. A malformation frequency of 4.3% was noted in diabetic pregnancies versus 3.0% in all births with the excess accounted for by cardiovascular and central nervous system abnormalities. The defects were not completely spelled out and their association with perinatal death was unclear; which was no doubt of some importance since perinatal death decreased appreciably during these years, from 17.7 to 6.1%. Also, while the diabetes was usually present before pregnancy, the proportion insulin dependent was unknown, this fact not being included on the registration record.

Similar difficulties were present in a report of outcomes of diabetic pregnancy in the general population in 1982–1990, with an apparently high 6.4% major malformation frequency noted (Apeland et al. 1992). Detailed consideration of the findings was precluded however because the article was in Norwegian, only an inadequate English summary being available (my ignorance of the language to be blamed on a typically inadequate American education).

A recent account of congenital malformations in newborns of women with type 1 diabetes in 1999–2004 noted a 5.7% frequency, not otherwise described but excluding minor anomalies defined according to the EUROCAT system, the predominant defects being of the cardiovascular system, 3.2% (Eidem et al. 2010). No information was given regarding the proportion of the defects occurring in perinatal or other mortalties.

Australian Birth Registers

A survey of the association of maternal diabetes and congenital malformations was conducted in Aboriginal and nonaboriginal individuals in Western Australia in 1980–1984 (Stanley et al. 1985; Bower et al. 1992). The distinctness of the two groups was shown by the 18 times greater proportion of noninsulin-dependent pregestational diabetes in the former than in the latter; the probable explanation being that the Aboriginals were prone to precocious insulin dependent type 2 diabetes, resembling in this respect the Pima Indians discussed elsewhere in this work. This supposition was supported by the almost seven times greater prevalence among them of what was called gestational diabetes, which however apparently consisted mostly of glucose intolerance.

Analysis of the congenital malformations was barred by their not being named in detail and by the unclear tabulation of the findings. This was clarified by the enumeration Dr. Carol Bower kindly sent me of the abnormalities in the affected children born during these years; which indicated that the conditions in one-third of them were diagnosed at postneonatal ages up to 3 years, and that many others had inadmissible defects (congenital hip dislocation, hypospadias, trisomy 21, congenital hypothyroidism), or were misdiagnosed. Almost 40% of the defective offspring were Aboriginals, with a frequency of 15.3%, while in nonaboriginals it was 7.3%. In sum it was not possible to calculate the frequency of acceptable congenital abnormality for either group. It is regrettable that the enumeration of malformations was less clear and complete than in a contemporary review of perinatal death (Bower et al. 1984).

A publication from South Australia was equally confused (Sharpe et al. 2005). It dealt with live- and stillbirths in 1986–2000 of women with preexistent diabetes and gestational diabetes or impaired glucose tolerance, with prevalences respectively of 3.4 per 1000 and 23.9 per 1000 (the latter of course meaningless). Defects consisted of those diagnosed before the age of 5 years, so it is not surprising that their frequency was high, 10.9%. The defects that it can be taken for granted were present at birth were limb reduction defects, renal agenesis, transposition of great vessels, orofacial clefts, tracheoesophageal and anorectal atresia, neural tube defects, etc., with a total of 1.6%.

An account of births in a maternity hospital in Melbourne in 1971–1988 to women with "established" (82% insulin dependent) and gestational diabetic pregnancies was largely limited to reporting congenital malformations in the perinatal mortalities of the gestational diabetic women (White and Beischer 1990). For what it may be worth, five of the 15 mortalities had defects such as anencephalus, acrania, and spina bifida, which were obviously unrelated to the maternal condition, being present before the diabetes developed, a matter unacknowledged by the authors. Gestational diabetes was almost 20 times as common as the so-called established form, while the perinatal death rate though quite low was three times as common in the latter as in the former. The ethnic composition of the population, a subject of some importance in gestational diabetes, was disregarded.

A report of the outcome of pregnancies of type 1 and type 2 diabetic women in 1989–1998 was based on notes in a hospital in Sydney, New South Wales (Gunton et al. 2000). Though both were called pregestational, type 1 women were apparently insulin dependent while those with type 2 were not. Not surprising, a far larger proportion of the former were Caucasian than the latter. Strangely, there were said to have been no perinatal deaths at all, and not so strange, no major abnormalities in type 2. Some of congenital malformations called major cannot be considered such at all, namely epilepsy and cerebral palsy, while some cardiovascular conditions, e.g. partial anomalous pulmonary venous drainage, may not be serious.

One additional consideration. Ultrasonography detected an anencephalus and a spina bifida at 16 weeks gestation, both aborted, with no reason stated for the procedure in the first place. Discounting small sample size, compared with population statistics, this number seems to be beyond expectation (Mathers and Field 1983). It must be remembered however that New South Wales apparently did not have a mechanism for reporting early termination of pregnancy (Lancaster and Hurst 2001), and hence this may only be an apparent elevation.

Hesse Birth Register

Like some others the study in Hesse drew on the records of so many hospitals and covered so large a fraction of the population, about 78% of all born in 1982–1986, that it could be considered the equivalent of a conventional population study (Lang and Künzel 1989). The use of the omnibus term diabetes mellitus permitted 446 diabetic pregnancies to be identified, some unknown number of which were not the pregestational form. Congenital malformation data were vague and nonspecific, the total being 2.8% in diabetic cases and 0.5% in controls. Supposedly guiding the diagnosis was a computerized listing of many individual malformations, which however were not specified nor seemed to have been followed. The only thing to say for this project is that even a large population sample all by itself is not in the least a guarantee of definitive results.

Maine Birth Register

Pregnancies of pregestational diabetic women in 1987–1990 were identified through a regional network of private and hospital-based physicians (Willhoite et al. 1993). Of the 185 pregnancies 30 (16.2%) ended in fetal or neonatal death and 9 of the survivors (5.8%) were congenitally malformed, none of the defects named. In the approximately one-third of women who received preconception education to prevent adverse outcomes of pregnancy the malformation frequency was 1.7% and in the others it was 8.2%. Aside from the one defect in the former group, said to be major, none was characterized; but according to the authors the frequency difference was not significant. These results will be considered further in the section dealing with attempts to prevent malformations by counseling before or early in pregnancy.

Iceland Birth Register

Since 1974 all diabetic patients in Iceland have been cared for in the National University Hospital in Reykjavík, containing the only diabetic clinic in the country. This centralization enabled a validated prevalence of 1.4 per 1000 of type 1 diabetes to be determined, the lowest of any Nordic country (Hreidarsson et al. 1993). It also permitted identification of all pregnancies of diabetic women in Iceland; in 1981–1990 there were 86 such occurrences, two-thirds type 1 and one-third type 2, glucose intolerant, or gestational diabetics. In all of which there were two fetal anomalies, both cardiac, one occurring in the two perinatal mortalities, the other successfully surgically repaired. Assuming the worst case—that both malformed children were offspring of the 57 type 1 diabetic women—the frequency of the abnormalities was 3.5%, close to that expected for populations as a whole. Perhaps this survey done in a small island nation came closest to a definitive answer to a perplexing question. It might have been clinched had a control been included.

English Birth Registers

The outcome of births of diabetic women in 1994 in hospitals in a northern region of England, most of whom were pregestationally insulin dependent, was briefly, not to mention confusingly, described (Hawthorne et al. 1997). Of 113 pregnancies 29 were said to have had adverse outcomes, presumably including those not reaching the 24th week of pregnancy. The perinatal death rate was 4.6%; the majority being malformed left but a few of uncertain number among the survivors. The congenital malformation rate was 8.2% (9/109; 6 of the 9 fatalities) were not named. From the point of view of this work, a nearly worthless report.

The outcomes of 462 pregnancies in 1990–1994 of pregestational insulin-dependent diabetic women in maternity units in a northwest region of England were well depicted (Casson et al. 1997); 16.9% of the pregnancies spontaneously aborted, the vast majority in the 1st trimester, not an unusual total proportion; and again not unusually, a small number, 1.3%, were congenitally malformed. Quite different were the induced abortuses, comprising 5.2% of all pregnancies, 37.5% of which were malformed, the malformations unnamed however. Of the nonabortuses 3.6%

were perinatal mortalities, another 0.83% died postneonatally, 50.0% congenitally malformed. Of the survivors 27 were said to be malformed, a seemingly high 7.8%. Unfortunately the important matter of what malformations the survivors had was glossed over, not being well spelled out.

Of those named, cardiovascular defects were commonest, occurring in all of the perinatal mortalities as well as 2.5 per 1000 of the liveborn. The other defects mentioned were unnamed, renal and skeletal malformations and hypospadias, but relatively few and probably none major. As elsewhere therefore, malformations did not occur beyond the frequency expected for mortalities and survivors.

One further matter must be noted, that in the total of 462 pregnancies not one anencephaus was mentioned, in an area in which this conspicuous anomaly is not rare (Kalter 2009). However a considerable number of pregnancies were "terminated because of a congenital malformation." Strangely, none was named. Were any of them anencephalus?

By contrast was a brief note regarding pregnancies in Norwich in the east of type 1 diabetic women in 1991–2000 (Temple et al. 2002). There were 7.4% spontaneous abortions, 2.5% perinatal mortalities, and 3.6% congenital malformations, three-quarters of which were neural tube defects, obviously in the perinatal mortalities; all in all not an unusual outcome.

Case-Control Studies

We move now to case-control studies, a type of population-based examination of the association of maternal conditions and congenital malformations, which has a relatively young history.

Finland Study

The earliest such study of diabetic pregnancy appears to have been conducted in 1965–1973 by the Finnish Register of Congenital Malformations, which examined the prevalence of "diabetes mellitus," various infectious diseases, and other problems in women who gave birth to infants with central nervous system malformations (Granroth 1978).

Based on the finding that 1.5% of the 710 cases of all central nevous system defects occurred in offspring of women with diabetes and that none of the controls was diabetic, it was considered that the defects were significantly associated with the maternal condition. Two facts weakened this assumption: first over one-third of the abnormalities on which it was based were hydrocephalus and microcephalus, two defects, as noted above, of mixed etiology and vague diagnostic criteria; and second the Finnish registry required the notification of all malformations detected not only at birth but during the 1st year of life (Saxén et al. 1974), diminishing the usefulness of the outcome for evaluating defects present at birth.

Japan Study

A novel variation of the case-control approach was taken by Matsunaga and Shiota (1980). They examined 3,474 well preserved, undamaged abortuses induced for sociomedical reasons, as permitted by Japanese law (Nishimura et al. 1968). The women undergoing the procedure were apparently a random sample and the morphological condition of the embryos was unknown to the gynecologists performing it. Six of the abortuses came from women with "diabetes mellitus," seemingly a low incidence of the disease, until it is recalled that Japan been reported to have a low prevalence of insulin dependent diabetes (Patrick et al. 1989; World Health Organization Multinational Project 1991). Only one of the 'diabetic' abortuses had a malformation, a myeloschisis, a frequency not significantly different from that in the entire sample.

Other Reports

In a study at the Children's Hospital in Philadelphia of 150 children with myelomeningocele and 22 with anencephalus, the mothers of none of the former and one of the latter was an "overt" diabetic (Eunpu et al. 1983), fewer than expected, according to a calculation made by the authors.

In a recently published study from Hungary of the occurrence of type 1 and 2 and gestational diabetes in women with malformed infants an occurrence greater than that in background data was found only in the first group, 0.35%, with few specific defects, unnamed cardiovascular malformations, etc. (Bánhidy et al. 2010).

Atlanta Study

Casting a wider net, a study was made of all "serious or major" malformations in liveborn infants diagnosed by 1 year of age of women with insulin dependent presumably pregestational diabetes in the five-county metropolitan Atlanta area in 1968–1980, relative to those in the background population (Becerra et al. 1990).

The absolute frequency of malformations in the case women was not stated, only the risk of defects relative to that of the population; this being 7.9, implying an 18% medically validated major malformation frequency in offspring of diabetic mothers, far greater than even the most convinced and enthusiastic believers in the teratogenicity of diabetes had ever claimed in recent times. Even larger risk ratios were calculated for certain specific malformations, especially of the central nervous and cardiovascular systems, even though the authors stated it seemed these infants were not "particularly prone to a characteristic pattern of defects."

The prevalence of insulin dependent diabetes in the case and control mothers was 5.3 per 1000 and 0.7 per 1000 respectively, the latter extraordinarily low. Positive replies by case mothers to the question "at any time before [date of index birth] were you ever diagnosed as having diabetes or sugar diabetes?" were not medically validated; negative replies by the control mothers were not. The authors defended this inconsistency by asserting that the possible underascertainment of insulin dependent diabetes should have been negligible; but then themselves explained it by the absence of routine intensive diabetes screening of the area's population during the study period.

All information was gathered from interviews of both parents, which consisted of a large number of questions, expected to take 45 minutes for each (Erickson et al. 1984b). This was undoubtedly a burden to all, but without doubt considered more intrusive by parents of normal than malformed children and, as it has often been found, were probably answered less patiently, fully, and accurately by the former than the latter.

Other problems and weaknesses besetting the study can also be mentioned. Control mothers were selected from birth certificates of children "without defects;" the accuracy of which with regard to the recording of malformations has frequently been found wanting (e.g. Gittelsohn and Milham 1965; Mackeprang et al. 1972; Hexter and Harris 1991). The case infants included stillbirths as well as live births; the controls only live births. An unstated number of the malformed case infants were diagnosed postneonatally, as revealed by the list of defects given by Erickson et al. (1984a); there was no opportunity for doing so in controls. This list also revealed that a substantial number of the defects were either not major malformations or had a known or probable etiology. The relative risks were based principally on occurrence of individual malformations, not on that of malformed infants.

It was also mentioned incidentally that the study included a relatively small proportion of women with gestational diabetes, whose children had a risk of malformations that was found to be as great as those of insulin dependent ones, a matter that alone casts doubt on the project as a whole.

Further comments: The material had originally been gathered for the purpose of assessing the risk of US Vietnam veterans for fathering children with congenital malformations, and may have suffered to some extent from the constraint the original investigation was under to "be completed as quickly as possible" (Erickson et al. 1984a).

Finally, information regarding many aspects of maternal health before and during the index pregnancy were obtained from mothers of the malformed and matched control children by telephone interview 2–3 years after the births (Erickson et al. 1984b). Not all parents were located or cooperated, and for only about 70% of the eligible individuals in each group were interviews completed. Participation was lower for nonwhite than white mothers, who formed one- and two-thirds respectively of all births.

Baltimore-Washington Infant Study

Recent case-control studies were generally more ambitious than the few earlier ones. Typifying them was the Baltimore-Washington study. This was a survey of liveborn children with cardiovascular malformations whose purpose was to examine its association with maternal diabetes (Ferencz et al. 1987). The malformed children were identified through a search of the records of 53 hospitals in Maryland, the District of Columbia, and five northern Virginia counties, supplemented by hospital pathology and vital statistics death records. The malformations of concern were those identified at birth or confirmed before 1 year of age by autopsy or various diagnostic procedures performed at six pediatric cardiology centers. From these numerous and diverse sources infants with various malformations of the heart and great vessels born in 1981–1987 were identified.

The mothers of the malformed children and those of a randomly selected control group were interviewed in their homes some months after the births, at which time whether or not they were diabetic or had diabetes apparently from before or only during the index pregnancy was ascertained, statements that were not confirmed medically. Significantly more case mothers claimed to be pregestational diabetics than controls (1.5% vs 0.5%). Gestational diabetes was also increased in the former, but not significantly. An analysis of individual types of cardiovascular malformations indicated that only a few were significantly increased (double outlet right ventricle, truncus arteriosus, tetralogy of Fallot, ventricular septal defect), while many others were not.

The study had several shortcomings, which detracted from its impressiveness, the most serious and obvious being its entire reliance on unconfirmed maternal recall at unstated, perhaps delayed, times after the births. As the authors admitted, this probably led to "misclassification of true overt and gestational diabetes." At least as serious is the well known difficulty, as McKeown (1988, p. 104) put it, that "... mothers who have had an abnormal child report a higher frequency of many occurrences than mothers whose children are normal." Evidence of this was the elevated frequency of many sorts of cardiovascular malformations in children of gestational diabetic mothers.

Perinatal death is another matter of concern. Some of the abnormal infants died perinatally and were diagnosed postmortem; but the proportion of all instances that these composed was not stated. [Cardiovascular malformations were found in 1.5–2.7% of background perinatal deaths (Hoffman and Christianson 1978), and formed a sizable proportion of all such defects found perinatally.] Also many malformed infants may not have been included in the study since a large fraction of infants with congenital cardiovascular malformations die in infancy without their condition being recognized (Abu-Harb et al. 1994).

Findings at postneonatal ages were included, which is relevant since an important fraction of cardiovascular malformations are found in later months of infancy (e.g. Hoffman and Christianson 1978). In an earlier Baltimore-Washington report the authors themselves reported that 80% of septal defects were diagnosed after the

1st month of life (Ferencz et al. 1985). Although the practice of considering older ages may be necessary for depicting a fuller picture of the cardiovascular situation it debases the value such studies may have for clarifying the principal question the present monograph is grappling with.

Finally and most strangely, malformed offspring with abnormalities whose etiology was more or less clearly known to have nothing to do with maternal diabetes were not excluded from consideration, as was done in other case-control studies described below. These included various recognized syndromes, and especially those with conditions due to chromosomal aberrations, which comprised a large fraction of the entire sample. Failure to exclude the latter is particularly relevant in Down syndrome since it is often associated with congenital cardiovascular malformations, especially ventricular septal defect (Park et al. 1977; Hyett et al. 1995). This failure further weakened any conclusion that the study claimed about the relation of diabetes and the malformations.

Heart Defect Studies in Sweden

A study of major congenital cardiovascular malformations in offspring of diabetic women in 1981–1986 used data collected by the Swedish Registry of Congenital Malformations and the Child Cardiology Registry (Pradat 1992a). The focus was still- and liveborn children with such defects identified in the first postnatal week or at autopsy within the first year of age, excluding those with chromosomal aberrations.

Cases were compared with nonmalformed matched controls of normal birth weight surviving the neonatal period randomly selected from the Medical Birth Registry; which also provided the facts regarding the maternal characteristics whose possible association with the malformations was examined. These sources noted that 22 of the 1,324 case offspring and 17 of the 2,648 controls had mothers with "diabetes mellitus," giving an odds ratio of 2.7. This was regarded this as a "strong correlation" with the disease, but the association was significant only for septal defects. Judging from the 6.4 per 1000 prevalence of the maternal condition in the controls it is likely that the diabetes ascertained was of the pregestational variety.

Two difficulties with the study impaired its usefulness for the purposes of the present work. The number of case perinatal mortalities and their malformation frequency and the number of the 22 cases with diabetic mothers diagnosed after the neonatal period were not stated. As for the significance of the results per se this will be evaluated in the section below devoted to the studies in which children of diabetic mothers were followed postnatally.

In an overlapping survey the increased malformation risk noted by numerous health registries in several counties in a southeast region in 1982–1996 was found to be largely accounted for by a variety of conditions mislabeled major malformations (Blomberg et al. 2000). In one of the counties however, compared to other regions, there was an increased risk of major cardiovascular malformations of variable severity and significance diagnosed by the age of 1 year. No reason was broached for this apparent geographic limitation.

A prospective study during the same period and in the same area looked into possible risk factors affecting the frequency of cardiovascular malformations at birth (Cedergren et al. 2002). A search of various health registers, omitting those with known chromosomal anomalies, persistent ductus arteriosis, and single umbilical artery, left a frequency with specified heart defects of 13 per 1000 births, almost one-quarter of them ventricular septum however, and as commented previously, the high proportion probably due to overdiagnosis.

A child cardiology register, identifying those referred with severe defects before age 1 noted 1.6 per 1000 births and only maternal diabetes mellitus to be associated with them. Strangely, in a detailed study that examined various possibly related situations, no specific indication was given of the type of the maternal diabetes.

CDC Congenital Renal Disease Study

An investigation bearing a remote likeness to a case-control study can be mentioned here. Data gathered in 1970–1984 by the Birth Defects Monitoring Program of the Centers for Disease Control, made primarily to examine the temporal trend of renal absence and renal dysgenesis, were incidentally used to search for an associations of these defects with an unstated number of maternal conditions or exposures. This led to the discovery that maternal diabetes was noted in the records of 20 of 709 infants with the former of these abnormalities, suggesting that they were associated (Stroup et al. 1990).

The things that can be criticized about this study are legion, not to speak of the vagueness of the designation of the maternal illness. The Program being a passive system was based on newborn hospital discharge diagnoses made by physicians and other staff and not routinely checked for accuracy; thus may have included irrelevant renal abnormalities as well as Potter syndrome and other conditions of recognized or suspected etiology. Not all hospitals contacted participated and not all records requested were received. Maternal history was abstracted from the infants' medical records, a source open to incompleteness and inaccuracy. The resemblance of the study to a case-control one however totally breaks down because the search for associations apparently almost having been an afterthought there was no control. Clearly, no credence can be given to the finding of an association of these renal conditions and diabetes.

Miscellaneous Studies

A study in two Belgrade University obstetrics clinics noted 591 children with congenital malformations born in 1986–1988, a considerable number with minor malformations and those of genetic etiology being omitted. Two of the mothers had diabetes during pregnancy versus none of the controls, a nonsignificant difference (Ananijevic-Pandey et al. 1992).

A case-control study in Spain monitoring about 10% of the live births in the country in 1976–1985 was part of a collaborative study of congenital malformations (Ramos-Arroyo et al. 1992). During this period 2.0% of all births were found to be malformed in the first 3 days of life, including nearly 40% minor types and those due to single genes and chromosomal aberrations. The ascertainment of maternal insulin dependent diabetes was suspect, the prevalence in mothers of case infants being 1.1 per 1000 and in controls 0.2 per 1000; a 5.5-fold difference, meaningless if for no other reason than it was based on the total of all malformations. The odds ratio for major malformations alone was large, 8.7, but misleading because of the severe underascertainment of the maternal condition; and also because the unit of analysis, as in the Atlanta study discussed above, was the individual abnormality, and not the abnormal infant. That alone invalidated the study, if only because it exaggerated the statistical significance by inflating sample size.

A registry of births in Alsace in 1979–1987 permitted a case-control study of the relation of congenital hydrocephalus to maternal diabetes (Stoll et al. 1992). Instances of the condition secondary to trauma, due to chromosomal aberrations, and part of recognized syndromes were omitted, leaving 76 occurrences discovered in the first year of life. Three of the mothers had "diabetes," as did two of the mothers of the matched controls, making for an insignificant difference.

A malformation surveillance program at the Brigham and Women's Hospital in Boston in 1972–1974 and 1979–1990 identified insulin dependent diabetes in the mothers of 11 of 147 (7.5%) offspring with neural tube defects (Holmes 1994). A control was not obtained. The prevalence of the defects in those years was 1.2 per 1000, rather low for a presumably largely white patient load in an area a significant part of whose population had a greater than average proneness to such defects (Naggan and MacMahon 1967).

It may not be amiss to note another article of appropriateness here. A retrospective study of 22 families each with a child with sacral absence found a 5% recurrence rate and a similar rate of association with (an undesignated type of) maternal diabetes (Magnus et al. 1983), making it equally likely (or unlikely) that the condition had a genetic as an environmental provenance. Also cited were reports of an association of this abnormality with paternal diabetes, for which evidence of teratogenicity has not been found (e.g. Koller 1953; Rubin and Murphy 1958; Chung and Myrianthopoulos 1975b; Theile et al. 1985). Apropos of this study it is appropriate to note the virtual nonexistence of studies of the frequency and type of congenital malformations in the families of women with diabetes.

National Birth Defects Prevention Study

A study of the outcome of pregnancy in 1997–2003 of women with pregestational diabetes (types 1 and 2 combined) and gestational diabetes utilized data from ten congenital malformation surveillance systems throughout the US (Correa et al. 2008). The type of diabetes was not medically validated, but relied on maternal self report, as was true of a previous population-based study (Becerra et al. 1990), and hence probably led to some misclassification. As in the former study information was obtained by interviewing mothers up to 2 years after delivery. The prevalence of each form of pregestational diabetes being noted separately, it was revealed that that of type 1 was an extraordinarily low 1.1%, far less than the often found 5%. Finally, although not made clear, it was alleged that gestational diabetes was associated with some unstated frequency of malformations.

Nova Scotia Study

A study was made of the outcome of pregestational insulin-dependent diabetic women (85% White classes B and C) referred to maternity clinics after 20 weeks of gestation throughout the province in 1988–2002 (Yang et al. 2006). There were 516 births of which 1.7% died peri- and neonatally; and 9.7% had congenital anomalies, said to be severe, but of which the great majority survived; an overblown report, fully but irrelevantly detailed and of minimal significance.

A Multi-center Study

Women with type 1 diabetes studied at 63 centers in 18 countries in 2002–2005 were randomized to receive a rapid-acting insulin analog or human insulin (Hod et al. 2008). There were 35 fetal losses, 37 peri- and neonatal deaths, and 268 live births; 15 with malformations (3 in 4 of the terminations); but defects in the 27 "miscarriages" was not mentioned). No difference was noted between the two treatment regimens in any of these mishaps. All in all an apparently infrequent set of them; but much was left unsaid, the emphasis having been on a comparison of the two regimens.

Chapter 16
Specific Congenital Malformations

Among those who harbor no doubt that diabetes and malformations are associated some have held that the disease is associated with an increased frequency of all congenital malformations whereas others believe the increase is limited to some particular ones, especially or even the latter only. The former school was represented by Pedersen (1977, p. 196) although somewhat equivocally, when he said that "no specific defect is peculiar to diabetes, but severe congenital heart disease and skeletal deformity are characteristic." The latter school, less hesitantly, favored a number of abnormalities, among them of course caudal dysplasia, but also holoprosencephaly, neural tube defects, and cardiovascular malformations. This chapter will look into these assertions.

Caudal Dysplasia

There have been many reports of the occurrence of caudal abnormalities in offspring of diabetic women. One form or another of such conditions was mentioned in numerous articles, the earliest from 60 years ago (Peel and Oakley 1949). Increased awareness of them and growing belief in their association with diabetes no doubt accounts for the majority of the publications mentioning them having appeared since 1980.

It has aptly been said that it is "difficult to make a good case for caudal agenesis as a diabetic embryopathy mainly because of the poor definition of the syndrome…." (Chung and Myrianthopoulos 1975b). Ever since Duhamel (1961) included malformations of the lumbosacral spine as an element in his "syndrome of caudal regression" the use of this term has been confused and abused. As explained elsewhere in this work Duhamel defined this syndrome as including not only vertebral defects but also in "variable proportion anomalies of the rectum, of the urinary and genital systems…and of the lower limbs." This scheme was the culmination of his attempts to explain the frequent association of anorectal with other abnormalities, especially of the lower vertebral column (Duhamel 1959, 1961), which led him to theorize that since these were the very abnormalities found most often in sirenomelia they must

H. Kalter, *A History of Diabetes in Pregnancy*,
DOI 10.1007/978-94-007-1557-8_16, © Springer Science+Business Media B.V. 2012

form a syndrome of graded and variable content. Opposing the extension of this theory to diabetic pregnancy however was the frequent observation that in sirenomelia the sacrum, though often dysplastic, was seldom absent.

But it is absence of the sacrum that is the specific feature of the so-called caudal dysplasia syndrome, if such a syndrome exists at all, contrary to the attempted revision of the nomenclature (e.g. Welch and Aterman 1984). Nevertheless Duhamel's concept has made analysis of the conjectured association of diabetes and sacral abnormalities difficult.

The reason for this difficulty is that many of the nonvertebral malformations—anal, femoral, etc.—said to be part of the caudal dysgenesis syndrome ["…an absolutely obnoxious term" (Benirschke 1987)] has each by itself often been taken as denoting it. Thus when, as is often the case, infants of diabetic women labeled as having *the* syndrome or one or another of its variant designations, without clear-cut description of the abnormalities that are present, it is impossible to know whether sacral absence, the malformation thought by Benirschke (1987) and others to be "characteristic for the offspring of maternal diabetics," was truly present or not. The few crystal-clear examples of the misuse invited by this term only hint at other such instances masked by vague and imprecise terminology.

The syndrome has been equated with "…reduction defects of the legs with or without agenesis of the lower segments of the spinal column…" (Soler et al. 1976). An infant said to have caudal dysplasia was thus described, "Une radiographe post mortem montre qu'il existe 6 vertèbres lombaire; *le sacrum est normal* [emphasis added], ainsi que le reste du squelette" (Kubryk et al. 1981). Others mislabeled had severe defects of the lower limbs (Assemany et al. 1972), femoral and humeral defects and fistulae on the sacrum (Berstein 1978), and bilateral femoral hypoplasia alone (Hitti et al. 1994).

Two of the many further examples of the potential confusion caused by such imprecision will be cited to illustrate the widespread misinterpretation it encourages. Amendt et al. (1974) observed six instances of what were called "caudal regression," only three of which had sacral absence and the others defects of the pelvis alone or combined with vertebral defects. Likewise, Ballard et al. (1984) observed three of "caudal dysplasia," though only one had sacral absence, another unspecified sacral vertebral abnormalities, and the last defects of the long bones of the legs; and Miodovnik et al. (1988) three of "caudal dysplasia," but of none was it explicitly said that the sacrum was absent.

Finally, of the three instances of sacral dysplasia noted in 1950–1974 in children of diabetic women at the diabetes clinic of the General Hospital in Birmingham, England (incidentally, identified neonatally no doubt only because they were multiply and lethally malformed) only one apparently lacked sacral vertebrae, though this fact was detailed in one report (Malins 1979) but not in another (Soler et al. 1976). Thus the designation sacral or caudal regression or dysgenesis or dysplasia did not necessarily mean that the sacrum was absent.

Nor have animal experimenters, out of their depth, been immune to this misconception. In one report hindgut malformations, one of the many types of abnormalities induced in mice by the potent vitamin analogue retinoic acid, was equated with caudal dysplasia; which compounding the misconception was then erroneously stated to be associated with gestational diabetes (Alles and Sulik 1993). [With greater justification thymic absence induced in fetal mice by excess vitamin A (Kalter and Warkany 1961) was considered completely analogous to a human condition, the DiGeorge syndrome (DiGeorge 1968; Lammer and Opitz 1986), a rare affliction with immunological consequences (Warkany 1971, pp. 739–740).]

Therefore, if the proposition that caudal abnormalities are associated with maternal diabetes is to be taken seriously only clear-cut instances of sacral absence must enter into the consideration. It is to be remembered that absence of the sacrum failed to be discovered in the neonatal period in many affected children, owing to absense of external indication (Van Dyke et al. 1995), and usually only first came to medical attention months or even years later, when urological and other difficulties surfaced. For example, a sacral aplasia was only discovered when detected by a radiograph of a 5.5-year-old child (Manzke et al. 1977). Such late-detected instances cannot be included in an analysis of phenomena found at birth.

Reports of Caudal Abnormalities

The facts as they are can now be put into focus. All told offspring with caudal abnormalities mentioned in articles since about 1960 (none identified most recently) amounted to a prevalence of 5.6 per 1000 births (Kalter 2000, p. 165). But for only about a third was it explicitly stated that the sacrum was absent, and the age the condition was first diagnosed was not always clearly stated. About 17% died perinatally, at least 31% survived the neonatal period, and the fate of 52% was not mentioned at all. Assuming then, based on these figures, that about half of these instances was detected neonatally, it may be estimated that over the years the mean prevalence of the condition at birth was about 4.4 per 1000. [At this point it is important to know that the estimates arrived at did not consider the reports of malformations in several thousand offspring of diabetic women in which, whether because they were overlooked or not present, no such spinal malformations were mentioned.]

What is known of the frequency of sacral absence in the general population with which this tentative figure may be compared, especially that discovered at birth? Very little. In a search of nearly one million birth registrations in Czechoslovakia in 1961–1964, five cases of agenesis of the lower spine were located (Kučera and Lenz 1967), a low frequency it would seem. The fact that these registrations recorded an overall congenital malformation frequency of only 1.4% and that not all instances of the spinal malformation are detected at birth make the number hardly credible.

A survey of still- and live births in hospitals in Spain during about a 15-year period uncovered frequencies of 4.5 per 1000 and 0.2 per 1000 respectively of "caudal dysgenesis (any degree)" (Martínez-Frías et al. 1994). But these figures cannot be taken seriously, since the surveyed conditions included "urinary, genital, and/or anal anomalies, and/or those with lumbosacral spine defects (including the most severe anomalies of the caudal region such as sirenomelia)…."

That most children with such conditions survive the neonatal period was indicated by a single instance of sacral absence being found in 2145 autopsied perinatal mortalities, i.e. 0.47 per 1000 (Holmes et al. 1976). A radiological analysis of the spines of 700 children of postneonatal ages examined in 1940–1955 gave a more realistic assessment: four had absent infralumbar vertebrae, for a frequency of 5.7 per 1000 (Shands and Bundens 1966), about 30% more than the one calculated for diabetic births noted above.

It is not amiss to note that the frequency of congenital sacral absence surmised above is a far cry from the estimate made years ago—over 200 times greater—of lower spinal abnormalities in children of diabetic mothers (Passarge and Lenz 1966); nor to note that the latter was uncritically cited not long ago (Feigenbaum et al. 1996). The data in the few publications relating to the overall frequency of sacral absence in perinatal mortalities and older children thus pointed to the small likelihood of this malformation being increased in frequency in the offspring of diabetic women.

The major source of the belief that sacral absence is associated with diabetes are case reports of their concurrence. But case studies do not prove relationships. To paraphrase Leck (1993), the most that they can show is that a proportion of cases of a type of defect has occurred after exposure to some factor such as disease or medication of the mother during early pregnancy, not that exposure has occurred in a higher proportion of cases than of all pregnancies and therefore cannot be regarded as proof that this exposure is even a risk factor for the defect let alone a cause.

Central Nervous System Malformations

The congenital central nervous system malformations anencephalus, meningocele/encephalocele, and spina bifida, sometimes aggregated under the heading neural tube defects, have often been said to be among the anomalies that are especially increased in frequency in the offspring of diabetic women. Many fetuses with these defects die prenatally, but of those surviving to birth anencephalus being markedly conspicuous and invariably lethal has gotten much attention (Lemire et al. 1978).

A startling feature of anencephalus is that despite this lethality it reappears generation after generation; which must mean that the etiology of nonsyndromic anencephaly, despite some tendency to familial recurrence, is either overwhelmingly environmental or multifactorial.

Consequently anencephalus has been extensively studied, with a great deal of information regarding its prevalence and worldwide distribution being at hand (Kalter 2009). Inciting and enabling investigation is the harsh reality that in many parts of the world anencephalus is among the commonest of the major congenital malformations. This plus its extraordinary variations in frequency—racial, ethnic, temporal, socioeconomic, geographic, as well as the still unexplained fact of its being commoner in girls than boys (Elwood and Elwood 1980; Little and Elwood 1991)—have piqued the interest of geneticists, epidemiologists, and many others in this condition for decades (Penrose 1957). Nor to be forgotten is that its relative frequency in fetal death has surged with the steady decline in the stillbirth rate from the mid-twentieth century (Anon. 1965).

Though these variables are certainly relevant to the relation of neural tube defects and maternal diabetes, except for geography and an occasional mention of ethnicity or race, such aspects have been almost totally ignored by the numerous investigators studying the pregnancies of diabetic women. Even such elemental facts, of significance to patterns of occurrence, as the sex of affected infants or its incidence in previous pregnancies or other close family members have seldom been considered. The possible impact of such matters on the epidemiology of this malformation has thus been largely closed to analysis.

While anencephalus is the most glaring of the neural tube defects and thus almost impossible to overlook, infants with others, spina bifida especially, though often stillborn (Martin et al. 1983; Sadovnik and Baird 1985), seldom fail to be registered in hospital and vital records. It is the putative association of these defects with maternal diabetes that is considered here.

It can be taken for granted that in diabetic pregnancies, closely monitored as they usually are, the conspicuousness and frequent lethality of neural tube defects assure that in virtually every case the defects were noticed and recorded. Therefore in determining their frequency all reports of pregestational diabetic pregnancies were considered, not only those in which malformations, central nervous system or others, were noted and enumerated, but those reports as well in which it was explicitly stated or could be taken as implied that no malformations were found; with the exclusion only of those that noted malformations but did not specifically name them.

Neural Tube Defects in Diabetic Pregnancy

The record of the occurrence of neural tube defects in offspring of diabetic women is sparse. A summary shows that its mean rate in the final six decades of the last century was 5.2 per 1000 in America and 6.4 per 1000 in Europe (Kalter 2000). These are the records of what were most certainly only a small percentage of all diabetic pregnancies during these years. In the US alone, with about 4 million births annually, in this period pregestationally diabetic women had over three-quarters of a million births. The conclusion is unavoidable that the small fraction of them that entered into published series was undoubtedly a selected and intensively observed set, and as such their outcomes must be suspected of not being entirely representative.

These figures are to be compared with population estimates of the prevalence of neural tube defects. Except that it is necessary to remember that their background frequency has varied widely geographically and temporally, and therefore that no one statistic will answer the question. In Europe e.g. it ranged from as high as 8.7 per 1000 births in 1964–1968 in Belfast (Elwood and Nevin (1973) and 7.7 per 1000 in 1956–1962 in South Wales (Laurence et al. 1967) to a low of 0.5 per 1000 in France in 1945–1955 (Frézal et al. 1964), clear disparities conforming to the

United Kingdom and Ireland generally being a high-rate neural tube defect region and Europe on the whole a lower one (Penrose 1957; Dolk et al. 1991; Little and Elwood 1991; Kalter 2009). In North America an east-west gradient was in effect, superimposed upon which there was an overall decline in later decades (Mathers and Field 1983; Yen et al. 1992). And generally an increasing portion of the decline was the result of prenatal diagnosis and elimination of defective specimens (EUROCAT 1991; Chan et al. 1993; Limb and Holmes 1994); in England and Wales steadily declining from 1964 to 1990, remaining rather constant afterward (Morris and Wald 2007).

These statistics indicate that in past decades, when the level of neural tube defects was more or less constant, diabetic pregnancy was not associated with higher frequencies than occurred in the general population; shortage of relevant information from more recent studies precluded up to date comparison. This reading must be accepted cautiously however, since several considerations may challenge it. For example in addition to "nonuniformity in the duration and diligence of case ascertainment" (Borman and Cryer 1990), the data from diabetic pregnancies came from hospital series, while most of the overall prevalences were based on population series, which left the door open to the possibility of a possible excess partly owing to biases stemming from referral and self-selection of diabetic women. Again, familial occurrence of neural tube defects, known to be associated with increased risk of recurrence (Little and Elwood 1991), may have led to the high level of anencephalus detected in diabetic women prenatally screened by the alphafetoprotein assay (Milunsky et al. 1982); although absence of details about the women and their histories and how they came to be cared for at large hospitals made this surmise speculative.

Perinatal Death

Uncertainty that may linger can be clarified by another calculation, that of the frequency of anencephalus in diabetic perinatal deaths, a definitive account of which may be gathered from reports listing all the malformations that occurred in them. As expected the frequencies of perinatal death and anencephalus were inversely related; clearly depicted by the trends showing that as the former decreased the latter increased.

Overall population data to compare these figures with are scarce. Those from an assessment of the fetuses of 12,620 high-risk pregnancies of various sorts over a 4.5-year period may be useful (Manning et al. 1985). Two percent of the pregnancies were of insulin dependent diabetic women (which incidentally is about four times the overall prevalence of the condition, and illustrates the selective proclivities of large medical centers). Ninety-three of the offspring were perinatal mortalities, 0.7%, 15 with anencephalus, 16.1%. The number of the mortalities that occurred in the diabetic pregnancies and the number anencephalic were not stated, but omitting the probable number of the latter reduced the frequency of the malformations in the nondiabetic remainder to 15.2%, indicating that the frequency in the diabetic mortalities was not excessive.

Can such high-risk pregnancies be suitable for comparison with diabetic ones? Yes, because these supposedly high-risk Canadian pregnancies, it turned out, had a lower mean perinatal death rate than did the white population of the US during a comparable period (Powell-Griner 1989). It may be acceptable therefore to take the anencephalus frequency in mortalities as representative of the overall population, and to conclude that the frequencies in the most recent diabetic pregnancies were not out of line with them.

Cardiovascular Malformations

Another species of congenital malformations, those of the heart and great vessels—cardiovascular malformations—were found to be increased in frequency in infants of type 1 diabetic women, and in fact usually to be their commonest abnormalities. Because this is a subject of much complexity, it is best to consider these abnormalities separately in the general population and in infants of diabetic women. First in the former.

Vexing questions have confounded observations of these malformations, because of frequent difficulties of ascertainment and multiplicity of malformation type—in distinction e.g. to defects of the central nervous system. As Kenna et al. (1975) commented "…congenital heart disease is…possibly the most difficult group of defects to ascertain with any accuracy…[because many] affected infants show no abnormal symptoms or signs at birth…[and] 'congenital heart disease' is not a single entity, but comprises a large number of anatomically distinct lesions…."

In addition cardiovascular malformations are among the commonest of all congenital malformations. Years ago they composed about 10% of all congenital malformations (Rowe et al. 1981, p. 110), but later rose to perhaps 20% or more (e.g. Roth et al. 1987), and to about 40% in all neonatal and infant deaths associated with malformations (Berry et al. 1987; Kalter 1991).

Their reported frequency varied greatly however, for several reasons as well as uncertainties of ascertainment. Sometimes only live births were considered and the appreciable number in stillbirths excluded (Hoffman 1990). Because they are not all detected at birth the cumulative frequency has varied with the diligence and extent of postnatal follow up. Furthermore time has brought more refined diagnostic methods, which yielded expanded estimates (Anderson 1991). It was no doubt these new procedures, as well as more intense and longitudinal efforts, allowing detection of types and degrees of abnormalities once less apparent, that led to the increases discovered, usually up to 1 year of age but also beyond, from 3 to 5 per 1000 live births in older studies (Rowe et al. 1981, p. 111) to 8–10 per 1000 and more found more recently (Hoffman 1990; Meberg et al. 1994; Wren et al. 2003). These prevalences will be of particular interest later in this work, when the health of older children of diabetic women is discussed.

Ventricular Septal Defects

All types of cardiovascular malformations are not equally numerous. Almost invariably the most prevalent are ventricular septal defects, once composing about one-quarter to one-third of all cardiovascular malformations in liveborn children (Hoffman and Christianson 1978; Anderson 1984), and more recently usually as much as 45–57%, the increase almost certainly due to surged recognition (Spooner et al. 1988; Anon. 1994; Meberg et al. 1994). Further, it is likely that the increase may be due in large part, if not entirely, to the great jump in that of ventricular septal defects (Newman 1985; Fixler et al. 1989; Martin et al. 1989). This was made especially obvious by the lack of a significant increase between 1982–1985 and 1986–1991 in any cardiovascular malformations but ventricular septal defects (Meberg et al. 1994).

Although it was unclear at first whether this 'epidemic' of ventricular septal defects, as it was called (Layde et al. 1980), was an artifact due to refined diagnosis, the evidence indicated that the increase was due to the detection of small, isolated septal defects of the sorts largely overlooked by past less precise methods of diagnosis (Laursen 1980; Newman 1985; Spooner et al. 1988; Martin et al. 1989; Fixler et al. 1989; Anon. 1994; Meberg et al. 1994). It must not be neglected, however, that most of them are of the sorts that close spontaneously in a large proportion of cases and hence are without physiological consequence (Evans et al. 1960; Mitchell et al. 1967; Anderson et al. 1984). In a recent period this repair occurred in almost 70% by 1 year of age (Meberg et al. 1994)!

But the cumulative rate of cardiovascular malformations is not the item of interest here. It is instead the frequency discovered in the neonatal period, since it is during the first days and weeks of life that the vast majority of children of diabetic women have been examined for congenital defects.

Heart Defects in Perinatal Death

Information about the frequency of cardiovascular malformations in the neonatal period comes most definitively from perinatal death, yet this source presents ambiguities tied to inconsistent stillbirth definition and variable rates of perinatal death and autopsy. In addition such data are scarce, especially owing to the recent decrease in the rate of autopsy. Nevertheless it is clear that the frequency of cardiovascular malformations in mortalities is appreciable. Older studies of stillbirths and neonatal deaths all or almost all of which were autopsied noted a mean of 3.5 and 12.5% respectively (Richards et al. 1955; Mitchell et al. 1971b; Kenna et al. 1975; Hoffman and Christianson 1978), giving a combined population frequency for the years before 1980 of about 6–8%. Comparing this with later years is difficult, more recent data being scarce to nonexistent, as alluded because of the infreqency of autopsy.

Heart Defects in Survivors

Population studies have given only indirect and uncertain information about cardiovascular malformations in newborns, the estimates having varied widely, e.g. 36–66% (Hoffman 1968, 1987; Stoll et al. 1989). Data regarding survivors (i.e. live births diagnosed neonatally) are even scarcer than for perinatal deaths.

Examination of infants has yielded uncertain estimates. A carefully conducted survey found a frequency of about 5 per 1000 neonates (Hoffman and Christianson 1978), about the same as the 6 per 1000 diagnosed by 1 year of age during earlier decades (Richards et al. 1955). It must be understood that a sizable proportion of infants with cardiovascular malformations, at least at one time, died in the postneonatal period, 11.3% in one survey (Mitchell et al. 1971b), which may mean that some ascertained frequencies were serious underestimates.

Nevertheless, estimates of the frequency of cardiovascular malformations in surviving offspring were atttempted. An unequivocal diagnosis of ventricular septal defect was made in 49 infants in Seattle in 10,476 live births in 1981–1986, of whom at least 47 survived the neonatal period, i.e. 4.5 per 1000 for this one type of heart defect alone, the only one reported (Moe and Gunderoth 1987). From this it can be extrapolated that the overall cardiovascular malformation frequency was about 9 per 1000. Spontaneous closure occurred in 45% of these cases by a mean of 12 months.

From somewhat ambiguous figures it can be deduced that cardiovascular malformations were noted in 489 surviving infants diagnosed by the 1st week in 105,330 live births in 1979–1986 in Strasbourg, i.e. 4.6 per 1000 (Stoll et al. 1989). In Oslo 224 infants with cardiovascular malformations were noted in 22,810 live births in 1982–1991, perhaps 92% of whom, i.e. 9.0 per 1000 survived the neonatal period, about 57% ventricular septal defect, i.e. about 5.1 per 1000; again many, over 69%, closed by the 1st year (Meberg et al. 1994).

A recent study of a different type of population, 29,154 chromosomally normal fetuses of 10–14 weeks of pregnancy, examining fetal nuchal translucently thickness, found a 2.0% prevalence of major cardiovascular malformations (Hyett et al. 1999); which as the authors commented "is similar to that found in pregnancies affected by maternal diabetes mellitus…."

Heart Defects and Diabetes

Several epidemiological studies have paid particular attention to the association of cardiovascular malformations and maternal diabetes (Mitchell et al. 1971a; Ferencz et al. 1987; Pradat 1992a). Conducted or participated in by pediatric cardiologists, they presented a full enumeration and description of the types of such malformations found. But because of the nature of the studies the frequencies reported were based on abnormalities diagnosed at various, sometimes extended, childhood ages, and hence cannot entirely serve the principal purpose of this inquiry, namely, to determine whether the frequency of malformations found in the neonatal period was greater in the children of diabetic women than in the general population. For this purpose information about children examined at birth or in the earliest weeks afterward must be used, i.e. reports of hospital series of diabetic pregnancy, where such information, though sometimes imperfect, may be found.

In an early attempt to grapple with such questions, Kučera (1971a), compiling the information given in a large number of reports of hospital-based series, found that heart anomalies were about five times more frequent in diabetic pregnancy than in a large population sample. But, as was well noted, the validity of this wide difference was imperiled by numerous confounding factors, which may have led not only to overestimating the former frequency but also to underestimating the latter.

But even more to the point, having found as discussed above that the frequencies of cardiovascular malformations differ so greatly in perinatal mortalities and survivors, it can be seen that total findings did not address the question validly.

Heart Defects in Diabetic Perinatal Death

Studies in about 1940–1960 of cardiovascular malformations in perinatal deaths of diabetic women noted frequencies of 4–14% with a mean of about 10% (Rowe et al. 1981, pp. 675–680). Fuller information yielded about 7–8%, which was about the same as the frequency at the time in the overall population; as much as possible this figure was based only on autopsied diabetic mortalities (see Kalter 2000, Table 14.4, p. 174). Comparable population data for later years appear to be scarce.

The increase in recent years in the frequency of cardiovascular malformations in diabetic mortalities, is no doubt part of the relative increase in the congenital malformation frequency associated with the reduction in rate of offspring death (Kalter 1991). Whether widened diagnosis may also have contributed is unclear.

Cardiovascular Malformations in Survivors

Earlier studies in the US and Europe found the frequency of cardiovascular malformations increased beyond background levels in surviving offspring of diabetic pregnancies, while more recent data, though scarce, seemed to indicate that the increase had modified in Europe but not in the US (Moe and Gunderoth 1987; Stoll et al. 1989; Meberg et al. 1994; Lisowski et al. 2010), the regional difference due perhaps to greater temporal changes in one than the other.

While the background frequency increased in later years to approximately the same extent in both regions, from 0.2–0.3 to 0.9%, the diabetic cardiovascular malformation frequency increased only slightly in Europe (1.6–2.0%), but somewhat more so in America (0.9–2.9%), raising them both however to about the same level.

What the difference may have been due to is unclear; but zealousness of diagnosis, as discussed below, cannot be disregarded in interpreting these data.

No persuasive analysis could be made of the type or types of cardiovascular malformations that might have accounted for the increased frequency in diabetic pregnancy, the number of cases being small and the number in which the defects were specified few. Many consisted of venricular septal defect, apparently amounting to a larger frequency than that in the general population (Hoffman and Christianson 1968). It must not be forgotten, however, that the frequency of venricular septal defect in all live births was substantial, amounting in recent findings to 3.5–5.1 per 1000 (Moe and Gunderoth 1987; Meberg et al. 1994; Graham and Gutgesell 1995).

This dominance was confirmed by a summary of the types of cardiovascular malformation reported by studies of diabetic pregnancies in 1964–2003, which found that the commonest defect by far, at 28%, was indeed venricular septal defect, with transposition of the great vessels a poor second, at 14% (Wren et al. 2003).

A similar effort widened the study to comparing cardiovascular malformation type in offspring of three groups of diabetic women in 1988–2000 with that in nondiabetic pregnancies from a Eurocat registry (Lisowski et al. 2010). The total cardiovascular malformation frequency in the former varied from 2.5 to 6.1%, differences probably owing to the heterogeneous methodology. The commonest anomaly, in both, was ventricular septal defect, at just under 30%, maternal diabetes thus appearing to play no part in its occurrence. As for the other numerous varieties of defects those apparently appearing more significantly often in the diabetic than the nondiabetic group were mostly of the conotruncal sort. But the heterogeneity of the material precluded definitive judgment. An incidental component of the survey found little or no difference in glycemic level between mothers of affected and non-affected offspring in the diabetic groups.

As recent studies have shown, intense examination of children leads to elevated discovery of cardiovascular malformations, so its apparent excess in surviving children of diabetic women may also have resulted in part from such close attention, especially in America. In any case, venricular septal defect, the predominant lesion, has long been considered to have little clinical importance, since "most cases are clinically insignificant" (Carlgren 1959) and "with small defects, the clinical course is benign" (Graham and Gutgesell 1995). Furthermore many sooner or later close spontaneously (Anderson et al. 1984; Moe and Gunderoth 1987; Meberg et al. 1994; Tegnander et al. 1995).

The temporal increase in the cardiovascular malformation frequency in survivors, in contrast with that in the mortalities, was inconsistent, being statistically insignificant in Europe but more real in America. A difference perhaps due to venricular septal defect forming a larger proportion of cardiovascular malformations in the latter, resulting, as in the general population, from earlier and more intense diagnosis of smaller defects (Bound and Logan 1977; Laursen 1980; Spooner et al. 1988; Fixler et al. 1989).

The cardiovascular malformation picture in diabetic births thus may be summed up as follows. For perinatal death the record clearly showed that its occurrence was not increased; in fact in the earlier period some population groups had larger frequencies than the diabetic cases; and the increase in later years was probably the by-product of the greatly lowered mortality rate together with improved methods of detection. The story in the neonatal period in survivors was inconsistent, being apparently increased only in America, possibly indicating more intense diagnosis, especially of venricular septal defects, which compose a dominant fraction of all cardiovascular malformations.

Prenatal Diagnosis

This section ends with studies of major cardiovascular malformations in fetuses of women with pregestational insulin dependent diabetes detected by ultrasound or echocardiography examination during the mid-second trimester. In the last 20 or so years many such studies were conducted (Gomez et al. 1988; Pijlman et al. 1989; Wheller et al. 1990; Greene and Benacerraf 1991; Brown et al. 1992; Maher et al. 1994; Albert et al. 1996; Meyer-Wittkopf et al. 1996; Gladman et al. 1997; Smith et al. 1997; Bernard et al. 1009; Lisowski et al. 2010; Sekhavat et al. 2010). Others with insufficient details were ignored here. Cardiovascular malformation was diagnosed in about 4% of the fetuses screened, which may be an overestimate since it probably included inadmissible or questionable conditions as well as some type 2 and other diabetic pregnancies.

Comparing this figure with the cardiovascular malformation frequency of 0.66% found in prenatal screening of nearly 150,000 low-risk and unselected patients in 1991–1995 (Kirk et al. 1997), the diabetic risk is seen to be about three times that found by the survey. While this suggested that diabetic pregnancy poses an increased fetal risk for cardiovascular malformations, without information regarding the pre- and perinatal death fate of abnormal fetuses a comparison with the situation in surviving neonatal offspring is difficult.

A few incidental findings: Not all the defects were successfuly detected prenatally in the population study. Nor were all the defects considered structural or "critical" (i.e. probably requiring surgical or medical intervention), as evidenced by only about half of the abnormal fetuses in one study having structural defects (Wheller et al. 1990), while in another only about one-quarter required surgical repair (Tegnander et al. 1995). Also revealed was that none of the mothers with defective offspring had abnormal recurrences (Meyer-Wittkopf et al. 1996). And finally, glycemic level findings were inconsistent, being higher in one study in cases with than without cardiovascular malformation (Bernard et al. 2009) but not in another (Lisowski et al. 2010).

Chapter 17
Preventing Malformations

Soon after the beginning of the insulin era it became a firm tenet that the infants of pregnant diabetic women were at increased risk of congenital malformations. Addressing this consensus the causes and prevention of these abnormalities were the subject of countless scholarly publications. From early on innumerable etiological factors—genetic, metabolic, teratologic—were considered as the possible basis of this risk (e.g. Gabbe 1977; Simpson 1978). But for prevention the most promising path to pursue seemed the metabolic one, since as was reasoned, "if perturbations in the maternal metabolic milieu…cause anomalies in offspring, then strict diabetic control should lower the anomaly rates…" (Ober and Simpson 1986)

Hyperglycemia and Congenital Malformations

It was the success in lowering the rate of perintal death, achieved in part by controlling the maternal blood glucose level, that led to the belief that by this route the malformation frequency would also be lowered; an expectation that was frustrated since it did not result in a lowered malformation frequency. But the ultimate misunderstanding was to focus on the glyemic level in the last weeks of pregnancy, when it could not have had any relation to embryonic development (Karlsson and Kjellmer 1972).

An apparent clue as to where attention should have been focused instead came from the insight that "malformations in infants of diabetic mothers occur before the seventh gestational week" (Mills et al. 1979). This pronouncement, novel to many diabetologists, led many studies to direct attention to maternal blood glucose in the earliest weeks of pregnancy. Recognizing at the same time that a longitudinal perspective was called for investigations turned to the recently discovered entity, glycosylated hemoglobin, to provide that view.

Studies of the relation of the outcome of pregnancy and level of glycosylated hemoglobin (HbA_1) in the 1st trimester of pregnant diabetic women, as noted above, began in the late 1970s. Not only directed at spontaneous abortion they also turned to studies of the glycemic level in mothers of congenitally malformed children,

H. Kalter, *A History of Diabetes in Pregnancy*,
DOI 10.1007/978-94-007-1557-8_17, © Springer Science+Business Media B.V. 2012

which it was noted exceeded the range for well-controlled diabetics and suggested an association with maldevelopment (Leslie et al. 1978).

Further studies duplicated the finding of higher mean levels in mothers of malformed than in those of nonmalformed children, with rough dose-response relations between glycemic level malformation frequency (Miller et al. 1981; Jovanovic et al. 1981; Reid et al. 1984; Ylinen et al. 1984).

But, as often happens, further studies clouded the picture. In almost all instances the relation between glycemic level and malformation rate was not statistically significant or at best was of borderline significance (Shields et al. 1993; Greene et al. 1995). Compounding the uncertainties was some contamination of the data by inclusion of defects not major and of diabetic women not pregestationally insulin dependent.

Others also found similar mean glycemic levels in mothers of children with minor as well as major malformations (Greene et al. 1989; Lucas et al. 1989; Hanson et al. 1990); and even a dose-response relation with glycemic level (Reid et al. 1984; Ylinen et al. 1984; Greene et al. 1989; Hanson et al. 1990)—the reason for which undoubtedly being a nonspecific factor common to glycemic level and malformation.

It should be noted that the fraction of diabetic women with the highest glycemic levels, at the right end of a skewed distribution, was far larger in hospital-based studies, with a mean of 20.2% than in a population study, with 6.2% (Hanson et al. 1990); which may mean that women attending, i.e. usually referred to, diabetes clinics early in pregnancy were more severely affected than diabetic women generally. But despite this relative diabetic severity there was little unambiguous evidence of an association of glycemic level and congenital malformation.

Finally, should it be surprising that studies pursuing the leads of earlier ones often largely contradict them? It is after all only positive findings that are followed up, which then sometime turn out to have been deceptive.

Preconception Control and Malformation

Despite these contradictions and inconsistencies studies continued unabated—flogging a dead horse, as it were—with attempts to reduce the occurrence of malformations and spontaneous abortions, by instituting rigorous control before conception.

Copenhagen Study

Whose possible efficacy was looked into by comparing outcomes of pregnancies of diabetic women in 1966–1977 attending hospitals in the Copenhagen area, assumed to be in good glycemic control, with those of women with irregular or little care attending hospitals outside the area (Pedersen and Mølsted-Pedersen 1978). Comparison was impossible however because the findings were vague and inconclusive, and the congenital malformations unspecified and defined obscurely to begin with (see appraisal of this study above).

Edinburgh Study

Studies begun in 1977 at a clinic in Edinburgh proposed to prevent malformations by obtaining "optimum diabetic control at the time of conception" (Steel et al. 1980). The final report of this effort compared the outcomes of the insulin dependent diabetic pregnancies of 143 attenders of the clinic and 96 nonattenders (Steel et al. 1990). Two offspring of the former (1.4%) and 10 of the latter (10.4%) had major malformations, a statistically significant difference indicating that preconception metabolic control had successfully reduced the frequency.

Before accepting this conclusion the methodology of the study must be examined. As Steel et al. (1990) agreed, the attenders and nonattenders were not selected randomly, a logistical and ethical impossibility perhaps. Instead the groups were formed in the following manner. All insulin dependent women registered in the Diabetic Department of the Edinburgh Royal Infirmary were sent letters announcing the imminent establishment of a clinic to counsel diabetic women contemplating becoming pregnant, and inviting them to attend. In addition the clinic was advertised in notices displayed in the department and in the clinic newsletter; colleagues were asked to refer appropriate patients; and it was brought to the notice of young women during personal contact at the diabetic units of the Infirmary and the Hospital for Sick Children (Steel et al. 1982; 1984a, b).

The women reponding to these notices and attending the prepregnancy clinic were mostly self-selected, had planned pregnancies, and were highly motivated. The nonattenders were ignorant of the clinic's existence, had no desire to attend, or were not originally department patients.

The composition of the nonattending group can be challenged. Several of them were seen before the prepregnancy clinic came into existence (Steel et al. 1980, 1982), and their malformed offspring (Steel and Johnstone 1992) therefore should not have been included among the offspring of the true nonattenders. Also improperly included were children whose malformations were not recognized till after the first few weeks of life, including a sacral agenesis diagnosed at the age of 3 years (Steel et al. 1982; Steel and Johnstone 1992). These should be excluded because, among other things, no assurance was given that all the children were as closely followed postnatally for this length of time. Other features by which the two groups differed were in age, education, etc.

To curtail this overlong tale, omitting the malformed offspring of the incorrectly included nonattenders and those diagnosed at older ages, leaves the following: 2/143 (1.4%) in the attenders and 3/80 (3.8%) in the nonattenders, a nonsignificant difference. And this was so despite the significantly lower 1st trimester glycohemoglobin level in the attenders.

Karlsburg Study

Another center studying the effect of preconception glycemic control on prenatal maldevelopment, located in Karlsburg in what was then the German Democratic Republic, was attended by about half of all pregnant diabetics in the country.

Detailed reports were made of the 620 insulin dependent women delivering in 1977–1983 (Fuhrmann et al. 1983, 1984). Of them 184 were willing to take part in the demanding metabolic and dietary regimen, commencing before 8 weeks of pregnancy. The remaining 436 women did not submit to the regimen and began metabolic control later than at this time. About 84% of the former and far fewer of the latter had normoglycemia during the early weeks of pregnancy. Glycosylated hemoglobin was not measured.

A total of 17 offspring had major congenital malformations diagnosed in the first 3 weeks of life, two from the preconception-controlled women and 15 from the late-entering ones. Omitting the five inadmissible defects from the latter gives frequencies not statistically significantly different from eachother (2/184, 1.1% vs 10/436, 2.3%).

Although the narrative need go no further, other elements will be discussed to note differences between the two groups, as an illustration of possible biasing factors that must be recognized and discounted if such efforts are ever to attain legitimacy.

Less than 30% of women elected to undergo the strenuous metabolic and dietary requirements of the program, in part because of the distances necessary to travel for the frequent consultations and lengthy preconception hospitalizations; suggesting inordinate motivation, perhaps having to do with poor previous perinatal outcomes (Fuhrmann 1982; Fuhrmann et al. 1983, 1986). Patient self selection of one sort or another can introduce potent biasing factors. A minority of insulin dependent diabetic women in areas offering these programs participated in them (Gabbe and Landon 1989; Holing et al. 1998), and those getting such attention differed in many ways from those not doing so. The possible importance of the background and motives of those who do should not be minimized in evaluating the outcome of studies wishing to understand the bases of their findings. Until such influences are sorted out there can be no clear resolution of the basis of the favorable pregnancy outcome found in some preconception studies.

National Institutes of Health Study

The challenge was met by a multicenter collaborative study, discussed in part above, conducted prospectively in 1980–1985 under the auspices of the National Institutes of Health (Mills et al. 1983). The large sample needed to address the question satisfactorily it seemed could only be supplied by a joint effort. A control was included whose role was limited to the spontaneous abortion part of the study (Mills et al. 1988a) with none in the part discussed here (Mills et al. 1988b).

The original intention, only partly fulfilled, was to recruit insulin dependent diabetic women before conception to insure early diagnosis of pregnancy. Thus included were two groups, an early entry group enrolled before conception or up to 21 days afterward, considered collectively; and a late-entry group, women enrolled later in conception. No uniform standard for management of the early-entry group was imposed upon the several centers participating in the study, and no metabolic data were obtained for the late-entry group.

Children were examined for congenital malformations on the 3rd postnatal day only, and the 4.9% frequency of all malformations in the children of the early-entry group was found to be significantly smaller than that, 9.0%, in the late-entry group. But if the defects in both groups that were minor or dubious were omitted (viz. labial fusion, paraurethral cyst, and strawberry hemangioma in the early-entry group, and clubfoot, inguinal hernia, cryptorchidism, and Hirschsprung disease in the late-entry group; see table 2 in Mills et al. 1988b), the frequencies became 4.0 and 6.8% respectively, and no longer significantly different. Also, ventricular septal defects were among the abnormalities in both groups, which often close in later infancy (e.g. Tegnander et al. 1995), whose fate thus could not be determined by a single early postnatal examination. Omitting them further lessened the statistical significance of the difference in malformation frequency.

The mean glycosylated hemoglobin level early in pregnancy of early-entry women was no higher in those with malformed children than without, nor were different degrees of hyperglycemia associated with malformation frequency.

For the sake of argument let us accept the interpretation made by the examiners of the children at the five different centers collaborating in this study, that the plan of the study succeeded in analyzing the separate putative roles of maternal self selection and strict periconceptional diabetic control in leading to a favorable pregnancy outcome.

Unfortunately this goal was a chimera from the beginning, since motivational factors could not be nullified. Clear evidence of which was the fact that early-entry women were significantly older than the late-entry ones [incidentally the same was seen in many like studies (Goldman et al. 1986; Steel et al. 1990; Rosenn et al. 1991; Willhoite et al. 1993; Holing et al. 1998)], which undoubtedly pointed to their greater concern because of untoward outcomes in previous pregnancies, such as had been documented e.g. by Fuhrmann et al. (1986).

The finding by Mills et al. (1988b) of no correlation between glycemic level and malformation frequency raised a small storm of protest. A Lancet leader writer (Anon. 1988), echoing the conventional wisdom, asserted that "there is unquestionably an increased incidence of major congenital abnormalities in the infants of diabetic mothers." Thus, in comparing the malformation frequency in the early- and late-entry groups, he or she, accepting the reported malformation data, pronounced that the "findings are in complete accord" with received gospel, which totally missed the point, since the negative judgment of the Mills et al. study came not from a comparison of these two groups but of the women in the early-entry group who did and did not have malformed children.

Other critics (see Lancet 319:647–648, 1988) had a variety of complaints, none of which seriously undermined Mills and colleagues' findings. Another charged that since comparing the mothers of malformed and nonmalformed offspring was not a primary aim of the study it was improper to make such a post hoc analysis (Skyler 1989). But a reading of the paper outlining the National Institutes of Health study design (Mills et al. 1983) revealed nothing that debarred retrospective analyses, and indeed mentioned an example of when such would be carried out.

Much was also made of the fact that the malformation frequency in the early-entry group was higher than in the control, which was interpreted to mean that the metabolic control of these women was suboptimal. The foundation of this point can also be challenged by returning to table 2 in Mills et al. (1988b), mentioned above, where it can be seen that none of the children of the 389 control women had a major congenital malformation (with the possible exception of one with a condition vaguely labeled an "anatomical brain lesion"). It seems likely that these children were not as thoroughly examined as the children of the diabetic mothers were, or were a most unusual group, and thus no argument can be based on the supposed difference in malformation frequency between them.

Other Preconception Control Studies

Aiming at preconception glycemic normalization of diabetic women, a multicenter study in California registered diabetic women none of whom had children, and in contrast pregestational diabetic women enrolled some time after conception 23 of whose 347 children (6.6%) had congenital malformations. Nothing was said about how they were diagnosed, but in addition to fatal and surgery-requiring abnormalities significant psychological conditions were defined as major defects. First-trimester glycosylated hemoglobin levels were measured, but data were not presented for women entering the program before and after conception (Cousins 1991c). Little of any clear value came out of this study

A more modest study from California was presented clearly (Kitzmiller et al. 1991). By means of announcements in various media, word of mouth, or physician referral, diabetic women were recruited in 1982–1988 to participate in a program of preconception instruction and rigorous glycemic control. Others who were already pregnant were similarly registered for metabolic management at different times during gestation, nearly half at as early as 6–8 weeks, but many as late as 21–32 weeks. About 65% of the women in both groups were insulin dependent. An apparent selection bias was shown by the former group, though of approximately the same age as the latter, having an earlier disease onset.

One of the 84 offspring of women in the preconception group with viable pregnancies and 12 of the 110 in the postconception group were malformed. Omitting inadmissible abnormalities left none in the first and nine in the second. Four of the latter were ventricular septal defects (only one of whose mothers had a glycohemoglobin level above 10%). All surviving children were reexamined at 1 year of age, but the number with septal defects still present at that time was not stated.

There was a stepwise increase in the frequency of the accepted major malformations in the postconception group with increased maternal glycohemoglobin level, but predominantly the increase was beyond the 10.6% level. There were no data of course regarding the glycemic state of the postconception groups in the earliest weeks of pregnancy; such information would have helped in interpreting one of the malformations, holoprosencephaly, since it arises as early as at 5 weeks of gestation (Müller and O'Rahilly 1989).

The data indicated a possible relation between hyperglycemia in early pregnancy and fetal maldevelopment [it is noteworthy that in an earlier study of a management program instituted in the first trimester, conducted by one of the authors of this article (Jovanovic et al. 1981), it seems no major or minor congenital malformations were found]. It is unfortunate that the possible existence of more anterior etiological factors, as were hinted at in studies discussed above, indicated by the simultaneous association of major and minor congenital malformations with hyperglycemia, was overlooked by this study in not recording all minor congenital malformations.

A meta-analysis of studies published from 1990 to 2005 of teratogenesis associated with preexisting and other sorts of diabetes concluded ambiguously that all conduced to "increased awareness of fetal abnormalities," which was not to be taken seriously since it included gestational diabetes as causing malformations (Allen et al. 2007).

A recent report of the benefits of a preconception care regimen made no mention of its supposed efficacy in preventing congenital malformations (Kitzmiller et al. 2010). This was the culmination, to the present, of a large number of studies of this subject; 11 of which considered appropriate were subjected to meta-analysis (Wahabi et al. 2010). In no instance did close reading of them clearly support the contention that preconception counseling prevents fetal maldevelopment (see my summary and critique of these 11 elsewhere in this book).

A study in Cincinnati in 1984–1989 was designed to optimize the glycemic state of diabetic women planning to become pregnant (Rosenn et al. 1991). After a large number of women removed themselves from the program, perhaps finding the regimen too difficult to comply with, 28 randomly selected pregnancies of the remaining women, some of whom had entered the program more than once, comprised the preconception study group. A similarly selected group of 71 pregnancies of diabetic women that enrolled within 9 weeks following conception comprised the control. The mean glycohemoglobin level of the control at the first prenatal visit was significantly higher than that of the study women, despite which the malformation frequencies in the infants of both were similar and very low. No satisfactory explanation was attempted for this result, which seemed to contradict strongly held beliefs.

A statewide program of preconception counseling for pregestational diabetic women was conducted in Maine in 1987–1990 (Willhoite et al. 1993). During this time 185 pregnancies (64% type 1, 35% type 2) were reported by 150 counselors (physicians, nurses, dieticians), 62 in women seen before conceiving, predominantly in a nonhospital setting, and 123 not (percentages with type 1 and 2 diabetes in each group not disclosed). Major congenital malformations were reported in one child of the former group and eight of the latter, a suggestive but not statistically significant difference. No metabolic data were included. The abnormalities were not all fully described, and the methodology of their diagnosis was not mentioned.

These failings call for a brief aside. Much naivety regarding fetal maldevelopment was true to one extent or another of some of the studies discussed in this section, and others elsewhere, in glaring contrast to the frequent abundance of detail about the diabetic state and metabolic management of the patients, unbalanced approaches that obviously stemmed from the predominant professional interests of the investigators. But this neglect often diminished the value of the studies in the eyes of a teratologist.

The completeness of the ascertainment of diabetes accomplished by the Maine statewide program must be considered. Publications of the National Center for Health Statistics indicated that during the 4-year period of the program 76,072 live births occurred in Maine. According to the expectation of about five pregestational insulin dependent diabetic births per 1000 pregnancies, not including perinatal deaths there should have been approximately 335 such pregnancies in these years, almost three times as many type 1 diabetic pregnancies alone as were the subjects of the report. A shortage of this size must have implications regarding representativeness and selection of subjects.

Temporal Trends

Several studies compared pregnancy outcome in two periods during which different management of diabetic pregnancy was practiced or presumably practiced. For example, studies in the Birmingham Maternity Hospital extended over many years, in the course of which it is likely that management improved. Conforming to expectation, as the rate of perinatal death decreased the frequency of lethal congenital malformations increased, but that of all malformations did also (Soler et al. 1976). The latter, however, was clouded by the inclusion of various minor and other inadmissible defects, and so cannot be credited. The comparison of two periods made by Ballard et al. (1984) was discussed earlier. In a report from the Mayo Clinic a chart depicting pregnancy outcome over a 30-year period showed that the frequency of congenital defects increased decade by decade, from about 8 to 15%, while that in the control remained constant at about 2–3% (Lufkin et al. 1984). Specific data for these periods were not given; but nearly half of the malformations listed in the diabetic cases were minor or otherwise inadmissible.

An extensive set of observations in Copenhagen over the 20 years 1967–1986 noted a constant 7–8% major congenital malformations in the first 15 years and a decline in the last 5 years to 2.7% (Damm and Mølsted-Pedersen 1989). This gratifying outcome was thought to be due to improved diabetic care and metabolic control during the latter years, which were facilitated by the high frequency of planned pregnancies in that period. This belief seems to be contradicted however by the data presented, which showed that the mean glycohemoglobin levels before 13 weeks of pregnancy in women with planned and unplanned pregnancies were very much alike (7.1 vs 7.3%), even though the malformation frequency in the former was significantly less than in the latter, and with no correlation between HbA_{1c} and malformations. The glycohemoglobin similarity should perhaps have been expected, since the outpatient department of the Copenhagen Diabetes Center had given advice for optimal metabolic control since 1976. The improved malformation record therefore continued unexplained, but may possibly be explained by the later inclusion of infants of less that 1000 g birth weight, since lighter babies are at reduced risk for malformations (Kalter 1991). The presentation of weight-specific data regarding malformation frequency would have been useful in examining this possibility.

A report comparing 1971–1977 and 1978–1985 noted that in the first period no women were enrolled in a "systematic preconception program," while in the second 18% were (Tchobroutsky et al. 1991). There was no difference in the malformation frequency between the two periods however, perhaps because the number enrolled was insufficient to have made any impact. Also, the efficacy of the program in controlling blood sugar was not documented.

I close by mentioning an all-encompassing review and summarization of studies of the outcome of preconception care on congenital malformations and spontaneous abortions—including a novelty, animal studies—with 324 references, up to the mid-1990s (Kitzmiller et al. 1996). Covering every imaginable aspect of the subject, relevant and irrelelvant, the only thing missing unfortunately was an evaluation of any sort of the effectiveness of such care. This judgment is perhaps unfair since the stated purpose of this technical review was not to judge but merely to provide a background for a professional guideline. Nevertheless it is regrettable that the impression given was total agreement with the usefulness of such care.

A Matter of Puzzlement

Despite the findings detailed above it was repeatedly and dogmatically echoed "that there is no doubt that congenital malformations occur more frequently in the offspring of diabetic mothers…[that] studies of glycosylated hemoglobin during the 1st trimester have demonstrated a significant relationship between poor metabolic control in diabetic pregnancy and the likelihood of congenital malformations," and that diabetic pregnancy is teratogenic in animals (Coustan 1998)—citing for the last asseveration experimental studies that had been discredited in an obstetrics journal itself (Kalter 1997).

It is always the lazier course merely to follow where others have led, but which as the sheep found in Hardy's Far From the Madding Crowd often leads to peril.

I close with a glance at what was called a meta-analysis of studies published in 1970–2000 reporting the effect of preconception care in reducing congenital malformations in children of women with diabetes (Ray et al. 2001). Of the 154 citations of some relevance that were identified the analysis made use of only 16, the rational for whose selection was only meagerly explained. In the greater picture of this effort the putative role of glycemic control was hardly of consequence and will be set aside and the malformation picture solely attended to.

The authors mentioned some flaws that may have disturbed the analysis, but failed to mention other more serious ones. First, the outcomes of type 1 and type 2 pregnancies, forms of the disease that are hardly to be equated in their repercussions on fetal development, were indiscriminately lumped together. Second, though the type and frequency of congenital malformations that occurred in perinatal deaths differed starkly from those in surviving offspring, they were not considered separately, preventing meaningful analysis. In the absence of any recognition of these and other matters the entire analysis turns out to be valueless.

Over the course of some time there appeared a number of original articles or meta-analyses dealing with preconception care and its purported beneficial fetal consequences, (see e.g. Garcia-Patterson et al. 1997). See below for a further consideration of this subject.

Chapter 18
Prenatal and Follow-up Studies

Fetal Growth Delay

Most fetal problems associated with diabetic pregnancy—perinatal mortality, congenital malformations, macrosomia, preterm birth—are prominent and have long been recognized. In contrast another presumed manifestation of diabetic pregnancy, retarded prenatal growth, is covert and perhaps was for that reason only recently brought to attention.

It was uncovered fortuitously in the course of an ultrasound study. In searching for the possible early prenatal origins of neonatal overgrowth in offspring of insulin dependent diabetic women, Pedersen and Mølsted-Pedersen (1979) noted instead that many early fetuses were considerably smaller than normal, and reasoned that the delay was probably of embryonic origin. Furthermore the smallest of the retarded fetuses weighed significantly less at birth than others, and seemed at increased risk of malformation. Confirmatory reports strengthened this indication, and for good measure noted that small fetal size was correlated with maternal 1st-trimester glycemic state (Pedersen and Mølsted-Pedersen 1981; Pedersen et al. 1984; Tchobroutsky et al. 1985; Visser et al. 1985).

Growth-retarded fetuses were not restricted to insulin dependent diabetic pregnancies however, but also occurred in those of class A diabetics, i.e., in noninsulin dependent pregestational diabetes, and even in gestational diabetic women (Sutherland et al. 1981). These findings call for a new interpretation, since they must mean that the growth delay in and of itself could not be related to fetal maldevelopment; because, as was often noted above, malformation frequency is not increased in class A or gestational diabetes. Thus if retarded growth and risk of maldevelopment are associated it must be due to both being the outcome of antecedent or ancillary conditions, as Little et al. (1979) and Spiers (1982) suggested.

But an even more fundamental doubt was raised, that of the accuracy of the observation of delayed fetal growth itself, based on the likelihood of mistaken dating of conception owing to inaccurate estimation of ovulation (Little et al. 1979; Steel et al. 1984b, 1995).

Sad to relate, but too common merely to be a curiosity, the provocative early findings and the attractive theories they fathered were not long afterward refuted by

H. Kalter, *A History of Diabetes in Pregnancy*,
DOI 10.1007/978-94-007-1557-8_18, © Springer Science+Business Media B.V. 2012

sonographic studies in early pregnancy. Cousins et al. (1988), employing rigorous obstetric dating criteria, relative to controls found no delayed fetal growth in insulin dependent diabetic pregnancies; Reece et al. (1990), comparing diabetic and non-diabetic pregnancies, no statistically significant difference in size and growth rate of the early fetal head; and Brown et al. (1992) no difference in early fetal growth rate between diabetic and nondiabetic pregnancies. Note that in all three of these studies nondiabetic pregnancies were included, controls, in such investigations at least, if not in other sorts, having correctly been considered mandatory for credible interpretation.

Fetal Detection of Malformations

The prenatal visualization of congenital malformations became truly effective with the development of real-time ultrasonography. This permitted many different structural abnormalities to be detected in the 2nd trimester (Campbell and Pearce 1983; Hegge et al. 1990); and incidentally provided the possibility of altering the prevalence of some of these conditions at birth by fetal elimination (Julian-Reynier et al. 1994).

Such sonographic studies in diabetic pregnancies were prompted by the finding of early fetal growth retardation. Up to the present relatively few have been made (Szabó et al. 1986; Gomez et al. 1988; Pijlman et al. 1989; Greene and Benacerraf 1991; Brown et al. 1992; Albert et al. 1996), and their purpose has varied: to provide obstetric guidance, maternal counseling and choice, and examine the relation of maldevelopment to fetal retardation, glycemic control, and alphafetoprotein level. But they have accomplished little, perhaps because they were beset by the familiar inadequacies and failures: biased ascertainment, no control (an even more than usual necessity in prenatal studies, as realized by those conducting the studies described in the previous section), and lack of discrimination between true major malformations and minor and otherwise questionable ones.

Prenatal detection of CVM is discussed in the chapter dealing with specific malformations.

Follow-up of Children

We leap from features of embryos of diabetic women to postnatal physical and developmental characteristics of their children, especially congenital malformations, height and weight, neurological state, and intellectual ability. Children of various ages beyond infancy, usually of early school age, were examined or their parents questioned about these matters. The shortcomings of these studies will be set forth below.

Congenital Malformations

Almost all the earliest follow-up studies and many of the later ones took malformations discovered at various older ages for their outcome subject. Malformations or deformities were defined variably; and interestingly, when they included controls, the children of diabetic men and prediabetic women were used for this purpose (Koller 1953; White et al. 1953; Claye and Craig 1959; Dekaban 1959; Hagbard et al. 1959). The largest study, part of an early multicenter project, gathered data through questionnaires sent to mothers (Hagbard et al. 1959). If even a generous view is taken of what constitutes a deformity, the total frequency of the defects discovered in the neonatal period and afterward was not significantly larger in the children born after the women developed diabetes than in those born before, i.e., in the prediabetic period. The same nonsignificant difference occurred in a study from a nearby country (Hiekkala and Koskenoja 1961).

In the next decade two relatively large studies following children for many years found abnormality frequencies of 8–9% respectively, but included as major defects various inconsequential abnormalities (Breidahl 1966), and found no difference from the control (Farquhar 1965, 1969).

Degen et al (1970) were surprised, they said, to find no additional pathologies, physical or neurological, in children examined at ages 1–13 years. White (1971), amplifying an earlier report (White et al. 1953), noted that the frequency of congenital anomalies was almost identical in the older children of diabetic women and diabetic men. Essex et al. (1973) cited an unpublished doctoral dissertation (Watson 1970) that noted that the frequency of malformations in children of diabetic women was not statistically different from that in a control group. A Danish study reported that 4.9% of a large number of children of diabetic women examined at 15–26 years of age had major malformations and 6.2% minor ones (Yssing 1975). The study lacked controls and none of the abnormalities, an appreciable proportion of which were said to run in the families, was named. Other studies apparently found no additional malformations in children of various ages beyond those discovered at birth (Amendt 1975; Stehbens et al. 1977; Cummins and Norrish 1980). Similarly, in another, children followed for 1–27 years, discounting dubious conditions, had a maximum of 3.2% malformations (Schwaninger 1973).

Cardiovascular malformations (CVM) were the subject of a study of children examined at several ages up to 7 years (Rowland et al. 1973). All together 19 cases were diagnosed (3.8%), 14 of which had occurred in perinatal mortalities. Which defects were present in the latter unfortunately was not stated, since four of them—three ventricular septal defects and a patent ductus arteriosus—were conditions that often vanish in time. Nevertheless, the frequency of CVM was far greater than the usual population rate.

A doubt lingers whether at least some of this excess was related to the mothers of the children being a highly select sample of diabetic women attending the Joslin Clinic and the children themselves undergoing intensive serial examinations when "signs or symptoms suggesting heart disease prompted referral" to the hospital for evaluation. This doubt might have been quelled had a proper control been employed rather than the wholly inappropriate one. In an early study, of the physical and mental development of 123 children of diabetic women, only one child with a malformation, a CVM, was found (Fredrikson et al. 1957).

A late study found 15% malformations during a 3-year follow-up in the children of insulin dependent diabetic women, about twice that in controls (Sells et al. 1994). Some of the abnormalities were obviously already present in neonates, but the age others, like ventricular septal defects, were discovered was not mentioned, an important consideration since this condition very often spontaneously closes by 1 year of age (e.g., Moe and Guntheroth 1987). It was not clear therefore whether the frequency at older ages was different from that at birth. This study was an offshoot of the Mills et al. (1988) multicenter study, and some of the other doubts about the congenital malformation findings will be found in a previous chapter where the latter is discussed. Finally, it may be mentioned as apropos to this section that dental development was found to be delayed in one study (Amendt 1975) but normal in another (Adler et al. 1977).

Height and Weight

The children of diabetic women in the past were very often excessively heavy at birth (Hsia and Gellis 1957), and in fact this serious complication, macrosomia, is not uncommon even today (see above). Since birth weight may influence postnatal growth (see Bergmann et al. 1984 for citations), among the questions about the prognosis of children of diabetic women awaiting resolution was whether and how neonatal and later size were related, though the question was rarely put in these explicit terms, Instead for the most part investigators simply sought to establish whether later height and weight were within normal limits or not.

The diverse findings at best reflect the absence of a standard approach to the question. It was found that at various later ages the children (often as compared with national standards of the time and place) were taller and heavier than normal (White et al. 1953), shorter but heavier (Hagbard et al. 1959), of normal height and weight (Komrower and Langley 1961), normally distributed in height (Hiekkala and Koskenoja 1961; Farquhar 1969a; Amendt 1975), often above the 90th percentile for height and weight (Breidahl 1966), tended to be heavier than normal (Weitz and Laron 1976); and most recently again were significantly taller and heavier, which, since it was not true of the children of diabetic fathers, was concluded to be evidence of the lasting effect of intrauterine environmental factors on later body build (Bergmann et al. 1984).

Also, to compound the confusion, some children proportionately large at birth were significantly heavier and taller at 4 years of age than others not large or disproportionately large at birth (Jährig et al. 1993), and others, obese at birth, but of normal weight and length at 1 year of age, had increased weight and height at later ages, effects that were correlated with various maternal and fetal characteristics

(Silverman et al. 1991). In this study the outcome in children of women with gestational and type 1 diabetes were reported collectively; how this may have vitiated the observations is unclear. [This commingling also damaged any validity other studies may have had (Rizzo et al. 1994, 1995; Yamashita et al. 1996)].

If the majority wins, then greater height, at times accompanied by greater weight, comes closest to the consensus; but discordant findings cannot be discounted. A definitive examination of the question is still awaited, one that will be discriminating in its choice of mothers whose children are to be longitudinally followed, will take an agreed-upon approach, and that for comparison will not rely entirely on sometimes outdated and inappropriate population standards.

Neurological Development and Intelligence

It is not surprising that the birth traumas and neonatal morbidities children of diabetic women often experienced, and still occasionally experience, led to asking whether these events had long-term psychological and related consequences. In fact many follow-up studies of such children were directed to these considerations. Here too, not surprisingly, the results were mixed, probably because as it hardly seems necessary to reiterate, most of the studies were beset by the usual shortcomings of limited sample size, diverse follow-up procedures, varied and seldom entirely appropriate 'controls' (and others well enumerated by Goldstein et al. 1991); and hence that some investigators found an increased incidence of mental and neurological impairment and others did not.

The pioneering effort of this sort (only a brief summary of which as far as can be determined was ever reported) found that at examination at 6 months to 15 years of age, 86 of 91 children of 'diabetic' women had "developed perfectly normally, mentally and physically," and of the four others still alive, two had "oligophrenia," one diabetes mellitus, and the last a congenital heart lesion (Pedersen and Schondel 1949).

An early greatly detailed study, a Swedish multicenter project, gave negative results (Hagbard et al. 1959), but another large-scale survey, the Collaborative Study, found that children of diabetic women with ketonuria during pregnancy had a mean IQ of 93, significantly less than the score of 102 of children of mothers without ketonuria, or the 101 of controls (Churchill et al. 1969). Curiously, the reduction was true of children of class A mothers as of more severe degrees of diabetes. Later studies, however, noted no relation between maternal ketonuria and IQ, nor any abnormal neurological development or diminished IQ in children of insulin dependent or gestational diabetic women; on the contrary, in some studies the majority had IQs over 100 (Persson et al. 1984; Persson and Gentz 1984; Silverman et al. 1991). Most recently significant IQ impairment was found at about 4 years of age; the data, however, coming from children of mothers with insulin dependent, noninsulin dependent, and gestational diabetes all mixed together, cannot be taken seriously (Yamashita et al. 1996).

Applying other criteria of intellectual and neurological development, most older studies reported deficits to one extent or another (Francois et al. 1974b; Haworth et al. 1976; Manzke et al. 1977; Stehbens et al. 1977), but not all (Watson 1970), whereas almost all of the more recent ones found little or no such outcome (Cummins and Norrish 1980; Hadden et al. 1984; Olofsson et al. 1984; Ornoy et al. 1994; Rizzo et al. 1994; Sells et al. 1994; Kimmerle et al. 1995). One dissenting voice found that children who had been growth retarded as early fetuses performed worse on certain developmental tests than controls, and thus that children of diabetic women were at risk of psychomotor developmental problems (Petersen et al. 1988; Petersen 1989). Considering the possibly flawed means of relating fetal size and age mentioned above, this finding too may be suspect. The other noted an inverse relation between IQ and maternal lipid metabolic factors in late pregnancy (Silverman et al. 1991). Another noted a positive coorelation, of psychomotor development at 6–9 years with maternal late trimester beta-hydroxybutyrate, a measure of maternal metabolic state; but as mentioned it was flawed by not considering children of mothers with insulin dependent and gestational diabetes separately (Rizzo et al. 1995).

Discrepancies in the relation between features in children and maternal states, such as that of cognitive ability and toxemia, might have been due to the recent great reduction in severity or occurrence of that maternal condition (Cordero and Landon 1993). But it is not likely that anything of this sort can explain the wide variability found in congenital malformation frequency and type.

A Comment

A striking means of commenting on these studies of the later consequences of being born to insulin dependent pregestationally diabetic women, and by indirection on much of the diabetes work discussed in this work till now, is to compare their execution with one generally similar to them: an investigation of the putative developmental consequences in children of women who had hypertension during pregnancy (Ounsted et al. 1984). The sine qua non for validity of studies of human reactions to given situations is that the subjects be a fair sample of the entire group from which they are drawn, and that the experimental procedures be strictly defined.

In the words of the statistician-philosopher Fisher (1934), "It is a statistical commonplace that the interpretation of a body of data requires a knowledge of how it was obtained. Equally, it is usually understood that the conclusions drawn from experimental results must rest on a detailed knowledge of the experimental procedure actually employed." These requirements were met by the Ounsted study: the ascertainment of the pregnant subjects was detailed and the maternal risk situation and the means of evaluating the developmental state of the children were strictly defined.

On the contrary, in the diabetes studies the primary essential ingredient of a representative sample was ignored or unestablished, and the second sometimes flouted, with the collective inclusion of pregnant women with different types of diabetes—insulin dependent, noninsulin requiring, and gestationally diabetic women, as well as some whose diabetes type was not specified at all.

In the hypertension study the follow-up procedure consisted of ascertaining the relation between numerous maternal factors and the intellectual state of children of a specific age as evaluated by standardized tests. The former included social class, birth rank, maternal smoking status, preeclampsia, spontaneous or other delivery, breast or bottle feeding, birthweight for gestation age, fetal distress, and various others, all of which affected the several test scores in different ways, some being associated negatively, some positively, some not at all.

Again, by contrast, the diabetes studies were directed toward diverse ends diversely investigated. Of course, they were not conducted by one group at one period of time. That explains and should in part excuse the heterogeneity of their findings and their consequent overall inconclusiveness. But it does not excuse the great majority of them neglecting the consideration of many factors that may have been relevant in their studies, especially serious obstetric problems that often attend diabetic pregnancies—hypertension, ketoacidosis, preterm delivery, etc. (Cousins, 1987; Beaufils 1990; Siddiqi et al. 1991). Thus what is not yet satisfied is the need for an indisputable answer to the question of what can be expected to be the physical and mental development of children of mothers type 1 diabetes, the form of diabetes that is most worrisome.

Solace can be taken, however, in the findings of the hypertension study, since all in all they indicated that "children who survive a highly adverse intrauterine environment with subsequent complications at delivery and in the neonatal period are no more likely to have developmental problems in childhood than those whose early biographies had been much less hazardous."

Chapter 19
Diabetic Pregnancy in Animals I

It is reasonable to believe that human beings and other animals share propensities and adverse responses to diseases. If this is so human diseases may be advantageously studied by turning to animals afflicted with conditions mimicking them i.e. by the use of so-called animal models. Pregestational insulin dependent diabetes is one of these conditions, presenting not entirely resolved problems which were felt might benefit from animal investigation.

It is to the unraveling of unanswered questions left in the wake of the belief that this type of diabetes leads to congenital malformation that much of the experimental investigation discussed below was directed. Such studies depended on the occurrence of diabetes in laboratory animals, the several kinds of which, both experimentally induced and spontaneously occurring, provided opportunities for investigating in the laboratory many aspects of this complicated disease associated with human pregnancy.

The original method of producing diabetes experimentally—partial or total pancreatectomy—in that case in dogs, was, as is well known, the one that led to the discovery of insulin (Banting and Best 1923). It was also the earliest method used in pregnant animals but with variable success in producing the disease.

Experimentally Induced Diabetes

In what was perhaps the last such pancreatectomy study female rats were operated on at various times during pregnancy and insulin then administered (Hultquist 1950). Almost half died and most conceptuses in the remainder were resorbed. Of those reaching term many soon died, especially those with excessive birth weight, but in others on the contrary birth weight was reduced. Such inconsistent apparently contradictory results continued in later studies.

In this as in many early studies almost all attention was given to offspring survival and weight, not surprisingly since, as was seen above, these were among the features of most concern in pregnant diabetic women in those days. Malformations were regarded as contributing little to these outcomes, which seemed to be con-

H. Kalter, *A History of Diabetes in Pregnancy*,
DOI 10.1007/978-94-007-1557-8_19,

firmed by this study, since only one offspring in several hundred had a congenital defect, a cleft palate.

Alloxan

Even earlier, pancreatectomy had been replaced by a less traumatic way of inducing diabetes, i.e. by injecting the diabetogenic chemical alloxan, the first agent with this property discovered (Henry 1937; Dunn and McLetchie 1943), followed by steptozotocin, not long afterward (Rakieten et al. 1963). These, plus hereditary forms of the disease (Rerup 1970; Salans and Graham 1982; Bone 1990), provided the techniques and material for pursuing studies of the fetal effects of diabetes in animals.

Alloxan caused diabetes by destroying beta cells of the pancreatic islets. But it also caused kidney damage, wherein lay the problem. While the nephrotoxic effects were generally caused by larger doses than the diabetogenic ones, the dose ranges overlapped making it necessary to moderate the dosage and consequently limit the severity and duration of the induced diabetes; a limitation to be accepted until streptozotocin became available.

Two of alloxan's other features were important. Because it had an extremely short half it was most effective when given intravenously. Also, sensitivity to its diabetogenic property varied widely within and between species (Rerup 1970; Lukens 1948; Martinez et al. 1954; Cohn and Cerami 1979), whose meaning was little appreciated; and its neglect will be commented on below.

Rats

Studies of alloxan's diabetogenic effects on reproduction and pregnancy, made mostly with rats, began soon after the discovery of this property. Injection before or soon after conception frequently caused whole-litter resorption (i.e. early prenatal death) and stillbirth, while treatment later in pregnancy led mostly to increased fetal death, but with the viability of survivors little impaired.

Gross congenital abnormalities did not occur in the earliest studies (e.g. Miller 1947), except for minor and negligible ones (Bartelheimer and Kloos 1952; Kreshover et al. 1953). Effects on weight and size were infrequent, much of which were prevented by insulin. Many of the studies were summarized by Angervall (1959).

Incomprehensibly, such studies continued for 20 years, with the same assortment of outcomes—infertility, abortion, increased offspring death, inconsistent effect on newborn weight, and no gross malformations (Angervall and Stevenson 1960; Lawrence and Contopoulos 1960; Lazarow and Heggestad 1970).

A number of abnormalities, major and minor, occurred in a small percent of offspring in later studies after injection in early fetal stages—exencephaly, cleft lip or palate, cataract, hydronephrosis, some skeletal defects, but no absent or delayed development of the lower vertebrae, i.e. an unrelated assortment of defects (Takano and Nishimura 1967). The same was true with other breeds of animals and other treatment regimens (Ward and Readhead 1970; Ellison and Maren 1972; Khera 1984).

In a different procedure some fetuses examined 2 days after treatment on the 10th day of pregnancy had what later became clear was delayed closure of the neural folds, but whose later fate was unclear since older fetuses were not examinened (Deuchar 1977). Later examination of effects of alloxan treatment at an early stage found a wide variety of internal and external congenital malformations, each of 2–4% in frequencty, including decreased but transient ossification of sternebrae and caudal vertebrae, with severity of hyperglycemia unrelated to malformation frequency (Wilson et al. 1985).

Streptozotocin was no more successful. Female rats made severely diabetic by injection on day 5 of life were mated on day 90, and offspring examined on day 21 of pregnancy. The only developmental consequence mentioned was "growth restriction,"—all in all, much sound, little significance (Kiss et al. 2009).

In sum, in only two of the studies did major congenital malformations occur, with very few offspring affected, and they were diverse and without any pattern that could be considered a syndrome. There were also some minor defects, especially at certain skeletal sites, which probably represented retarded development.

Mice

These unimpressive teratological results led to turning to mice, a first experiment with alloxan however yielding no greater success in causing malformations (Koskenoja 1961). Others were more successful, but muddied the picture. Injection in midpregnancy caused gross malformations varying in composition according to the day treated, the great majority cleft palate and most of the remainder limb defects (Watanabe and Ingalls 1963). But treatment before or soon after conception had confusing results, mostly not causing malformations at all or seldom various ones such as agnathia, craniorachischisis, and other neural tube defects (Endo 1966), outcomes distinct from those following treatment during embryogenesis. This may have meant that while the former set was due to the diabetogenic action of the drug, the latter to its immediate effects on the embryo. But the relation was a loose one, since although the mean blood glucose level was significantly higher in females with than without malformed fetuses the levels overlapped widely. It was thus probable that hyperglycemia was not the cause of the malformations.

Attempted preventive studies followed. Mice were given alloxan prior to implantation and soon after insulin repeatedly till later gestation, the controls the drug only. In the latter, offspring had a malformation frequency of 5.0%, with neural tube defects and cleft palate predominating, while in the insulin exposed ones the frequency was 0.2% (Horii et al. 1966). Insulin was thus interpreted as preventing the malformations, but its basis was clouded.

This was so because while the blood glucose level was greatly reduced in the insulin-treated females, in the controls the mean level during midpregnancy in females bearing normal offspring was virtually identical to that in females bearing malformed ones. These seemingly irreconcilable results meant that hyperglycemia alone could not have been responsible for the malformations, and thus that alleviation of the hyperglycemia was not by itself responsible for their prevention, conclusions reached by the authors themselves.

Almost all these studies had low malformation frequencies compared with those induced in experimental teratology studies. The suggested reason for which was that the malformations stemmed from "extensive disturbance of metabolic homeostasis," and if malformation frequency were related to degree of such disturbance, any greater degree of the latter—as would be caused by even larger doses of alloxan—would be lethal to most pregnant females (Horii et al. 1966); as was noted in early investigations of the dose-resonse relations of the chemical (Lukens 1948 and in others cited above), and would thus close the door to greater malformation frequency.

This possible basis of at least of some of the limitations of the teratological consequences of induced diabetes is reminiscent of early studies of the teratogenicity of nutritionally deficient diets. In the days before vitamin antagonists existed such experiments required a balance between a degree of malnutrition so extreme as to impair growth and development of animals and one permitting them to mature, maintain fertility, and produce surviving congenitally malformed offspring (Warkany and Nelson 1941).

Streptozotocin

With the advent of the 1970s alloxan virtually ceased being used in studies of the effects of diabetes on reproduction and fetal development; replaced by streptozotocin because of its supposed advantageous features: more specific beta cell toxicity, reduced nephrotoxicity, generally larger margins between diabetogenic and general toxic and lethal dosages, and less need of insulin for greater maternal survival. What was enabled was easier and more specific induction of diabetes, expected to facilitate teratological study (Junod 1967).

Again rats were favored for experiments with the drug. And again, in the many studies made with it in the final 30 years or so of the last century, the record of the induction of congenital malformations was inconsistent. The number reporting them being far outweighed by those noting their absence or failing to mention them at all, signifying the negligible teratological potential of streptozotocin-induced maternal diabetes in animals.

Matched against this preponderance were the few occurrences of congenital malformations. The first teratology study of streptozotocin-induced diabetes, it turned out, was one of the few in which abnormalities occurred (Deuchar 1977). Female rats were given the drug intravenously some days before or on the day of conception and fetuses examined at midgestation or near the end of gestation. Abnormalities in the former consisted of variable degrees of failure of the neural tube to close and distortion or reduction in one or more cardiac chambers. Both types of abnormalities were also present in controls, but the the frequency of the former was greater in test animals than in the latter (10.0 vs 2.8%), as was the rate of fetal resorption. In any case, neither defect was present in near-term fetuses; which perhaps means they were not malformations, but simply expressions of developmental delay. This phenomenon will be explored below.

Near-term fetuses also had abnormalities, which were entirely different from those in the younger ones, i.e. omphalocele, micrognathia, and incomplete ossification of sacral vertebrae; the last in offspring of females with greatly elevated blood glucose, but also some with lesser levels.

The transitory phenomena in the fetuses and absent ossification in the term offspring raised a difficult question in teratology. Small size is not necessarily evidence of developmental retardation, yet when coupled with missing and incomplete ossification probably indicates nonspecific fetal growth retardation (Fritz and Hess 1970). Which may indicate that delayed skeletal maturation resulted from toxic effects of a situation stressful to the pregnant female, an accepted concept in reproductive toxicology (Aliverti et al. 1979; Khera 1984).

The results of this study, and of similar ones examining fetuses of streptozotocin-treated mice (Kawaguchi 1994; Tatewaki 1995), may be contrasted with multi-stage studies. For example, younger fetuses showed neural tube nonclosure or delayed development of various features, while older ones had no such abnormalities (Zusman and Ornoy 1986). The authors, however, missed the opportunity of offering an obvious explanation of this discrepancy—that of transient retarded development—and held instead that the abnormalities were no longer found because many of the abnormal fetuses had died and been resorbed. But the facts contradicted this, since the resorption rates at the oldest stages were similar to those in the controls. Which must leave the conclusion that whatever irregularities were present in the earliest stages had recovered with time, and a brief time at that.

Malformation vs Developmental Delay

Among the studies in which insulin was administered for the purpose of modifying the prenatal effects of diabetes two were of particular interest. Both were directed at examining the belief that strict management of diabetic women from early pregnancy prevented fetal maldevelopment (Reece and Hobbins 1986); with the supposition in mind that the lumbosacral abnormalities in offspring of diabetic animals were analogous to the human lumbosacral defects held to be associated with maternal diabetes.

In one study rats were given streptozotocin on an earlier or later day in mid-gestation, and insulin administered to those given it earlier (Baker et al. 1981). Two types of defects were noted in the lumbosacral area, but only in offspring of the earlier treated animals: failure of "neural tube fusion...(spina bifida occulta)" and lack of ossification. Both very likely entailing no more than delayed skeletal maturation at different sites, a likelihood supported by the near-term offspring weighing far less than controls.

Insulin decreased the frequency of the defects, but did not abolish them. Only with increased insulin and the glucose level further reduced did the frequency return to the control level; though fetal weight was not restored to normal, being roughly related to defect frequency. The question thus comes down to the nature of the relation between maternal hyperglycemia, fetal weight impairment, and defect frequency. Whatever this may be—and only multifactorial analysis might have disentangled it—the point the authors were at pains to make was that "meticulous control of diabetes during organogenesis" produced the mitigation; and hence that early control in diabetic women would prevent the sacral abnormality in their children. The argument being predicated on the animal and human abnormalities being analogous is clearly indefensible.

The second study, hypothesizing that the developmental delay masked the occurrence of true malformations, tried to separate these phenomena (Eriksson et al. 1982, 1989). Rats made diabetic by streptozotocin before conception were given insulin throughout pregnancy and late fetal offspring examined. Abnormalities seen were skeletal anomalies and malformations: minor departures from normal patterns of ossification in various sites and minor abnormalities such as extra ribs, etc.; and micrognathia and caudal dysgenesis, i.e. "lack of the tail" and "failing ossification of the caudal vertebrae." Evidence however made it apparent that the former designation was an exaggeration, especially since imperforate anus was not reported along with the supposed absent tail; which is unusual since anal imperforation almost always included taillessness (e.g. Gillman et al. 1948; Kalter and Warkany 1961; Grüneberg 1963). Incidentally, in an earlier study gross external malformations were not noted in routine inspection of several hundred late fetuses and newborn offspring of diabetic rats (Eriksson et al. 1980).

Turning to other findings, diabetes was correlated with increased fetal resorption and fetal retardation, indicated by reduced ossification in older fetuses, but greatly restored in neonates. Insulin improved all fetal conditions, largely preventing the malformations and ameliorating the anomalies. In a sense one of the objects of the study was met, dissevering the two sorts of abnormalities—anomalies and malformations—since one was remedied and the other not. Another goal—clarifying the teratogenic mechanisms in diabetic pregnancy, whatever that means—failed to be achieved, perhaps because insulin was given throughout pregnancy.

Teratological Mechanism

As part of investigating teratological mechanism, studies were made to learn when during pregnancy the maternal diabetic state exerted its effects (Eriksson et al. 1983, 1989). Thus insulin given intermittently usually reduced the frequency of the malformations, indicating that they were determined during the early to middle embryonic period.

It is important to recall however that the definition of malformation was broadened, making comparison with previous studies difficult. Finally, as elsewhere, the maternal glycemic state seemed irrelevant to the teratological outcome, since the serum glucose levels did not differ in rats with and without malformed offspring; and uninterpretable variations in beta-hydroxybutyrate concentrations were of no help in understanding the etiology of the defects. Thus, understanding mechanism once more proved elusive.

Rat Stock Studies

The findings in studies using different rat stocks will be briefly summarized. Severe hyperglycemia induced in females of Sprague-Dawley and Wistar rats resulted in fetal weight and growth impairment, but very few offspring of the former and none of the latter had external abnormalities (Uriu-Hare et al. 1985). Growth retardation, indicated by fewer ossification centers, occurred at several sites including caudal vertebrae, in Wistar usually to a greater extent than in Sprague-Dawley offspring. Thus none of the external malformations were seen that were reported by Eriksson et al. (1982); on the contrary, various minor skeletal abnormalities occurred not seen previously, but infrequently.

In contrast two long separated Sprague-Dawley sublines displayed some varibility, one but not the other having micrognathia and caudal dysgenesis, depite having similar degrees of induced hyperglycemia (Eriksson et al. 1986). For want of a better explanation it may be that the difference originated in a single gene mutation, as was likely the case for the difference in susceptibility to streptozotocin-induced diabetes between two inbred mouse strains (Kaku et al. 1989). But the outcomes of a cross-breeding experiment made this unlikely (Eriksson 1988), a situation reminiscent of the findings in a long-ago study of the genetics of cortisone-induced cleft palate with inbred strains of mice (Kalter 1954).

Another study examining early fetuses of the two sublines found similar frequencies of features, such as those seen previously (Deuchar 1977)—malrotation, open neural tube, heart hypertrophy—in both lines (Styrud et al. 1995). The explanation advanced for this unexpected finding was convoluted and unconvincing, but was admitted in the end to be unknown. It was clear that the apparent discrepancy showed that the developmental delay was nonspecific and unrelated to induction of major malformations.

Another largely negative study again found that the lines seemed to be of two discrete populations, one showing moderate and the other severe degrees of hyperglycemia, with no overlap, and with no or very little difference in fetal consequence between them (Giavini et al. 1986).

Still another study revealed inconsistency, a wide variety of external and internal defects but with no specificity to the time of treatment, and mostly of unimpressive incidence (Padmanabhan and Al-Zuhair 1988). Among the many types were two that appeared in other studies—omphalocele and micrognathia—as well as cardiac septal defects, that were seldom seen in near-term fetuses. The latter, the most frequent defect, also appeared in controls. but its diagnosis was unreliable. Insulin reduced all skeletal defects, contradicting another study (Eriksson et al. 1982). Finally, compounding the confusion, it was noted that insulin increased skeletal anomalies, perhaps by causing maternal hypoglycemia (Tanigawa et al. 1991).

Nutrition and Diabetes

Trace element metabolism appeared to be disturbed in diabetic animals (Eriksson 1984; Uriu-Hare et al. 1989). This might have been of significance since maternal nutrition had long been known to have a vital role in prenatal development, experimental studies having found that severe vitamin and mineral deficiency caused fetal growth retardation and congenital malformations (Kalter and Warkany 1959; Hurley 1977).

First came the discovery that fetuses of diabetic rats were deficient in zinc, despite the pregnant animals having elevated mineral levels. This led to attempts to prevent the fetal effects by zinc supplementation (Eriksson et al. 1984), which was unhelpful since the fetal zinc level remained reduced, growth was unimproved, and the abnormality rate was unchanged.

Equally negative was the evidence that deficiency of copper, magnesium, and protein had any part in the teratological effects of the maternal diabetes (Giavini et al. 1990, 1991, 1993; Jankowski et al. 1993); studies that revealed furthermore the limited ability of diabetes to cause major congenital malformations, and affirmed the nonspecificity of the teratological response to maternal diabetes.

A novel approach, whose description is much abbreviated here, was used in an attempt to prevent diabetes-associated embryopathy (Hagay et al. 1995). Mice homozygous for the human copper zinc superoxide dismutase transgene and those not possessing the gene were crossbred and administered streptozotocin at embryonic stages and embryos examined not long after. The findings—impaired size, certain anomalies—as would be expected from such young specimens, were unclear, although the transgenic state appeared to protect against the embryopathic changes, for which complicated explanations were given. Many of the defects however were similar to those transitory ones found in previous studies of embryos and young fetuses of diabetic animals, which were probably expressions of delayed development, and no doubt this was the case here as well.

Chapter 20
Diabetic Pregnancy in Animals II

Spontaneous Diabetes

The importance of spontaneous diabetes in animals for examining effects on prenatal development lies in the chance that it may offer a more valid model of the human condition than induced ones. Diabetes occurs in several animal species (Salans and Graham 1982), but pregnancy has been described in few of them.

Mouse Genes

Certain recessive genes in mice cause a diabetes syndrome, but most are maturity-onset states associated with obesity and sterility (Coleman 1982), and are not analogous to human type 1 diabetes. One that does not lead to sterility, the semidominant yellow (*Ay*), when incorporated into the KK inbred strain, which itself is prone to a noninsulin dependent diabetes, was briefly reported to cause external ear defects and various skeletal variations (Ooshima and Shiota 1991). Physical abnormalities did not occur in offspring of KK mice without the yellow gene (Reddi et al. 1975). In congenic inbred mice with the yellow gene there were no congenital malformations in offspring of pregnant hyperglycemic females (Teramoto et al. 1991).

Merely for the sake of leaving no stone unturned I mention a study with mice the basis of whose diabetes was not mentioned, one concerned solely with patterning defects in the neural tube, which deserves no further discussion (Dheen et al. 2009). [Buried in the article is a reference to one by this and other authors of mice made diabetic by streptozotocin; this was perhaps the basis of the diabetes in this paper as well.]

The NOD Mouse

Studies of the prenatal effects of spontaneously developing mouse diabetes have been made only with the NOD (nonobese diabetic) mouse strain. As with the BB

H. Kalter, *A History of Diabetes in Pregnancy*,
DOI 10.1007/978-94-007-1557-8_20, © Springer Science+Business Media B.V. 2012

rat, discussed below, its condition appeared to simulate the human type 1 form of the disease, and diabetic animals required maintenance doses of insulin (Makino et al. 1980; Leiter et al. 1987; Tochino 1987).

A teratology study found many fetuses dead, but the live and examinable ones had various defects, two predominating—a high frequency of exencephaly and a smaller one of spina bifida (Otani et al. 1991). All of the defects however also occurred in offspring of nondiabetic NOD females. A cross-transfer experiment attempted to clarify the maternal versus conceptal source of the teratogenic response, but no definitive conclusions were reached. Thus while in one experiment diabetes was associated with an increased frequency of malformation, in another maternal diabetic and nondiabetic backgrounds did not lead to different teratologic consequences, seemingly discrepant results difficult to interpret.

A different colony of NOD mice had a greater diversity of malformations, seen at later stages of pregnancy, many with abnormalities of the neural tube, face, tail, and ventral body wall, as well as complex viscero-cardiac malformations (Morishima et al. 1991). Some defects were also seen in a few offspring of nondiabetic NOD females, and many factors, such as differences in the glycemic state in females bearing and not bearing malformed offspring, made the results once more difficult to interpret.

Making the findings even more problematic was the fact that females of the NOD stock without overt diabetes also had offspring with malformations of the same sorts as occurred in those of diabetic ones. What this might mean respecting the etiology of the malformations in the diabetic group was left in mid-air.

The BB Rat

The study of spontaneous diabetes in rats began with the discovery of the condition in an outbred Wistar line, given the name BB (Nakhooda et al. 1976), which displayed clinical and pathological features similar to those of the human early-onset insulin dependent form (Marliss et al. 1982). Soon after its abrupt onset at 2–6 months of age diabetic animals required insulin daily for survival.

Despite the promise the model offered of investigating the effects of diabetes on fetal development and testing whether tight control of maternal diabetes would reduce fetal morbidity and maldevelopment it has been little exploited for these purposes.

In one such study diabetic females receiving insulin bred to diabetic or nondiabetic BB males had offspring with eye and central nervous system malformations and undescribed skeletal defects, one of the latter erroneously said to resemble the human caudal regression syndrome. The size reduction indicated the skeletal defects to consist of delayed ossification—hardly malformations (Brownscheidle and Davis 1981; Brownscheidle 1986).

True malformations, anophthalmia, exencephaly, and gastroschisis, were seen in late fetal and newborn offspring (Brownscheidle et al. 1983). Other conditions were present at term, delayed ossification of cranial elements and vertebral centra and wavy and absent ribs, but since the offspring were not fostered on nondiabetic females their meaning is clouded. The postnatal progress of the offspring was followed, with several developmental milestones delayed in some cases.

Only one other reproduction/teratology study, it seems, was made with BB rats, diabetic females being bred to like males and usually given insulin daily throughout pregnancy (Eriksson et al. 1989). As for congenital malformations only two were seen in 47 surviving fetuses, the sparsity of which, in contrast with studies described above, was imputed to the resorption of malformed fetuses, for which however no evidence was presented.

Chinese Hamster

Reproduction studies were made in another species that developed diabetes spontaneously, Chinese hamster. In one, other than a slightly increased birth weight, there was no physical change (Heisig and Schall 1971). In another, preweaning mortality was increased, but its cause was not determined (Gerritsen et al. 1974).

A more extensive study used two related lines, one with a low and the other a high rate of diabetes, the latter produced by brother-sister inbreeding and selection (Funaki and Mikamo 1983). Near-term offspring of diabetic females of both lines had a low frequency of various gross malformations, such as agnathia and omphalocele. The latter defect, occurring in offspring of a nondiabetic female of the low-rate line, indicated that in the diabetic animals it may have been due to a synergism.

Various things were left unnoted. Whether the blood glucose level in the diabetic females that bore offspring with malformations was different from that of the others was not examined. The proportion of growth retarded fetuses of diabetic females was increased, but whether it coincided with maldevelopment was not mentioned. The matter is raised because it may be as relevant to omphalocele—the most frequent malformation—as retarded development is to skeletal abnormalities discussed above.

A photograph in this publication displayed an abnormality mentioned in no other article on induced or spontaneous animal diabetes I am aware of. This was a defect labeled "omphalocele"—a defect discussed below—seen often enough in offspring of diabetic animals to be suspected of constituting a characteristic abnormality. The photo afforded insight into the possible nature of the defect which could not be conjectured in its absence. This subject will be dealt with in detail in the critique section below.

Postnatal Studies

Studies of the postnatal growth and development of offspring of animals with streptozotocin-induced diabetes were limited, but also inconsistent, due perhaps to variations in levels of maternal hyperglycemia.

For example, postnatal weight gain was accelerated, perhaps only temporarily (Oh et al. 1988). Also the weight of 4-week-old offspring was conflicting (Linn et al. 1993). It is obviously important to know whether the developmental detriments noted in these and other studies were prenatal or postnatal in origin, but this was not addressed here.

This uncertainty was removed by cross-fostering studies and others showing that the deleterious effects on postnatal growth of having a diabetic mother stemmed from conditions present after and not before birth (Vasilenko et al. 1989); furthemore the effects progressively diminished with age (Grill et al. 1991).

Preimplantation Studies

The impact of induced maternal diabetes on embryos in the period before implantation, in contrast with that after birth, was clear and consistent, the sole finding being retarded blastocyst development (Diamond et al. 1989; Vercheval et al. 1990; Moley et al. 1991; Hertogh et al. 1992); exceptional in this regard were embryos of spontaneously diabetic hamsters (Funaki and Mikamo 1983). This early retardation was as little helpful however in understanding the supposed teratological repercussions of diabetes on the definitive embryo and fetus (as many of the authors of these article thought it could do) as is the form of developmental retardation found in near-term fetuses. Regardless of anything else, the early-pregnancy studies complemented those of later stages in pointing to the fact that maternal diabetes, at least the induced form, had the common effect of causing growth retardation at whatever prenatal stage it acted.

An apparently identical inhibition of blastocyst development was caused by heat-shocking mice on the 1st day of pregnancy (Elliott and Ulberg 1971). Of which various interpretations were offered, but which may simply have been a nonspecific consequence, due to heat, diabetes, viz., of a systemic dislocation of maternal well-being—whatever that may mean.

Other Species

The effects of experimentally induced diabetes on reproduction and prenatal development were examined in various other species. In an early study of female rabbits made diabetic by alloxan prior to conception most of the pregnancies aborted, a few ended in premature delivery or stillbirth, but congenital malformations were not seen in any offspring (Miller 1947). A study of uterine glycogen in alloxanized pregnant rabbits failed to mention the outcome in offspring (Vaes and Meyer 1957).

Another study of rabbits had more positive results (Barashnev 1964). Alloxan was given before conception or at three widely spaced times during pregnancy and fetuses were examined grossly and histologically. Most offspring were alive but immature and growth retarded. The brain, the only internal structure studied, was reduced in size, but in some also malformed, especially the cerebral hemispheres. Also a very few offspring of females treated before conception or during the embryonic stage had external malformations, of eyes and skull. Whether these consequences were related to diabetes severity and whether those escaping maldevelopment were among the offspring of females receiving insulin were not clarified.

Dogs of an unspecified breed given alloxan before conception had apparently morphologically normal offspring (Miller 1947). Studies with guinea pigs made diabetic by streptozotocin injection before conception were similarly negative (Saintonge and Côté 1983, 1984).

Malformations—Direct vs Indirect Origin

Several matters mentioned above must be considered further. The first concerns the basis of the prenatal harm of chemical-induced diabetes. The fetal abnormalities that result from an agent given during pregnancy may be due to direct or indirect action, the latter via some effect on the pregnant animal, e.g. hyperglycemia. This is an old problem in experimental teratology, often difficult to resolve (Khera 1984).

This question was raised in a study of mice getting alloxan during midpregnancy, in which several fetuses had a defect suggesting myeloencephalocele (Ross and Spector 1952). Since the dose was subdiabetogenic and the maternal blood glucose level was normal it was suggested that the maldevelopment may have been due to histotoxic effects of the alloxan rather than its diabetogenic qualities.

The question is whether, despite their brief presence, the diabetogenic chemicals act on the conceptus directly or indirectly through the maternal organism. The argument that since such chemicals have extremely short half lives (Patterson et al. 1949; Kerunanayake et al. 1976) their prenatal consequences must be indirect, through induction of maternal diabetes, overlooks the consideration that if the brief moment of their potency is not too short to permit it to reach and destroy insulin-producing cells of the maternal pancreas, why should they not also be able during such a short spell to reach embryos to harm them directly. Other chemicals, of established teratogenicity, share this attribute of brief existence (Nau 1987). What the question perhaps calls for is a comparison of the fetal consequences of these chemicals administered before and at various times during pregnancy.

Malformations—Pre- or Postimplantation Origin

Do diabetogenic chemicals harm conceptuses by acting upon them directly or via the maternal disease state? Although their action in destroying beta cells is rapid the hyperglycemic consequences take time to be expressed. Therefore, when the chemicals are administered during embryonic stages, some of the embryotoxic effects may be due to direct, i.e., immediate, action because diabetes may not yet have developed. It follows that the malformations thus caused will be of specific types associated with the teratologic vulnerability of the time of treatment.

When, on the other hand, a chemical is administered before or at the time of conception, sufficient time will usually have passed for diabetes to be established when embryogenesis begins, and the anomalies induced will be due to the chronic maternal disease state. With these matters in mind, it can be asked whether the *true* malformations induced by these different etiologic avenues were distinct from each other.

True malformations did occur, although mostly in limited assortment and relatively low frequency. In mice, after alloxan, they were almost entirely of the neural tube, palate, and lower jaw; the same usually among the commonest in rats after alloxan. On the contrary, streptozotocin in rats led to a narrow array of defects, with those of the neural tube, jaw, and ventral body wall predominating. The overall impression, with few exceptions, is of a patternless miscellany.

Nevertheless, there seemed to be clear differences between the effects of direct and indirect action, despite the few overlaps that blurred the distinction. Strongly implicating direct action were the time-related specificities following treatment in midgestation, but with some defects occurring only after postimplantation treatment, e.g. digital and renal abnormalities (Wilson et al. 1985; Watanabe and Ingalls 1963; Takano et al. 1965; Takano and Nishimura 1967; Padmanabhan and Al-Zuhair 1988). In contrast, indirect action was indicated by agnathia and micrognathia occurring only after preconception treatment, and neural tube defects and omphalocele after preconception and early postimplantation treatment. Other malformations, especially facial clefts, were shared by almost all the studies, regardless of treatment time.

Fetal Growth Retardation

Since maternal diabetes retards development in the blastocyst as well as the embryonic stage—perhaps throughout prenatal existence—it is possible that this retardation is the feature underlying many of the defects in offspring of diabetic animals. Thus being the most prevalent and pervasive of its effects attempts were made to examine and explain it.

Signs of embryonic growth and developmental retardation were significantly reduced crown-rump length and somite number (Eriksson et al. 1984). This was hypothesized to be due to disturbed transfer of nutrients resulting from reduced utero-placental blood flow, a belief supported by measurements finding the total flow in the near-term placental circulation greatly decreased (Palacin et al. 1985; Eriksson and Jansson 1984; Chartrel et al. 1990). But this was cruelly negated by the contradictory finding that the flow in uterine and decidual tissue during midpregnancy was increased (Wentzel et al. 1995).

Attempts were made to reconcile these conflicting outcomes, to explain the connection to the so-called malformations (this qualification will be explained below). One, decreased blood flow could be related to the fetal growth retardation, but not to the malformations in near-term offspring, because the flow to malformed and nonmalformed fetuses was similar (a specious reasoning). Or, increased flow left the retarded growth unexplained, because of "increased delivery of oxidative substrates" (Styrud et al. 1995). Take your pick.

Why 'so-called' malformations? Altering a definition in midstream is unacceptable. In a preliminary study of growth-retarded embryos the most conspicuous and constant feature noted was posterior neuropore nonclosure, which "should take place" at an earlier stage of gestation than was examined (Eriksson et al. 1984). The delayed closure was thus wisely refrained from being labeled a malformation. Later however the same features that were earlier accepted as representing retardation—"neural tube closure abnormalities or rotational defects"—were called malformations, and the above fanciful explanation of their supposed occurrence was invoked (Styrud et al. 1995).

Therefore, except for a vague 'maternal nutritional inadequacy' the growth retardation caused by animal diabetes remains unexplained, as does its putative connection to malformations.

Missing Lower Vertebral Elements

The connection between prenatal retardation and the anomalies of the lower vertebrae reported in several studies is not difficult to see. These anomalies were of particular interest because they were said to be the counterpart of the caudal dysplasia syndrome claimed to occur frequently in children of women with diabetes, a syndrome typically consisting of absent sacral vertebrae. The lower vertebral bodies missing in defective offspring of diabetic rats were different in an important respect from the human abnormality. Though the latter were occasionally seen in newborn children, they were detected far more often only in older ones. In rats on the contrary the condition was noted in younger fetuses but not in older ones. The absence in rats was thus a consequence of temporary retardation which disappeared with catch-up growth.

This conclusion was supported by a detailed analysis of the "order, time, and rate of ossification" of the Wistar rat skeleton made years ago (Strong 1925), which noted that ossification in the first sacral arch began at 18 days and 10 hours of pregnancy, did not occur in more rostral arches till 22 days, i.e. the time of birth, and in caudal bodies did not begin till 3 days postnatal. The implication therefore is that were the offspring of diabetic rats allowed catch-up growth, and the skeleton examined postnatally, especially if allowed to be nursed by nondiabetic surrogate mothers, it would be found that the 'missing' elements had appeared. The analogy to the human abnormality was thus entirely spurious.

Omphalocele

Prenatal growth retardation may also be associated with omphalocele, one of the malformations that occurred in several studies of induced and spontaneous diabetes.

(In all but two instances the defect was labeled omphalocele, in the exceptions it was called gastroschisis. These are two different abnormalities, the latter the more serious one, but they are often confused and misnamed. This was probably the case with the exceptions).

Omphalocele consists of the presence at birth of intestine in the body stalk, due to partial or complete failure of the developing gut to return to the abdominal cavity during late 1st trimester, as it normally does. Although it is an abnormality when present at birth, in the embryo in the form of a transient umbilical herniation it is a normal phenomenon (deVries 1980).

Under certain conditions, however, e.g. growth disturbance, it may persist into later stages, and in some instances the omphalic sac may rupture before birth. Omphaloceles vary in size, and as commented "small and large omphaloceles should be distinguished because of their different nature and different prognosis" Warkany (1971, p. 759). A photograph of a fetus with what was labeled an omphalocele showed a specimen with intestine but no other abdominal organ extruded, which was probably a relatively small ruptured omphalocele (Funaki and Mikamo 1983). Such defects therefore were also probably an expression of the fetal growth-inhibiting influence of the maternal disease.

Conclusion

Animal models have been used to probe unresolved problems of human diabetic pregnancy, especially the one most regarded as still outstanding, the increased risk of congenital malformations in children of diabetic women. The current belief is that poor control of the maternal disease in early pregnancy is at its root, a belief that was supported by the beneficial fetal outcome apparently obtained by closely supervising the metabolic state of diabetic women from before or early in pregnancy (Steel et al. 1990).

This salutary result seemed to be complemented by findings of experimental studies in which insulin administration reduced the rate of malformations in offspring of diabetic animals. These and other outcomes, however, are not without difficulties of interpretation, and it is to these complications that attention now turns.

First to be considered are the aberrant conditions found in the embryos and fetuses of diabetic animals. These were of two sorts, which differ qualitatively from each other in a crucial attribute, namely, whether they are persistent or not. Persistent aberrations are present at birth and continue to exist into postnatal life. Transitory ones are those that are present at some time during prenatal life, but by the time birth approaches (or afterward in the case, e.g. of many ventricular septal defects, as discussed elsewhere in this work) have disappeared. The first consist of congenital malformations and the second of aberrant states of other sorts, described above.

The malformations comprised a relatively small variety; and could be almost completely divided into those caused by direct embryotoxic action of the chemical agents and those due indirectly to their diabetogenic repercussion. If any correspondence is to be sought between the human and animal effects of maternal diabetes, and insight gained into the fundamentals of their occurrence, it is only those of indirect origin that can be relevant. In studies in which malformations of this nature were produced the most often occurring, perhaps representing a characteristic cluster, were of the neural tube, ventral body wall, and mandible.

Many congenital malformations are said to be commoner, some of them far commoner, in the newborn children of women with diabetes than in those of normal pregnancies (e.g. Greene 1989; Combs and Kitzmiller 1991). [Parenthetically, these repeatedly cited statistics are largely based on a comparison of hospital series of diabetic pregnancies with wholly inappropriate and faulty control data (Kučera 1971a), and hence are untrustworthy, as often stated above.] Of this large variety of malformations only a small number however are held to be part of the constellation—the so-called diabetic embryopathy—that denotes it as diabetes-specific, prominent among them holoprosencephaly and certain lower vertebral defects. The first of these, or any of its varieties, was never reported in experimental studies of diabetic pregnancy. The second, on the other hand, occurred frequently.

The human malformation whose analogue the animal skeletal defects in question was assumed to be is absence of sacral vertebrae. It has the distinction of being considered the most common one; i.e. the ratio of its occurrence in diabetic vis-à-vis nondiabetic pregnancies is greatest of any defect; though it is far less so than universally cited (as detailed above). This malformation, held to be foremost among the hallmarks of the embyropathic effects of human maternal diabetes, was the focus of many of the experimental studies discussed above, in the endeavor to reproduce it in the offspring of the diabetic animals. But as was noted frequently, the analogy is false, since absence of lower vertebral elements in offspring of diabetic animals was invariably due to retarded fetal development, and with continued growth the supposedly missing ossification centers appeared by the time birth approached.

Insulin was administered to diabetic animals in several studies (Horii et al. 1966; Tanigawa et al. 1991; Baker et al. 1981; Eriksson et al. 1982; Wilson et al. 1985). In one, in which diabetes was induced before conception, insulin almost entirely prevented the defects produced by the maternal diabetes, micrognathia and what was termed caudal dysgenesis (Eriksson et al. 1982). The latter consisted of missing caudal vertebrae and "lack of the tail." But, as reasoned above, it is likely that it was absent only in the sense that no ossification sites were visible. That this defect was prevented by insulin was thus no doubt due to restored fetal growth. The prevention of the other defect, micrognathia, was apparently real. But its frequency in noninsulin-supplemented instances decreased with advancing fetal age, again indicating that it also had some growth-retarded aspects. In the other preconception study skeletal defects were not prevented, but on the contrary were induced, which was ascribed to the hypoglycemic effects of the insulin (Tanigawa et al. 1991).

In a study in which alloxan was given before implantation insulin prevented the very low percentage of various axial skeletal ones, and also all but prevented the neural tube and facial defects (Horii et al. 1966). Streptozotocin administered soon after implantation, i.e. at an early embryonic stage, apparently caused only defects of the lower vetebral column, and insulin, not surprisingly, since it improved fetal growth, lowered the frequency of the defects (Baker et al. 1981). Finally, following alloxan given soon after implantation, a single insulin treatment reversed the retarded ossification and mitigated the teratogenic effects (Wilson et al. 1985). Because at least some of the teratological results probably had an indirect basis their mitigation or prevention by insulin largely supported the separability of the direct and indirect effects of diabetogens.

Whether diabetes induced by cytotoxic chemicals in mice and rats is a suitable counterpart of human type 1 diabetes for studying and clarifying some of its outstanding problems has still not been fully agreed upon. What seemed indisputable is that the abnormalities of the vertebral column in offspring of animals with this diabetes were temporary by-products of fetal growth retardation, and did not correspond at all to the sacral abnormality in children of diabetic women. With respect to the malformations in the animals, most of the relatively small variety they consisted of were not among the ones occurring frequently in children. Even putting this fact aside, it is still to be proven whether these teratological experiments, indeed whether the diabetes induced, had any relevance for the investigation of human diabetic pregnancy.

So far as the experiments themselves are concerned, it is clear that the induction of diabetes by chemicals is often inefficient, and that when induced the diabetes was usually not teratogenic or only unclearly teratogenic. Finally, facts such as the poor relation between maternal blood glucose level and teratogenesis, and that animal stocks made equally hyperglycemic by diabetogens nevertheless differed in prenatal vulnerability, threw doubt on the concept that put upon hyperglycemia the entire blame for harming embryos and the belief that management of the human disease is the preventive formula.

A final word. It is hard to believe at this late date that elementary misconceptions are still prevalent. But they are. In an article called "animal models in diabetes and pregnancy" it was proposed that "experimental models of diabetes" can be useful for analyzing the induction of congenital malformations, etc., (Jawerbaum and White 2010). The thrust of the proposal, however, seemed to be about diabetes type 2—which the so-called animal models, such as those discussed above, were not afflicted with—and moreover that type of diabetes has not been accused of being teratogenic.

Chapter 21
Is Diabetes Teratogenic?

It is of use, from time to time, to take stock, so to speak, of our knowledge of a particular disease, to see exactly where we stand in regard to it, to inquire to what conclusions the accumulated facts seem to point, and to ascertain in what direction we may look for fruitful investigations in the future (Osler 1885).

Introduction

The basis of the supposed causation of congenital malformations by maternal diabetes, as the orderly mind conceives it, like everything in organic nature, must be either genetic or not genetic. Let us consider that the former is true. If so, the instrumentality may be construed as analogous to the hereditary pattern of insulin dependent diabetes mellitus itself, which probably has a multifactorial mode of transmission (Neel 1958; Vadheim et al. 1983). But serious inquiry into whether genetic factors play some role in the occurrence of these phenomena has never been made, e.g. by familial studies of malformations in sibs of affected individuals born before the clear advent of maternal diabetes, or of like patterns of malformations in offspring of maternal nondiabetic sibs, etc.

As it happens, a certain consistent finding overleaped the question and made speculation unnecessary, namely that the frequency of congenital malformations in the children of prediabetic women or, even more conclusively, in those of insulin dependent diabetic men does not exceed that in the overall population (Koller 1953; Rubin 1958; Hagbard et al. 1959; Neave 1967; White 1971; Chung and Myrianthopoulos 1975b; Theile et al. 1985). So, the reasoning goes, it cannot be the diabetes-related genes diabetic mothers transmit to their children that are the reason for the increased risk of congenital malformations, because children also inherit such genes from diabetic fathers (El-Hashimy et al. 1995). The proneness to maldevelopment must therefore be due to nongenetic i.e. environmental forces.

The knowledge that congenital malformations may be caused by environmental forces was only very recently acquired. Previously it was largely taken for granted

H. Kalter, *A History of Diabetes in Pregnancy*,
DOI 10.1007/978-94-007-1557-8_21, © Springer Science+Business Media B.V. 2012

that human and other mammalian embryos were sheltered from external damage, and that prenatal maldevelopment must be genetic in origin.

Observations of congenital malformations in human beings are as old as recorded history (Martin 1880; Ballantyne 1894; Warkany 1977); but extensive and detailed description and analysis of these phenomena, intermingled with inquiries into their origins, began only in the nineteenth century (Saint-Hilaire 1832; Ballantyne 1902; Schwalbe 1906; Mall 1908). Full realization of the fact that human maldevelopment can be caused extrinsically [aside from various superstitious notions (Glenister 1964)] only dawned with the discovery that therapeutic x-irradiation can be teratogenic (Goldstein and Murphy 1929; Murphy 1929). But this was little regarded, because that causative agency was felt to be unnatural and hence hardly physiologically relevant.

This attitude very soon greatly altered when it was revealed just a few years later that rubella, or German measles, a common infectious disease, and a long-standing part of humankind's everyday surroundings, an epidemic of which had struck wartime Australia, caused congenital abnormalities in offspring of infected pregnant women in that country (Gregg 1941). The final stroke, forcing the most reluctant skeptic to accept that environmental factors were capable of gravely damaging human embryos, came with the revelation that what had been considered to be a relatively harmless sedative, thalidomide, had caused devastating malformations (Lenz 1961; McBride 1961). In addition several other environmental agents and situations have been confirmed to be human teratogens, as noted in authoritative summaries of the contemporary understanding of the causation of congenital malformations in human beings (Kalter and Warkany 1983; Kalter 2010).

Diabetes and Malformations

Can type 1 diabetes mellitus cause malformations? Many authors have thought so; some exposing their naiveté have even written that "maternal diabetes is the only proven teratogen" (Kotzot et al. 1993). Some have provided a long list of defects so caused (e.g. Reece and Hobbins 1986) and loftily expounded on their etiology, mechanisms, and metabolic basis (Hoet 1986; Freinkel 1989; Cousins 1991b; Goto and Goldmann 1994; Sadler et al. 1995).

A number of authors, especially from older days, were more circumspect, and expressed doubt. They did this especially by noting the wide range of malformation frequencies, some not varying from normal, found by some studies of the outcomes of diabetic pregnancies (see Kyle 1963); and in trying to explain the reasons for this variability sounded their many weaknesses. Examples follow.

> Some authors may have included every trivial abnormality found on clinical examination, whereas others used technical aids to diagnosis or recorded only the lethal malformations discovered at autopsy. Some have mentioned only those anomalies which are obvious only in the first week whereas others have followed their cases and have added those malformations which were discovered later (Farquhar 1959).

> The figures vary with the source of information, the completeness of the clinical examination or autopsy, the age of the child at which the review is made, and the definition of a congenital abnormality (Breidahl 1966).

> Ces variations considérable tiennent aux moyens d'investigation mise en œuvre mais aussi et peut-être surtout à la définition des malformations congénitales, à l'âge du dépistage, à la possibilité de surveillance des infants (Mimouni 1972).

"Physicians would be remiss if they failed to appreciate the methodologic shortcomings in available studies. All studies lacked proper controls. Studies usually compared prevalences of anomalies studied prospectively in offspring of mothers with DM [diabetes mellitus] to prevalences in controls gathered retrospectively at different times by different investigators who may or may not have utilized identical criteria … no infants were examined in 'blind' fashion, i.e. by physicians unaware of whether their mother did or did not have DM. These represent quite serious objections and justify withholding definitive statements concerning the relationship between maternal diabetes and anomalies" (Simpson 1978). No recent findings have made it necessary to alter this declaration.

A further element, at least as capable of prejudicing the findings, is biased ascertainment, i.e. nonrandom selection of diabetic subjects. This is not a trivial matter but the importance of neutrality was almost never given due consideration. Unbiased ascertainment is the crux in the investigation of the etiology of congenital malformations (Little and Carr-Hill (1984)).

The Principles of Teratology

Of paramount importance in judging whether diabetes is teratogenic is determining whether this etiological factor conforms with teratological principles—principles formulated through studies with laboratory animals and which within the limitations imposed by human situations apply as well to people (Wilson 1973). In essence these entail: the basis and locus of teratogenic susceptability; the dependence of the adverse outcome on the prenatal stage exposed; the nature of the agent; and the degree and form of the expression of the harmful effects.

The question will focus on the relation between the malformations alleged to be caused by maternal insulin dependent diabetes and the excessive perinatal death rate in diabetic pregnancy.

Teratogens can be considered to be of two sorts, those the pregnant subject is exposed to once or intermittently and those present chronically, e.g. therapeutic pharmaceutical agents and environmental pollutants respectively.

Not all the principles are clearly applicable to human teratogens. Thus, there are but few explicit examples of the role played by genetics in affecting susceptibility. The experimental finding that agents causing maldevelopment at given dosages kill at larger ones (Kalter 1980) is inapplicable to humans, because teratogens have rarely been experienced by humans at levels that might be prenatally lethal; while those of specificity of timing and response are adhered to by teratogens as they act in humans, as illustrated by some examples.

Ionizing irradiation, medical or military, displayed target specificity by almost exclusively causing the single defect microcephaly; and its time-limitedness, by the relation of head circumference to maternal distance from the Hiroshima atomic-bomb hypocenter (Miller and Blot 1972; Miller and Mulvihill 1976).

Rubella viremia though protracted during pregnancy also displayed defect and time specificity by causing a particular combination of congenital abnormalities and those in most cases only by infection in the 1st trimester (e.g. Munro et al. 1987); the nature of the disease however did not allow a dose-response analysis of its consequences (Warkany and Kalter 1961; Warkany 1971, p. 62 et seq.).

Although suspicion fell early on thalidomide as the cause of an epidemic of limb malformations in several countries (Lenz 1961; McBride 1961) it took intense epidemiological study to establish the connection firmly (Weicker 1963, 1969). Various systems were affected but most frequent were unusual limb abnormalities (Smithells and Newman 1992). A precise time specificity existed as well, exposure on only the 35th to 50th days after the last menstrual period being teratogenic, with different parts affected at different times during this interval (Nowack 1965; Kreipe 1967).

Anticonvulsant drugs taken in the 1st trimester increased the risk of congenital malformation, with certain defects predominating. Primary risk factors were gestation exposure time, high drug dosage, and the particular anticonvulsant drug taken (Janz 1982; Bossi 1983; Kaneko and Kondo 1995).

Diabetes and Teratological Principles

Is genotype of influence? Type 1 diabetes is not always present during all of a woman's reproductive years. Yet seldom have the outcomes of the pregnancies of diabetic women preceding disease onset been considered. Some evidence may be pertinent.

Glasgow et al. (1979) saw two women who each twice delivered congenitally malformed children, one, first a baby with cardiovascular malformations and then a baby with an accessory auricle and tooth asymmetry (hardly major defects); and the second, successively a child with anencephaly, a normal one, one with transposition of the great vessels, and finally another without defects. Coustan et al. (1980) noted one child with an absent tibia who had an older sibling with the same defect (it was unstated whether the mother was also diabetic in the previous pregnancy). Small et al. (1986) reported two sets of malformed siblings, a pair with pyloric stenosis and pulmonary valve disease, and three children with cleft palate, anencephaly, and hypoplastic heart respectively. Stubbs et al. (1987) noted two women each with a malformed child who had each previously had a malformed baby, but the nature of the older children's defects and whether the mothers were diabetic during those pregnancies were not stated.

The possible intrinsic basis of some diabetes-associated malformations might have been examined by the simple means of studying the family histories of diabetic women. But such studies, to my knowledge, have never been made. Congenital malformations such as pulmonary stenosis, recorded several times as being due to diabetes, have long been known to have a significant familial rate of recurrence (e.g. Warkany 1971, p. 549). Numerous other malformations share this propensity.

Teratological Specificity

It has claimed by some, denied by others, and both claimed and denied successively by still others, that maternal diabetes is especially associated with an increased frequency of specific congenital malformations, namely cardiovascular malformations, particularly ventricular septal defect, anencephaly and certain other malformations of the central nervous system, and abnormalities of the caudal spinal column.

The present work has nullified such claims, with only the more modest belief remaining that there is a general increase in malformation incidence without a preponderance of any one type of abnormality. The rationale for a nonspecific outcome, as one author put it, is that "the diabetic state persists throughout pregnancy; thus one could reason that nonspecific anomalies of all organ systems would be expected, in contrast to the specific group of anomalies characteristic of drug- or virus-induced teratogenesis" (Simpson 1978).

This is specious reasoning, as a few examples attest. Thus, with respect to viral teratogenesis, fetuses may be infected with rubella throughout gestation, be born infected, and yet only have teratogenic effects related to the stage of gestation at the time of maternal infection (Ueda et al. 1979). Another, phenylketonuria, also a chronic or constitutional maternal disease, present throughout pregnancy, whose embryopathic effects yet show organ and time specificity (Koch et al. 1994).

As the previous pages showed however diabetes is not associated with specific congenital malformations, and especially departs in this respect from known human teratogens, whose analysis often related particular ones to susceptible periods of early gestation. Thus it does not adhere to the specificity tenet required for a teratogen.

Dose–Response Relation

The dosage of teratogens, as shown clearly by eperimental studies, determines the frequency and severity of the response. Dosages below a threshold level are without apparent harm to embryos; above it the teratological effects are progressively more frequent and severe until fetal death ensues. Death may be due to direct effects on fetal organs, specific or nonspecific, or to indirect effects of maternal toxicity; but in particular instances, even in experimental studies, it has not been easy to say which of these, or in fact any of them, is responsible for death (Kalter 1980).

Very early in the study of the outcome of diabetes in human pregnancy attempts were made to relate various features considered to indicate severity of the diabetic state to the high perinatal death rates of the day, such as maternal age at onset of the disease, the length of time it had endured, the dose of insulin required, pathological complications, sex hormone imbalance, etc. None of these was clearly tied to infant death. Still, closely supervised maternal care and its product, normal or nearly normal blood glucose levels, were noted to be related to improved survival.

The great decline in the infant death rate beginning in mid-twentieth century, in many parts of the world, turned attention to the most prominent remaining lethal factor, malformations, and here also attempts were made to find maternal correlates that would give insight to prevention. Taking a hint from certain beneficial effects of maternal glycemic control, studies were made of the association of malformation frequency and glucose level in early pregnancy.

If congenital malformations were caused by maternal diabetes, as mediated by maternal carbohydrate imbalance, then the degree (i.e. dosage) of this imbalance, gauged e.g. by level of glycosylated hemoglobin, should have been correlated with the intensity of the effect, at least above a threshold, as in adult diabetic complications (Viberti 1995). This proposition was tested by determining the frequency of congenital malformations in diabetic women with different mean levels of this component. But as noted above clear-cut consistent findings supporting the contention eluded investigators.

In experimental teratology the relation of malformation frequency and incidence of fetal death is complex. In some studies the malformation frequency due to larger doses was reduced by the death of abnormal fetuses; while in other studies the malformation frequency and death rate both increased with dosage, indicating nonspecific effects (Kalter 1980).

In diabetic pregnancy in women the perinatal death rate greatly decreased over time, probably partly owing to improved metabolic management (i.e. lowered dosage), but the malformation frequency, according to the results outlined above, remained constant in surviving offspring. Conforming to the first paradigm, ceteris paribus, the malformation rate should have increased, according to the second it should have decreased. It did neither. This would seem to be further indication of the nonteratogenicity of maternal diabetes.

A Summary of Sorts

In the present work, in order to determine whether insulin dependent diabetes can cause malformations in the offspring of diabetic women, perinatally surviving and nonsurviving offspring were considered separately. This was done to avoid the distortion introduced by the frequency of congenital malformations in perinatal mortalities—owing to their recalcitrance to prevention and the rates of malformation and mortality being inversely related—increasing significantly in the last years of the previous century.

Congenital malformations in perinatal mortalities are to be looked into first. The record for all mortalities gave an unambiguous picture. In each decade since early in the insulin era the frequency of congenital malformations in mortalities was not different from that in perinatal mortalities in the general population.

Supplementing this information was that from well examined autopsy material. When years ago Rubin and Murphy (1958) pointed to autopsies as a means of exploring the effects of maternal diabetes on pregnancy outcome they were able to identify only three reports of such data, with a mean malformation frequency in the 93 specimens of 22.6%. Time added many more such studies, but has not changed the outcome, the total number identified that have been autopsied stands about at present at 694, with a malformation frequency of 20.2%. Unfortunately in only four of the studies was the vital ingredient of controls examined as well, but the frequency in them of 17.4% provided no evidence that maternal diabetes led to an increased level of malformations.

It is unfortunate that the rate of autopsies of infants of diabetic pregnancies has greatly diminished in recent years. Of course the number of diabetic perinatal mortalities was greatly reduced also. But still the scarcity of autopsies is to be deplored because of the possible loss it entailed of further evidence regarding effects of diabetes on prenatal development. It may be wishful thinking, however, to expect clarification from this source, since the efficacy of autopsies for ferreting out the causes of death was, as always, rather poor (Cartlidge et al. 1995).

An unusual matter concerning malformations in autopsied infants from diabetic pregnancies is that, contrary to mortalities in general, there had been no increase over time in their frequency; that in earlier and later years were both about 20%, while malformations in general population mortalities showed a manyfold rise over the years. Thus the malformation frequency in autopsies did not vary with the perinatal death rate, as it had in overall mortalities. But why it did not is hard to say, except to guess that those autopsied were not always a random sample.

It is also unfortunate that, with rare exceptions, spontaneous abortuses of diabetic women have not been examined for structural abnormalities, despite the indication that the study of such material would surely yield answers to the question here pondered. One says this because of the abundance of abortuses, but especially because malformations in abortuses are far commoner than in neonates (Shiota 1993).

Last comes the issue of malformations in surviving offspring. The final account that has emerged from combing through the many studies of every variety that were published in the last 85 or more years was also unmistakable in its meaning. This too has told us that congenital malformations are not and never were increased in the children of diabetic women, despite the dramatically lowered perinatal death rate in such pregnancies; and thus the present 'lowered' levels were not the outcome of the great improvements in care of these women.

I have used sources from as many sides of this question as exist. As Gibbon put it long ago, the serious historian "is obliged to consult a variety of testimonies, each of which taken separately is perhaps imperfect and partial." And in sum their testimonies have obliged me to come to this conclusion, done at great peril. Research, someone once said, involves the shedding not the confirmation of our preconceptions.

The overwhelming majority of workers in the field of diabetic pregnancy—obstetricians, diabetologists, metabolists, clinical and experimental teratologists, medical geneticists, epidemiologists, and so on have seldom expressed the smallest doubt that type 1 maternal diabetes is teratogenic, that, on the contrary, as some have ventured and others parroted, it causes a two-fold or even greater elevation in the rate of defects beyond that occurring generally in the population (e.g. Fraser 1994; Garner 1995; Coustan 1998). And I—an outsider, as they may say—have the impudence to gainsay them all. But I have worked long and diligently and with much circumspection reached this conclusion, and any who will attempt to dispute it must turn their hands and heads to being as laborious.

Bibliography

Abell DA, Beischer NA (1975) Evaluation of the three-hour glucose tolerance test in detection of significant hyperglycemia and hypoglycemia in pregnancy. Diabetes 24:874–880

Aberg A, Westbom L, Källén B (2001) Congenital malformations among infants whose mothers had gestational diabetes or preexisting diabetes. Early Hum Dev 61:85–95

Abramovici A, Sporn J, Prager R et al (1978) Glycogen metabolism in the placenta of streptozotocin diabetic rats. Horm Metab Res 10:195–199

Abu-Harb M, Hey E, Wren C (1994) Death in infancy from unrecognised congenital heart disease. Arch Dis Child 71:3–7

Adashi EY, Pinto H, Tyson JE (1979) Impact of maternal euglycemia on fetal outcome in diabetic pregnancy. Am J Obstet Gynecol 133:268–274

Adler P, Fett KD, Bohatka L (1977) The influence of maternal diabetes on dental development of the non-diabetic offspring in the stage of dental transition. Acta Paediat Hung 18:181–195

Adra A, Cordero D, Mejides A et al (1994) Caudal regression syndrome: etiopathogenesis, prenatal diagnosis, and perinatal mangement. Obstet Gynecol 49:508–516

Airaksinen KE, Anttila LM, Linnaluoto MK et al (1990) Autonomic influence on pregnancy outcome in IDDM. Diabetes Care 13:756–761

Alberman E, Blatchley N, Botting B et al (1997) Medical causes on stillbirth certificates in England and Wales: distribution and results of hierarchical classifications tested by the Office for National Statistics. Br J Obstet Gynecol 104:1043–1049

Albert TJ, Landon MB, Wheller JJ et al (1996) Prenatal detection of fetal anomalies in pregnancies complicated by insulin-dependent diabetes mellitus. Am J Obstet Gynecol 174:1424–1428

Algert S, Shragg P, Hollingsworth DR (1985) Moderate caloric restriction in obese women with gestational diabetes. Obstet Gynecol 65(4):487–491

Aliverti V, Bonanomi L, Giavini E et al (1979) The extent of fetal ossification as an index of delayed development in teratogenic studies on the rat. Teratology 20:237–242

Allen, E (1939) The glycosurias of pregnancy. Am J Obstet Gynecol 38:982–992

Allen VM, Armson BA et al (2007) Teratogenicity associated with pre-existing and gestational diabetes. J Obstet Gynaecol Can 29:927–944

Alles AJ, Sulik KK (1993) A review of caudal dysgenesis and its pathogenesis as illustrated in an animal model. In: Opitz JM (ed) Blastogenesis: normal and abnormal, Wiley-Liss, New York, pp 83–102

Altemus LA, Ferguson AD (1965) Comparative incidence of birth defects in negro and white children. Pediatrics 36:56–61

Amankwah KS, Kaufmann R, Roller RW et al (1981) Incidence of congenital abnormalities in infants of gestational diabetic mothers. J Perinat Med 5:223–226

Amendt P (1975) Die somatisch-geistige Entwicklung von Kindern diabetischer Mütter: Ergebnisse Nachuntersuchung im Alter zwischen 4 bis 16 Jahren. Acta Paediat Acad Sci Hung 16:299–315

H. Kalter, *A History of Diabetes in Pregnancy*,
DOI 10.1007/978-94-007-1557-8, © Springer Science+Business Media B.V. 2012

Amendt P, Gödel E, Amendt U et al (1974) Missbildungen bei mütterlichem Diabetes mellitus unter besonderer Berücksichtigung des kaudalen Fehlbildungssyndroms. Zentrabl Gynakol 96:950–958

American Diabetes Association Workshop-Conference on Gestational Diabetes (1980) Summary and recommendations. Diabetes Care 3:499–501

Ananijevic-Pandey J, Jarebinski M, Kastratovic B et al (1992) Case-control study of congenital malformations. Eur J Epidemiol 8:871–874

Anderson RH (1991) Simplifying the understanding of congenital malformations of the heart. Int J Cardiol 32:131–142

Anderson RH, Lenox CC, Zuberbuhler JE (1984) The morphology of ventricular septal defects. Perspect Pediatr Pathol 8:235–268

Andersson B (1950) Diabetes and pregnancy. Acta Med Scand 138:259–278

Angervall L (1959) Alloxan diabetes and pregnancy in the rat:effects on the offspring. Acta Endocr 31(Suppl 44):1–86

Angervall RA, Stevenson JA (1960) Effects of alloxan-induced diabetes on the pregnancy of rats. Am J Obstet Gynecol 80:536–541

Anon (1963) Advance report: final natality statistics, 1962. Mon Vit Stat Rep 12(6):1–4 (Aug. 20, 1963)

Anon (1965) Congenital malformations of C.N.S. BMJ 2:1502–1503

Anon (1988) Congenital abnormalities in infants of diabetic mothers. Lancet 1:1313–1315

Anon (1989) Contribution of birth defects to infant mortality–United States, 1986. MMWR 38:633–635

Anon (1990) Cincinnati-Hamilton, OH. US census data. Database: C90STF3C1. Venus Lookup (1.4). http://venus.census.gov/cdrom

Anon (1991) Multicenter survey of diabetic pregnancy in France. Gestation and Diabetes in France Study Group 1991. Diabetes Care 14:994–1000

Anon (1992) Diagnosing congenital dislocation of the hip. BMJ 305:435–436

Anon (1994) Stratification by size in the epidemiology of ventricular septal defects. EUROCAT 8:1–2

Anon (1996) Pregnancy outcomes in the Diabetes Control and Complications Trial. Am J Obstet Gynecol 174:1343–1353

Anon (2009) Abstracts of Diabetes UK Annual Professional Conference 2009. Diabet Med 26(1):1–199

Apeland T, Bergrem H, Berget M (1992) Gravide diabetikere: en retrospektiv undersøkelse av svangerskap og fødsel hos type 1-diabetikere i Sør-Rogaland 1982–1990. T Norske Laegeforen 112:2520–2523

Arey JB (1949) Pathologic findings in the neonatal period. J Pediat 34:44–48

Armstrong D (1986) The invention of infant mortality. Sociol Health Illness 8:211–232

Artal R, Golde SH, Dorey F et al (1983) The effect of plasma glucose variability on neonatal outcome in the pregnant diabetic patient. Am J Obstet Gynecol 147:537–541

Artner J, Irsigler K, Ogris E et al (1981) Diabetes und Schwangerschaft. Z Geburtsh Perinat 185:125–136

Assemany SR, Muzzo S, Gardner LI (1972) Syndrome of phocomelic diabetic embryopathy (caudal dysplasia). Am J Dis Child 123:489–491

Aubertin E, Aubertin J, Gay J (1964) Importance de la valeur du traitement antidiabétique chez les diabétiques enceintes. J Med Bord 141:333–360

Aucott SW, Williams TG, Hertz RH et al (1994) Rigorous management of insulin-dependent diabetes mellitus during pregnancy. Acta Diabetol 31:126–129

Auinger W (1978) Diabetes und Schwangerschaft. 1. Mitteilung. Stoffwechselführung und Erfahrungen bei 90 manifest diabetischen Schwangerschaften. Wien Klin Wochensch 90:109–116

Ayromlooi J, Mann LI, Weiss RR et al (1977) Modern management of the diabetic pregnancy. Obstet Gynecol 49:137–143

Bachman C (1952) Diabetes mellitus and pregnancy with special reference to fetal and infantile loss. Am J Med 223:681–693

Bacigalupo G, Langner K, Saling E (1984) Glycosylated hemoglobin (HbA1), glucose tolerance and neonatal outcome in gestational diabetic and non-diabetic mothers. J Perinat Med.12(3):137–145

Baird D (1942) Discussion on stillbirth and neonatal mortality. Proc Roy Soc Med 36:59–60

Baird D, Walker J, Thomson AM (1954) The causes and prevention of stillbirths and first week deaths. Part III. A classification of deaths by clinical cause: the effect of age, parity and length of gestation on death rates by cause. J Obstet Gynecol Br Emp 61:433–448

Baker L, Egler JM, Klein SH et al (1981) Meticulous control of diabetes during organogenesis prevents congenital lumbosacral defects in rats. Diabetes 30:955–959

Bakketeig LS, Hoffman HJ, Oakley AR (1984) Perinatal death. In: Bracken MB (ed) Perinatal epidemiology, Oxford Univ, New York, pp 99–151

Balkau B, King H, Zimmet P et al (1985) Factors associated with the development of diabetes in the Micronesian population of Nauru. Am J Epidemiol 122:594–605

Ballantyne JW (1894) The teratological records of Chaldea. Teratologia 1:127–142

Ballantyne JW (1902) Manual of antenatal pathology and hygiene: the foetus. Green and Sons, Edinburgh

Ballantyne JW (1904) Manual of antenatal pathology: the embryo. Green and Sons, Edinburgh

Ballard JL, Holroyde J, Tsang RC et al (1984) High malformation rates and decreased mortality in infants of diabetic mothers managed after the first trimester of pregnancy (1956–1978). Am J Obstet Gynecol 148:1111–1117

Bánhidy F, Acs N, Puhó EH et al (2010) Congenital abnnormalities in the offspring of pregnant women with type 1, type 2 and gestational diabetes–a population-based case-control study. Congenit Anom (Kyoto) 50:115–121

Banta JV, Nichols O (1969) Sacral agenesis. J Bone Joint Surg 51A:693–703

Banting FG, Best CH (1923) The discovery and preparation of insulin. U Toronto Med J 1:94–98

Baptiste-Robert K, Barone BB, Gary TL et al (2009) Risk factors for type 2 diabetes among women with gestational diabetes: a systematic review. Am J Med 122:207–214

Barach JH (1928) Historical facts in diabetes. Ann Med Hist 10:387–401

Barashnev YI (1964) Malformations of the fetal brain resulting from alloxan diabetes in the mother. Ark Pat 26:T382–T386

Barlow TG (1962) Early diagnosis and treatment of congenital dislocation of the hip. J Bone Joint Surg 44B:292–301

Barnes HHF, Morgans ME (1949) Pregnancy complicated by diabetes melllitus. BMJ 1:51–54

Barnes PH (1961) Prediabetes and pregnancy. Can Med Assoc J 85:681–688

Barns HH (1941) Diabetes mellitus and pregnancy. J Obstet Gynecol Br Emp 48:707–725

Barns HH, Morgans ME (1948) Prediabetic pregnancy. J Obstet Gynecol Br Emp 55:449–454

Barr M, Burdi MM (1978) Arhinencephaly and polysplenia syndrome associated with maternal diabetes mellitus. Teratology 17:20A

Barr M, Hanson JW, Currey K et al (1983) Holoprosencephaly in infants of diabetic mothers. J Pediatr 102:565–568

Bartelheimer H, Kloos K (1952) Die Auswirkung des experimentellen Diabetes auf Gravidität und Nachkommenschaft. Z Ges Exp Med 119:246–265

Bass G (1970) Diabetes und Schwangerschaft. Schweiz Rundsch Med Prax 59:69–74

Beard RW, Hoet JJ (1982) Is gestational diabetes a clinical entity? Diabetologia 23:307–312

Beard RW, Oakley NW (1976) The fetus of the diabetic. In: Beard RW, Nathanielsz PW (eds) Fetal physiology and medicine: the basis of neonatology. Saunders, London, pp 137–157

Beaufils M (1990) Prise en charge de l'hypertension chez la femme enceinte diabétique:arterial blood pressure, pregnancy and diabetes. Diabete Metab 6:144–148

Becerra JE, Khoury MJ, Cordero JF et al (1990) Diabetes mellitus during pregnancy and risks for specific birth defects: a population-based case-control study. Pediatrics 85:1–9

Beischer NA, Oats JN, Henry OA et al (1991) Incidence and severity of gestational diabetes mellitus according to country of birth in women living in Australia. Diabetes 40:35–38

Bellamy L, Casas JP, Hingorani AD et al (2009) Type 2 diabetes mellitus after gestational diabetes: a systematic review and meta-analysis. Lancet 373:1773–1779

Benirschke K (1987) You need a sympathetic pathologist: the borderline of emryology and pathology revisited. Teratology 36:389–393

Benjamin E, Winters D, Mayfield J et al (1993) Diabetes in pregnancy in Zuni Indian women. Diabetes Care 16:1229–1235

Benjamin F, Wilson SJ, Deutsch S et al (1986) Effect of advancing pregnancy on the glucose tolerance test and on the 50-g oral glucose load screening test for gestational diabetes. Obstet Gynecol 68:362–365

Bennett PH, Burch TA, Miller M (1971) Diabetes mellitus in American (Pima) Indians. Lancet 2:125–128

Bennett PH, Webner C, Miller M (1978) Congenital anomalies and the diabetic and prediabetic pregnancy. Ciba Found Symp 63:207–225

Bennewitz HG (1824) De diabete mellito, graviditatis symptomate (diabetes mellitus: a symptom of pregnancy). Inaugural Dissertation in Medicine, Berlin

Berdon WE, Slovis TL, Campbell JB et al (1977) Neonatal small left colon syndrome: its relationship to aganglionosis and meconium plug syndrome. Radiology 125:457–462

Berendes HW, Weiss B (1970) The NIH collaborative study–a progress report. In: Fraser FC, McKusick VA (eds) Congenital malformations: proceedings of the third international conference. Excerpta Medica, Amsterdam, pp 293–298

Berg AT (1991) Menstrual cycle length and the calculation of gestational age. Am J Epidemiol 133:585–589

Bergmann RL, Bergmann KE, Eisenberg A (1984) Offspring of diabetic mothers have a higher risk for childhood overweight than offspring of diabetic fathers. Nutr Res 4:545–552

Bergqvist N (1954) The influence of pregnancy on diabetes. Acta Endocr 15:166–181

Bergstein NA (1978) The influence of preconceptional glucose values on the outcome of pregnancy. Ciba Found Symp 63:255–264

Berk MA, Mimouni F, Miodovnik M et al (1989) Macrosomia in infants of insulin-dependent diabetic mothers. Pediatrics 83:1029–1034

Berkeley C, Bonney V, MacLeod D (1938) The abnormal in obstetrics. Wood & Co., Baltimore

Berkowitz GS, Lapinski RH, Wein R et al (1992) Race/ethnicity and other risk factors for gestational diabetes. Am J Epidemiol 135:965–973

Berkowitz GS, Lapinski RH, Dolgin SE, Gazella JG, Bodian CA, Holzman IR (1993) Prevalence and natural history of cryptorchidism. Pediatrics 92(1):44–49

Berkus MD, Langer O (1993) Glucose tolerance test: degree of glucose abnormality correlates with neonatal outcome. Obstet Gynecol 81:344–348

Bernard LS, Ramos GA, Fines V et al (2009) Reducing the cost of detection of congenital heart disease in fetuses of women with pregestatinal diabetes mellitus. Ultrasound Obstet Gynecol 33:676–682

Bernard S, Delahaye-Plouvier G (1971) Pronostic foetal et réanimation néo-natale des enfants nés en milieu opératoire de mères diabétiques (à propos de 47 observations). Anesth Analg (Paris) 28:563–575

Berne C, Wibell L, Lindmark G (1985) Ten-year experience of insulin treatment in gestational diabetes. Acta Paediatr Scand Suppl 320:85–93

Berry RJ, Buehler JW, Strauss LT et al (1987) Birth weight-specific infant mortality due to congenital anomalies, 1960 and 1980. Public Health Rep 102:171–181

Bingley PJ, Gale EA (1989) Incidence of insulin dependent diabetes in England: a study in the Oxford region, 1985–2005. BMJ J 298:558–560

Birnbaum R (1912) A clinical manual of the malformations and congenital diseases of the fetus (trans Backer G). Churchill, London

Bix H (1933) Über Beziehungen zwischen mütterlichem Diabetes und Riesenkindern. Med Klin 29:50–52

Blank A, Grave GD, Metzger BE (1995) Effects of gestational diabetes on perinatal morbidity reassessed. Diabetes Care 18:127–129

Bliss M (1982) The discovery of insulin. Univ of Chicago, Chicago

Blomberg M, Selbing A, Källén B (2000) Congenital malformations in the southeast of Sweden–a registry study with validation. Acta Pediatr 89:1238–1243

Blot H (1856) De la glycosurie physiologique chez les femmes en couches, les nourrices, et un certain nombre de femmes enceintes. C R Acad Sci 43:676–678

Blumel J, Evans B, Eggers GW (1959) Partial and complete agenesis or malformation of the sacrum with associated anomalies: etiologic and clinical study with special reference to heredity: a preliminary report. J Bone Joint Surg 41A:497–518

Bone AJ (1990) Animal models of insulin-dependent diabetes. In: Pickup JC, Williams G (eds) Textbook of diabetes. Blackwell Scientific, London, pp 151–163

Böök J-A, Fraccaro M (1956) Research on congenital malformations. Étud Néonat 5:39–54

Borrelli M, Bruschin H, Nahas WC et al (1985) Sacral agenesis: why is it so frequently misdiagnosed? Urology 26:351–355

Boscq G (1979) Diabète et grossesse: réflexions sur la surveillance actuelle des grossesses des diabétiques. Rev Fr Gynecol 74:395–402

Bossi L (1983) Fetal effects of anticonvulsants. In: Morselli PL, Pippenger CE, Penry JK (eds) Antiepileptic drug therapy in pediatrics. Raven, New York, pp 37–64

Bottazzo GF (1993) Banting lecture. On the honey disease. A dialogue with Socrates. Diabetes 42:778–800

Bouchardat A (1887) De la glycosurie ou diabète sucré. Baillière, Paris.

Boué J, Boué A, Lazar P (1975) Retrospective and prospective epidemiological studies of 1500 karyotyped spontaneous human abortions. Teratology 12:11–26

Boulas MM (2009) Recognition of caudal regression syndrome. Adv Neonatal Care 9:61–69

Boulot P, Chabbert-Buffet N, d'Ercole C et al (2003) French multicentric survey of outcome of pregnancy in women with pregestational diabetes. Diabetes Care 26:2990–2993

Bound JP, Logan WF (1977) Incidence of congenital heart disease in Blackpool 1957–1971. Br Heart J 39:445–450

Bourbon RJ, Pignol B, Marin L et al (1985) Maturation of fetal rat lung in diabetic pregnancies of graduated severity. Diabetes 34:734–743

Bourgeois FJ, Duffer J (1990) Outpatient obstetric management of women with type-1 diabetes. Am J Obstet Gynecol 163:1065–1073

Boutte P, Valla J-S, Lambert J-C et al (1985) L'association vater chez un nouveau-né de mère diabétique. Pediatrie 40:219–222

Bowen BD, Heilbrun N (1932) Pregnancy and diabetes, with a report of 5 cases and a review of the literature. Am J Med Sci 32:780–811

Bower C, Hobbs M, Carney A et al (1984) Neural tube defects in Western Australia 1966–1981 and a review of Ausralian data 1942–1981. J Epidemiol Community Health 38:208–213

Bower C, Stanley F, Connell AF et al (1992) Birth defects in the infants of aboriginal and non-aboriginal mothers with diabetes in Western Australia. Med J Aust 156:520–524

Boyd ME, Usher RH, McLean FH (1983) Fetal macrosomia: prediction, risks, proposed management. Obstet Gynecol 61:715–722

Brandstrup E, Okkels H (1938) Pregnancy complicated with diabetes. Acta Obstet Gynecol Scand 18:136–163

Brearley BF (1975) The management of pregnancy in diabetes mellitus. Practitioner 215:644–652

Breidahl HD (1966) The growth and development of children born to mothers with diabetes. Med J Aust 1:268–270

Bronsteen RA, Wolfe HM, Zodor E et al (1987) Topics in perinatal ultrasonography. J Perinat 7:264–266

Brosco JP (1999) The early history of the infant mortality rate in America: "A reflection upon the past and a prophecy of the future." Pediatrics 103:478–505

Brown ZA, Mills JL, Metzger BE et al (1992) Early sonographic evaluation for fetal growth delay and congenital malformations in pregnancies complicated by insulin-requiring diabetes. Diabetes Care 15:613–619

Brownscheidle CM (1986) The BB rat: type I diabetes and congenital malformations. In: Jovanovic L, Peterson CM, Fuhrmann K (eds) Diabetes and pregnancy: teratology, toxicity and treatment. Praeger, New York, pp 15–36

Brownscheidle CM, Davis DL (1981) Diabetes in pregnancy: a preliminary study of the pancreas, placenta and malformations in the BB Wistar rat. Placenta Suppl 3:203–216

Brownscheidle CM, Wooten V, Mathieu MH et al (1983) The effects of maternal diabetes on fetal maturation and neonatal health. Metabolism 32:148–155

Bruce JH, Romaguera RL, Rodriguez MM et al (2009) Caudal dysplasia syndrome and sirenomelia: are they part of a spectrum? Fetal Pediatr Pathol 28:109–131

Brudenell M (1975) Care of the clinical diabetic woman in pregnancy and labour. In: Sutherland HW, Stowers JM (eds) Carbohydrate metabolism in pregnancy and the newborn. Churchill Livingstone, Edinburgh, pp 221–229

Buchanan TA (1991) Glucose metabolism during pregnancy: normal physiology and implications for diabetes mellitus. Isr J Med Sci 27:432–441

Budhraja M, Danel I (1986) Control of overt maternal diabetes during pregnancy in a county hospital. Arch Int Med 146:311–315

Bullen PK, Rankin JM, Robson SC (2001) Investigation of the epidemiology and prenatal diagnosis of holoprosencephaly in the North of England. Am J Obstet Gynecol 184:1256–1262

Bunn HF, Haney DN, Kamin S et al (1976) The biosynthesis of human hemoglobin A_{1c}: slow glycosylation of hemoglobin in vivo. J Clin Invest 57:1652–1659

Burck U, Riebel T, Held KR et al (1981) Bilateral femoral dysgenesis with micrognathia, cleft palate, anomalies of the spine and pelvis, and foot deformities. Helv Paediat Acta 36:473–482

Burkart W, Hanker JP, Schneider HPG (1988) Complications and fetal outcome in diabetic pregnancy: intensified conventional versus insulin pump therapy. Gynecol Obstet Invest 26:104–112

Burkart W, Fischer-Guntenhöner E, Standl E et al (1989) Menarche, Zyklus und Fertilität bei der Diabetikerin. Geburtsh Frauenh 49:149–154

Burt RL (1956) Peripheral utilization of glucose in pregnancy. III. Insulin tolerance. Obstet Gynecol 7:658–665

Burt RL (1960) Carbohydrate metabolism in pregnancy. Clin Obstet Gynecol 3:310–325

Butler NR, Alberman ED (eds) (1969) Perinatal problems: the second report of the 1958 British Perinatal Death Survey. Livingstone, Edinburgh

Butler NR, Bonham DG (1963) Perinatal death: the first report of the 1958 British Perinatal Death Survey. Livingstone, Edinburgh

Buyse ML (ed) (1990) Birth Defects Encyclopedia. Center for Birth Defects Information Services, Dover

Bye A, Henderson-Smart DJ, Storey B et al (1980) Incidence of the respiratory distress syndrome in infants of diabetic mothers: perinatal influences. Aust N Z J Obstet Gynecol 20:99–102

Calle EE, Khoury MJ (1991) Completeness of the discharge diagnoses as measure of birth defects recorded in the hospital birth record. Am J Epidemiol 134:69–77

Calzolari E, Colntidro MR, Roncarati E et al (1986) Aetiological factors in hypospadias. J Med Genet 23:333–337

Camerini-Davalos RA (1964) Prediabetes. In: Danowski TS (ed) Diabetes mellitus: diagnosis and treatment. American Diabetes Association, New York, pp 195–199

Campbell DM, Bewsher PD, Davidson JM et al (1974) Day-to-day variations in fasting plasma glucose and fasting plasma insulin levels in late normal pregnancy. J Obstet Gynecol Br Commonw 81:615–621

Campbell LV, Ashwell SM, Borkman M et al (1992) White coat hyperglycaemia: disparity between diabetes clinic and home blood glucose concentrations. BMJ 305:1194–1196

Campbell S, Pearce JM (1983) Ultrasound visualization of congenital malformations. Br Med Bull 39:322–331

Canavan JP, Goldspink DF (1988) Maternal diabetes in rats. II. Effects on fetal growth and protein turnover. Diabetes 37:1671–1707

Cardell BS (1953) The infants of diabetic mothers: a morphological study. J Obstet Gynecol Br Emp 60:834–853

Carmody D, Doyle A, Firth RG et al (2010) Teenage pregnancy in type 1 diabetes mellitus. Pediatr Diabetes 11:111–115

Carpenter MW, Coustan DR (1982) Criteria for screening tests for gestational diabetes. Am J Obstet Gynecol 144:768–773

Carr DH (1983) Cytogenetics of human reproductive wastage. In: Kalter H (ed) Issues and reviews in teratology, vol 1. Plenum, New York, pp 33–72

Carrington ER (1960) The effect of maternal prediabetes. Clin Obstet Gynecol 3:911–920

Carta Q, Meriggi E, Trossarelli GF et al (1986) Continuous subcutaneous insulin infusion versus intensive conventional insulin therapy in type I and type II diabetic pregnancy. Diabet Metab 12:121–129

Cartlidge PH, Dawson AT, Stewart JH et al (1995) Value and quality of perinatal and infant post-mortem examinations: cohort analysis of 400 consecutive deaths. BMJ 310:155–157

Case J, Willoughby D, Haley-Zitlin V et al (2009) Preventing type 2 diabetes after gestational diabetes. Diabetes Educ 32:877–886

Casson IF, Clarke CA, Howard CV et al (1997) Outcomes of pregnancy in insulin dependent diabetic women: results of a five year population cohort study. BMJ 315:275–278

Cedergren MI, Selbing AJ, Källén BA (2002) Risk factors for cardiovascular malformation–a study based on prospectively collected data. Scand J Work Environ Health 28:12–17

Chan A, Robertson EF, Haan EA et al (1993) Prevalence of neural tube defects in South Australia, 1966–1991: effectiveness and impact of prenatal diagnosis. BMJ 307:703–706

Chappard D, Lauras B, Fargier P et al (1983) Sirénomélie et dysplasie rénale multikystique. J Genet Hum 31:403–411

Chartrel NC, Clabaut MT, Boismare FA et al (1990) Uteroplacental hemodynamic disturbances in establishmnet of fetal growth retardation in streptozotocin-induced diabetic rats. Diabetes 39:743–746

Chase HC (1967) International comparison of perinatal and infant mortality: the United States and six west European countries. U.S. Government Printing Office, Washington

Chávez GF, Cordero JF, Becerra JE (1988) Leading major congenital malformations among minority groups in the United States, 1981–1986. MMWR CDC Surveill Summ 37(3):17–24

Chauhan SP, Perry KG Jr, McLaughlin BN et al (1996) Diabetic ketoacidosis complicating pregnancy. J Perinat 16:173–175

Christianson RE, Van Den Berg BJ, Milkovitch L et al (1981) Incidence of congenital anomalies among white and black live births with long-term follow-up. Am J Public Health 71:1333–1341

Chung CS, Myrianthopoulos NC (1975a) Factors affecting risks of congenital malformations. I. Epidemiological analysis. Birth Defects 11(10):1–22

Chung CS, Myrianthopoulos NC (1975b) Factors affecting the risks of congenital malformations. II. Effect of maternal diabetes on congenital malformations. Birth Defects 11(10):23–37

Churchill HA, Berendes HW, Nemore J (1969) Neuropsychological deficits in children of diabetic mothers: a report from the Collaborative Study of Cerebral Palsy. Am J Obstet Gynecol 105:257–268

Clausen TD, Mathiesen E, Ekbom P et al (2005) Poor pregnancy outcome in women with type 2 dabetes. Diabetes Care 28:323–328

Claye AM, Craig WS (1959) Pregnancy complicated by diabetes mellitus: a study in combined obstetric and paediatric management. Arch Dis Child 34:312–317

Clayton SG (1956) The pregnant diabetic: a report on 200 cases. J Obstet Gynecol Br Emp 63:532–541

Cobley JF, Lancaster HO (1955) Carbohydrate tolerance in pregnancy. Med J Aust 1:171–175

Cocilovo G (1989) Screening for gestational diabetes: an update. In: Morsiani M (ed) Epidemiology and screening of diabetes, CRC, Boca Raton, Fla, pp 69–75

Coffey VP (1974) Twenty-one years' study of anencephaly in Dublin. Ir Med J 67:553–558

Cohen MM (1989) Perspectives on holoprosencephaly. III. Spectra, distinctions, continuities and discontinuities. Am J Med Genet 34:271–288

Cohn JA, Cerami A (1979) The influence of genetic background on the susceptibility of mice to diabetes induced by alloxan and on recovery from alloxan diabetes. Diabetologia 17:187–191
Coleman DL (1982) Diabetes-obesity syndromes in mice. Diabetes 31(Suppl 1):1–6
Colwell KA, Baldwin VJ, Yong SL (1991) Sirenomelia and caudal regression–two distinct entities? Teratology 43:420
Combs CA, Kitzmiller JL (1991) Spontaneous abortion and congenital malformations in diabetes. Baillière Clin Obstet Gynecol 5:315–331
Comess LJ, Bennett PH, Burch TA et al (1969) Congenital anomalies and diabetes in the Pima Indians of Arizona. Diabetes 18:471–477
Conn JW, Fajans SS (1961) The prediabetic state: a concept of dynamic resistance to a genetic diabetogenic influence. Am J Med 31:839–850
Connell FA, Vadheim C, Emanuel I (1985) Diabetes in pregnancy: a population-based study of incidence, referral for care, and perinatal death. Am J Obstet Gynecol 151:598–603
Connor EJ (1967) Congenital malformations in offspring of diabetic mothers. Med Ann DC 36:465–507
Constam GR, Jost L, Rust T et al (1963) Diabetes und Schwangerschaft. Schweiz Med Wochensch 93:1611–1615, 1647–1653
Contreras-Soto J, Forsbach G, Vazquez-Rosales J et al (1991) Noninsulin dependent diabetes mellitus and pregnancy in Mexico. Int J Gynecol Obstet 34:205–210
Cooper WO, Hernandez-Diaz S, Gideon P et al (2008) Positive predictive value of computerized records for major congenital malformations. Pharmacoepidemiol Drug Safety 17:455–460
Cordero L, Landon MB (1993) Infant of the diabetic mother. Clin Perinat 20:635–648
Cormier CM, Landon MB, Lai Y et al (2010) White's classification of maternal diabetes and vaginal birth after cesarean delivery success in women undergoing a trial of labor. Obstet Gynecol 115:60–64
Correa A, Gilboa SM, Besser LM et al (2008) Diabetes mellitus and birth defects. Am J Obstet Gynecol 199:237.e1–237.e9
Corsello G, Buttitta P, Cammarata M, Lo Presti A, Maresi E, Zumpani L, Giuffrè L (1990) Holoprosencephaly: examples of clinical variability and etiologic heterogeneity. Am J Med Genet 37(2):244–249
Corwin RS (1979) Pregnancy complicated by diabetes mellitus in private practice: a review of ten years. Am J Obstet Gynecol 134:156–159
Cossard F, Horovitz J, Mage P et al (1982) La grossesse chez la diabétique. J Gynecol Obstet Biol Reprod 11:495–504
Cousins L (1987) Pregnancy complications among diabetic women: review 1965–1985. Obstet Gynecol Surv 42:140–149
Cousins L (1988) Obstetric complications. In: Reece EA, Coustan DR (eds) Diabetes mellitus in pregnancy: principles and practice. Churchill Livingstone, New York, pp 455–468
Cousins L (1991a) Insulin sensitivity in pregnancy. Diabetes 40:39–43
Cousins L (1991b) Etiology and prevention of congenital anomalies among infants of overt diabetic women. Clin Obstet Gynecol 34:481–493
Cousins L (1991c) The California Diabetes and Pregnancy Programme: a statewide collaborative programme for the pre-conception and prenatal care of diabetic women. Baillière Clin Obstet Gynecol 5:443–459
Cousins L, Dattel B, Hollingsworth D et al (1985) Screening for carbohydrate intolerance in pregnancy: a comparison of two tests and reassessment of a common approach. Am J Obstet Gynecol 153:381–385
Cousins L, Key TC, Schorzman L et al (1988) Ultrasonic assessment of early fetal growth insulin-treated diabetic pregnancies. Am J Obstet Gynecol 159:1186–1190
Coustan DR (1991) Diagnosis of gestational diabetes: what are our objectives? Diabetes 40:14–17
Coustan DR (1998) Pre-conception planning: the relationship's the thing. Diabetes Care 21:887–888
Coustan DR, Berkowitz R, Hobbins JC (1980) Tight metabolic control of overt diabetes in pregnancy. Am J Med 68:845–852

Coustan DR, Lewis SB (1978) Insulin therapy for gestational diabetes. Obstet Gynecol 51:306–310

Coustan DR, Nelson C, Carpenter MW et al (1989) Maternal age and screening for gestational diabetes: a population-based study. Obstet Gynecol 73:557–561

Coustan DR, Reece EA, Sherwin RS et al (1986) A randomized clinical trial of the insulin pump vs intensive conventional therapy in diabetic pregnancies. JAMA 255:631–636

Croen LA, Shaw GM, Lammer EJ (1996) Holoprosencephaly: epidemiologic and clinical characteristics of a California population. Am J Med Genet 64:465–472

Croen LA, Shaw GM, Lammer EJ (2000) Risk factors for cytogenetically normal holoprosencephaly in Californa: a population-based case-control study. Am J Med Genet 90:320–325

Crook A (1925) Incidence of glycosuria during pregnancy. Lancet 1:656–658

Crosse VM, Mackintosh JM (1954) Perinatal death. In: Recent advances in paediatrics. Little Brown, Boston, pp 63–86

Cruveiller J, Véron P, Benichou J-E (1977) Embryofoetopathie diabétique: à propos de cent observations. Sem Hôp 53:3217–3226

Cullimore J, Roland J, Turner G (1990) The mangement of diabetic pregnancy in a regional centre: a five year review. J Obstet Gynecol 10:171–175

Cummins M, Norrish M (1980) Follow-up of children of diabetic mothers. Arch Dis Child 55:259–264

Cundy T, Gamble G, Townend K et al (2000) Perinatal death in type 2 diabetes mellitus. Diabet Med 17:33–39

Cunningham GF, MacDonald PC, Leveno KJ et al (1993) William obstetrics. Appleton and Lange, Norwalk

Cunningham MD, McKean HE, Gillispie DH et al (1982) Improved prediction of fetal lung maturity in diabetic pregnancies: a comparison of chromatographic methods. Am J Obstet Gynecol 142:197–204

Curet LB, Izquierdo L, Gilson G et al (1992) Perinatal outcome and diabetes mellitus. Am J Obstet Gynecol 166:307

Cypryk K, Sobczak M, Pertyńska-Marczewska M et al (2004) Pregnancy complications and perinatal outcome in diabetic women treated with Humalog (insulin lispro) or regular human insulin during pregnancy. Med Sci Monit 10:P129–P132

Dabelea D, Hanson RL, Bennett PH et al (1998) Increasing prevalence of type II diabetes in American Indian children. Diabetologia 41:904–910

Daentl DL, Smith, DW, Scott CI et al (1975) Femoral hypoplasia-unusual facies syndrome. J Pediat 86:107–111

Damm P, Mølsted-Pedersen L (1989) Significant decrease in congenital malformations in newborn infants of an unselected population of diabetic women. Am J Obstet Gynecol 161:1163–1167

Dampeer TK (1958) Diabetes and pregnancy. J La St Med Soc 110:350–354

Damti A, Riakin-Mashiah S (2009) Preconception care and counseling for women with diabetes and those at risk for diabetes (in Hebrew). Harefuah 148:447–451, 475

Dandona P, Boag F, Fonseca V et al (1986) Diabetes mellitus and pregnancy. N Engl J Med 314:58–60

Dandrow RV, O'Sullivan JB (1966) Obstetric hazards of gestational diabetes. Am J Obstet Gynecol 96(8):1144–1147

Das S, Irigoyen M, Patterson B et al (2009) Neonatal outcomes of macrosomic births in diabetic and non-diabetic women. Arch Dis Child Fetal Neonatal Ed 94:F419–F422

David MP, Fein A (1974) Sirenomelia: report of a case with thoughts on the teratogenic mechanism. Obstet Gynecol 44:91–98

Davis EM, Peck JD, Thompson D et al (2010) Maternal diabetes and renal agenesis/dysgenesis. Birth Defect Res A 88:722–727

Davis WS, Campbell JB (1975) Neonatal small left colon syndrome: occurrence in asymptomatic infants of diabetic mothers. Am J Dis Child 129(9):1024–1027

Davis WS, Allen RP, Favara BE et al (1974) Neonatal small left colon syndrome. Am J Roentgen 120:322–329

Davison JM, Lovedale C (1974) The excretion of glucose during normal pregnancy and after delivery. J Obstet Gynecol 81:30–34

Daweke H, Hüter KA, Sachsse B et al (1970) Diabetes und Schwangerschaft: Ursachen und therapeutische Beeinflussbarkeit der kindlichen sterblichkeit. Dtsch Med Wochensch 95:1747–1755

Day RE, Insley J (1976) Maternal diabetes mellitus and congenital malformation: survey of 205 cases. Arch Dis Child 51:935–938

Degen R, Scholz G, Kunze C (1970) Die Früh- und Spätprognose von Kindern diabetischer Mütter. Pädiatrie 9:265–276

Dekaban AS (1959) The outcome of pregnancy in diabetic women. II. Analysis of clinical abnormalities and pathologic lesions in offspring of diabetic mothers. J Pediatr 55:767–776

Delaney JJ, Ptacek J (1970) Three decades of experience with diabetic pregnancies. Am J Obstet Gynecol 106:550–556

DeMyer W, Zeman W, Palmer CG (1964) The face predicts the brain: diagnostic significance of median facial anomalies for holoprosencephaly (arhinencephaly). Pediatrics 34:256–263

Depraetere M, Dehauwere R, Marien P et al (1995) Severe axial mesodermal dysplasia spectrum in an infant of a diabetic mother. Genet Couns 6:303–307

De Hertogh R, Vanderheyden I, Pampfer S et al (1992) Maternal insulin treatment improves preimplantation embryo development in diabetic rats. Diabetologia 35:406–408

D'Esopo DA, Marchetti AA (1942) The causes of fetal and neonatal mortality. Am J Obstet Gynecol 44:1–22

de Reu P, Van Diem M, Eskes M et al (2009) The Dutch Perinatal Audit Project: a feasibility study for nationwide perinatal audit in the Netherlands. Acta Obstet Gynecol Scand 66:1201–1208

Deuchar EM (1977) Embryonic malformations in rats, resulting from maternal diabetes: preliminary observations. J Embryol Exp Morphol 41:93–99

de Valk HW, van Nieuwaal NH, Visser GH (2006) Pregnancy outcome in type 2 diabetes mellitus: a retrospective analysis from the Netherlands. Rev Diabet Stud 3:134–142

deVries PA (1980) The pathogenesis of gastroschisis and omphalocele. J Pediatr Surg 15: 245–251

Dheen ST, Tay SS, Boran J et al (2009) Recent studies on neural tube defects in embryos of diabetic pregnancy: an overview. Curr Med Chem 16:2345–2354

Diabetic Pregnancy Study Group of the European Association for the Study of Diabetes (1989) A prospective multicentre study to determine the influence of pregnancy upon the 75-g oral glucose tolerance test (OGTT). In: Sutherland HW (eds) Carbohydrate metabolism in pregnancy and the newborn. V, Springer, New York, pp 209–226

Diamond MP, Moley KH, Pellicer A et al (1989) Effects of streptozotocin- and alloxan-induced diabetes mellitus on mouse follicular and early embryo development. J Reprod Fert 86:1–10

Diamond MP, Salyer SL, Vaugh WK et al (1984) Continuing neonatal mortality in infants of women with class A diabetes. South Med J 77:1386–1388, 1392

Dicker D, Feldberg D, Samuel N et al (1988) Spontaneous abortion in patients with insulin-dependent diabetes mellitus: the effect of preconceptional diabetic control. Am J Obstet Gynecol 158:1161–1164

DiGeorge AM (1968) Congenital absence of the thymus and its immunological consequences: concurrence with congenital hypoparathyroidism. Birth Defects 4(1):116–121

Dippel AL (1934) Death of foetus in utero. Bull Johns Hopkins Hosp 54:24–47

Doery JC, Edis K, Healy D et al (1989) Very high prevalence of gestational diabetes in Vietnamese and Cambodian women. Med J Aust 151:11

Dolger H, Bookman JJ, Nechemias C (1963) The management of diabetes in pregnancy. J Mt Sinai Hosp N Y 30:479–490

Dolk H, De Wals P, Gillerot Y et al (1991) Heterogeneity of neural tube defects in Europe: the significance of site of defects and presence of other major anomalies in relation to geographic differences in prevalence. Teratology 44:547–559

Dooley SL, Metzger BE, Cho NH (1991) Gestational diabetes mellitus: influence of race on disease prevalence and perinatal outcome in a U.S. population. Diabetes 40:25–29

Dornhorst A, Beard RW (1993) Gestational diabetes: a challenge for the future. Diabet Med 10:897–905
Dornhorst A, Rossi M (1998) Risk and prevention of type 2 diabetes in women with gestational diabetes. Diabetes Care 21(2):B43–B49
Downing DF, Goldberg H (1956a) Cardiac septal defects. I. Ventricular septal defect: analysis of one hundred cases studied during life. Dis Chest 29:475–491
Downing, DF, Goldberg H (1956b) Cardiac septal defects. II. Atrial septal defect: analysis of one hundred cases studied during life. Dis Chest 29:492–507
Dowse GK, Spark RA, Mavo B et al (1994) Extraordinary prevalence of non-insulin-dependent diabetes mellitus and bimodal plasma glucose in the Wanigela people of Papua New Guinea. Med J Aust 160:767–774
Drexel H, Bichler A, Sailer S et al (1988) Prevention of perinatal morbidity by tight metabolic control in gestational diabetes mellitus. Diabetes Care 11:761–768
Driscoll SG (1965) The pathology of pregnancy complicated by diabetes mellitus. Med Clin North Am 49:1053–1067
Driscoll SG (1966) Perspectives in human teratology 1965. Anesth Analg 45(1):9–14 (Jan-Feb)
Driscoll SG, Benirschke K, Curtis GW (1960) Neonatal deaths among infants of diabetic mothers: postmortem findings in ninety-five infants. Am J Dis Child 100:818–835
Drury MI (1961) Diabetes mellitus complicating pregnancy. Ir J Med Sci Driscoll SG:425–433
Drury MI (1966) Pregnancy in the diabetic. Diabetes 15:830–835
Drury MI (1979) Pregnancy in the clinical diabetic: a personal experience of 739 cases. Ir J Med Sci 148:75–79
Drury MI (1986) Management of the pregnant diabetic patient: are the pundits right? Diabetologia 29:10–12
Drury MI (1989) They give birth astride of a grave. Diabet Med 6:291–298
Drury MI, Greene AT, Stronge JM (1977) Pregnancy complicated by clinical diabetes mellitus: a study of 600 pregnancies. Obstet Gynecol 49:519–522
Drury MI, Stronge JM, Foley ME et al (1983) Pregnancy in the diabetic patient: timing and mode of delivery. Obstet Gynecol 62:279–282
Drury MI, Timoney FJ (1970) Latent diabetes in pregnancy. J Obstet Gynecol Br Comm 77:24–28
Drury TF, Powell AL (1987) Prevalence of known diabetes among black Americans. U.S. Public Health Service, Hyattsville
Duffty P, Lloyd DJ (1989) The infant of the diabetic mother: recent experience. In: Sutherland HW (eds) Carbohydrate metabolism in pregnancy in the newborn. IV. Springer, London, pp 327–332
Duhamel B (1959) Malformations ano-rectales et anomalies vertébrales. Arch Fr Pediat 16:534–540
Duhamel B (1961) From the mermaid to anal imperforation: the syndrome of caudal regression. Arch Dis Child 36:152–155
Duncan EH, Baird D, Thomson AM (1952) The causes and prevention of stillbirths and first week deaths. I. The evidence of vital statistics. J Obstet Gynecol Br Emp 59:183–196
Duncan JM (1882) On puerperal diabetes. Trans Obstet Soc Lond 24:256–285
Dundon S, Murphy A, Raftery J et al (1974) Infants of diabetic mothers. J Ir Med Assoc 67:371–375
Dunn JS, McLetchie NGB (1943) Experimental alloxan diabetes in the rat. Lancet 2:384–387
Dunn PM (1964) Congenital malformations and maternal diabetes. Lancet 2:644–645
Dunn PM (1989) Baron Dupuytren (1777–1835) and congenital dislocation of the hip. Arch Dis Child 64:969–970
Dunne FP, Avalos G, Durkan M et al (2009) ATLANTIC DIP: pregnancy outcome for women with pregestational diabetes along the Irish Atlantic seaboard. Diabetes Care 32:1205–1206
Dunne FP, Brydon PA, Proffitt M et al (2000) Fetal and maternal outcomes in Indo-Asian compared to Caucasian women with diabetes in pregnancy. QJM 93:813–818
Dunne FP, Brydon P, Smith T et al (1999b) Pre-conception diabetes care in insulin dependent diabetes mellitus. QJM 92:175–176

Dunne FP, Brydon PA, Smith K et al (2003) Pregnancy in women with type 2 diabetes: 12 years outcome data 1990–2002. Diabet Med 20:734–738

Dunne FP, Chowdhury TA, Hartland A et al (1999a) Pregnancy outcome in women with inbsulin-dependent diabetes mellitus complicated by nephropathy. QJM 92:451–454

Dyck R, Osgood N, Hsiang T et al (2010) Epidemiology of diabetes mellitus among First Nations and non-First Nations adults. Can Med Assoc J 182:249–256

Eastman JR, Escobar V (1978) Femoral hypoplasia-unusual facies syndrome: a genetic syndrome? Clin Genet 13:72–76

Eastman NJ (1946) Diabetes mellitus and pregnancy: a review. Obstet Gynecol Surv 1:3–31

Edmonds LD, Layde PM, James LM et al (1981) Congenital malformations surveillance: two American systems. Int J Epidemiol 10:247–252

Edouard L, Alberman E (1980) National trends in the certified causes of perinatal death, 1968 to 1978. Br J Obstet Gynecol 87:833–838

Edwards JH, Leck I, Record RG (1964) A classification of malformations. Acta Genet Stat Med 14:76–90

Ehrenfest H (1924) Carbohydrate metabolism during pregnancy and the value of insulin to the obstetrician. Am J Obstet Gynecol 8:685–709

Eidem I, Stene LC, Henriksen T et al (2010) Congenital anomalies in newborns of women with type 1 diabetes: nationwide population-based study in Norway, 1999–2004. Acta Obstet Gynecol Scand 89:1403–1411

Ekbom P, Damm P, Feldt-Rasmussen B et al (2001) Pregnancy outcome in type 1 diabetic women with microalbuminuria. Diabetes Care 24:1739–1744

Ekelund H, Kullander, S, Källén B (1970) Major and minor malformations in neborns and infants up to one year of age. Acta Paediat Scand 59:297–302

El-Hashimy M, Angelico MC, Martin BC et al (1995) Factors modifying the risk of IDDM in offspring of an IDDM parent. Diabetes 44:295–299

Elliott DS, Ulberg LC (1971) Early embryo development in the mammal. I. Effects of experimental alterations during first cell division in the mouse zygote. J Anim Sci 33:86–95

Ellison AC, Maren TH (1972) The effects of metabolic alterations on teratogenesis. Johns Hopkins Med J 130:87–94

Elwood JH (1970) Anencephalus in Belfast: incidence and secular and seasonal variations, 1950–1966. Br J Prev Soc Med 24:78–88

Elwood JH (1975) Secular trends in the incidence of anencephalus and spina bifida in Belfast and Dublin 1953–1973. Ir J Med Sci 144:388–394

Elwood JH, Elwood JM (1984) Investigation of area differences in the prevalence at birth of anencephalus in Belfast. Int J Epidemiol 13:45–52

Elwood JH, MacKenzie G (1971) Comparison of secular and seasonal variations in the incidence of anencephalus in Belfast and four Scottish cities 1956–1966. Br J Prev Soc Med 25: 17–25

Elwood JH, Nevin NC (1973) Anencephalus and spina bifida in Belfast (1964–1968). Ulster Med J 42(2):213–222

Elwood JM, Elwood JH (1980) Epidemiology of anencephalus and spina bifida. Oxford Univ, Oxford

Emanuel I (1993) Intergenerational factors in pregnancy outcome: implications for teratology? In: Kalter H (ed) Issues and reviews in teratology, vol 6. Plenum, New York, pp 47–84

Endo A (1966) Teratogenesis in diabetic mice treated with alloxan prior to conception. Arch Env Health 12:492–500

England LJ, Dietz PM, Njoroge T et al (2009) Preventing type 2 diabetes: public health implications for women with a history of gestational diabetes. Am J Obstet Gynecol 200:365.e1–365.e8

Engleson G, Lindberg T (1962) Detection of prediabetes by modified Exton-Rose glucose tolerance test sensitised by cortisone. Acta Obstet Gynecol Scand 41:321–327

Erhardt CL, Nelson FG (1964) Reported congenital malformations in New York City, 1958–1959. Am J Publ Health 54:1489–1506

Erickson JD (1976) Racial variations in the incidences of congenital malformations. Ann Hum Genet 39:315–320

Erickson JD (1991) Risk factors for birth defects: data from the Atlanta Birth Defects Case-Control Study. Teratology 43:41–51

Erickson JD, Mulinare J, McClain PW et al (1984a) Vietnam veterans' risk for fathering babies with birth defects. J Am Med Assoc 252:903–912

Erickson JD, Mulinare JD, McClain PW et al (1984b) Vietnam veterans' risk of fathering babies with birth defects. U.S. Department of Health and Human Services, Atlanta

Eriksson RS, Thunberg L, Eriksson UJ (1989) Effects of interrupted insulin treatment on fetal outcome of pregnant diabetic rats. Diabetes 38:764–772

Eriksson UJ (1984) Diabetes in pregnancy: retarded fetal growth, congenital malformations and feto-maternal concentrations of zinc, copper and manganese in the rat. J Nutr 114: 477–484

Eriksson UJ (1988) Importance of genetic predispostion and maternal environment for the occurrence of congenital malformations in offspring of diabetic rats. Teratology 37:365–374

Eriksson UJ, Andersson A, Effendic S et al (1980) Diabetes in pregnancy: effects on the foetal and newborn rat with particular regard to body weight, serum insulin concentration and pancreatic contents of insulin, glucagon and somatostatin. Acta Endocr 94:354–364

Eriksson UJ, Bone AJ, Turnbull DM et al (1989) Timed interruption of insulin therapy in diabetic BB/E rat pregnancy: effect on maternal metabolism and fetal outcome. Acta Endocr 120:800–810

Eriksson UJ, Dahlström E, Hellerström C (1983) Diabetes in pregnancy: skeletal malformations in the offspring of diabetic rats after intermittent withdrawal of insulin in early pregnancy. Diabetes 32:1141–1145

Eriksson UJ, Dahlström E, Larsson KS et al (1982) Increased incidence of congenital malformations in the offspring of diabetic rats and their prevention by maternal insulin therapy. Diabetes 31:1–6

Eriksson UJ, Dahlström VE, Lithell HO (1986) Diabetes in pregnancy: influence of genetic background and maternal diabetic state on the incidence of skeletal malformations in the fetal rat. Acta Endocr Suppl 277:66–73

Eriksson UJ, Jansson L (1984) Diabetes in pregnancy: decreased placental blood flow and disturbed fetal development in the rat. Pediatr Res 18:735–738

Eriksson UJ, Lewis NJ, Freinkel N (1984) Growth retardation during early organogenesis in embryos of experimentally diabetic rats. Diabetes 33:281–284

Eriksson UJ, Styrud J, Eriksson RS (1989) Diabetes in pregnancy: genetic and temporal relationships of maldevelopment in the offspring of diabetic rats. In: Sutherland HW, Stowers DW (eds) Carbohydrate metabolism in pregnancy and the newborn. IV. Springer, New York, pp 51–63

Eshai R, Gutberlet RL (1975) The infant of the diabetic mother. Pediatr Ann 4:318–322

Eshner AA (1907) The relations between diabetes and pregnancy: with the report of a case of diabetes in which the glycosuria disappeared with the inception of pregnancy and reappeared after delivery. Am J Med Sci 134:375–390

Essex NL (1976) Diabetes and pregnancy. Br J Hosp Med 15:333–344

Essex NL, Pyke DA (1979) Management of maternal diabetes in pregnancy. In: Sutherland HW, Stowers JM (eds) Carbohydrate metabolism in pregnancy and the newborn. Springer, Berlin, pp 357–368

Essex NL, Pyke DA, Watkins PJ, Brudenell JM, Gamsu HR (1973) Diabetic pregnancy. BMJ 4(5884):89–93

Eunpu DL, Zackai EH, Mennuti MT (1983) Neural tube defects, diabetes, and serum alpha-fetoprotein screening. Am J Obstet Gynecol 147(6):729–730

EUROCAT Working Group (1991) Prevalence of neural tube defects in 20 regions of Europe and the impact of prenatal diagnosis, 1980–1986. J Epidemiol Comm Health 45:52–58

Evans JR, Rowe RD, Keith JD (1960) Spontaneous closure of ventricular septal defects. Circulation 22:1044–1054

Evers IM, de Valk HW, Visser GH (2004) Risk of complications of pregnancy in women with type 1 diabetes: nationwide prospective study in the Netherlands. BMJ B:915–919

Fadel HE, Hammond SD (1982) Diabetes mellitus and pregnancy: management and results. J Reprod Med 27:56–66

Fadel HE, Hammond SD, Huff TA et al (1979) Glycosylated hemoglobins in normal pregnancy and gestational diabetes mellitus. Obstet Gynecol 54:322–326

Farmer G, Russell G (1984) Indices of fetal growth and neonatal morbidity in relation to glucose tolerance during pregnancy. In: Sutherland HW, Stowers JM (eds) Carbohdrate metabolism in pregnancy and the newborn. Churchill Livingstone, Edinburgh, pp 190–194

Farmer G, Russell G, Hamilton-Nicoli DR et al (1988) The influence of maternal glucose metabolism on fetal growth, development and morbidity in 917 singleton pregnancies in nondiabetic women. Diabetologia 31:134–141

Farquhar JW (1959) The child of the diabetic woman. Arch Dis Child 34:76–96

Farquhar JW (1965) The influence of maternal diabetes on foetus and child. In: Gairdner D (ed) Recent advances in paediatrics, 3rd edn. Little Brown, Boston, pp 121–153

Farquhar JW (1969a) The infant of the diabetic mother. Postgrad Med J Suppl 45:806–811

Farquhar JW (1969b) Prognosis for babies born to diabetic mothers in Edinburgh. Arch Dis Child 44:36–47

Farrell J, Forrest JM, Storey GN et al (1986) Gestational diabetes: infant malformations and subsequent maternal glucose tolerance. Aust N Z J Obstet Gynecol 26:11–16

Farrell T, Neale L, Cundy T (2002) Congenital anomalies in the offspring of women with type 1, type 2 and gestational diabetes. Diabet Med 19:322–326

Feig DS, Palda VA (2002) Type 2 diabetes in pregnancy: a growing concern. Lancet 359:1690–1692

Feigenbaum A, Chitayat D, Robinson B et al (1996) The expanding clinical phenotype of the tRNALeu(UUR) A→G mutation at np 3243 of mitochondrial DNA: diabetic embryopathy associated with mitochondrial cytopathy. Am J Med Genet 62:404–409

Feldt RH, Avasthey P, Yoshimasu F et al (1971) Incidence of congenital heart disease in children born to residents of Olmsted County, Minnesota, 1959–1969. Mayo Clin Proc 46:794–799

Feller A, Sternberg H (1931) Zur Kenntnis der Fehlbildungen der Wirbelsäule. III. Mitteilung. Über den vollständigen Mangel der unteren Wirbelsäulenabschnitte und seine Bedeutung für die formale Genese der Defektbildungen des hinteren Körperendes. Virchow Arch Path 280:649–692

Fenichel P, Hiéronimus S, Bourlon F et al (1990) Macrosomie du foetus de mère diabétique. Presse Méd 19:255–258

Ferencz C, Rubin JD, McCarter RJ et al (1985) Congenital heart disease: prevalence at livebirth: the Baltimore-Washington Infant Study. Am J Epidemiol 121:31–33

Ferencz C, Rubin JD, McCarter RJ et al (1987) Cardiac and noncardiac malformations: observations in a population-based study. Teratology 35:367–378

Figueroa C, Plasencia W, Equiluz I et al (2009) Prenatal diagnosis and tridimensional ultrasound features of bilateral femoral hypoplasia-unusual facies syndrome. J Matern Fetal Neonatal Med 22:936–939

Fink A (1955) Die perinatale Sterblichkeit (eine Übersicht über 55 300 Geburten der letzten 20 Jahre). Zentralbl Gynakol 77:1094–1104

Fischer L (1935) Riesenkinder bei mütterlichem Diabetes. Zentralbl Gynakol 59:249–260

Fisher RA (1934) The effect of methods of ascertainment upon the estimation of frequencies. Ann Eugen 6:13–25

Fixler DE, Paster P, Chamberlin M et al (1989) Trends in congenital heart disease in Dallas County births 1971–1984. Circulation 81:137–142

Flynn FV, Harper C, de Mayo P (1953) Lactosuria and glycosuria in pregnancy and the puerperium. Lancet 2:698–704

Forsbach G, Contreras-Soto JJ, Fong G et al (1988) Prevalence of gestational diabetes and macrosomic newborns in a Mexican population. Diabetes Care 11:235–238

François R, Picaud J-J, Ruitton-Ugliengo A et al (1974a) The newborn of diabetic mothers: observations on 154 cases, 1958–1972. Biol Neonat 24:1–31

François R, Picaud J-J, Ruitton-Ugliengo A et al (1974b) Le nouveau-né de mère diabétique (expérience de 168 cas 1958–1974). Diabète 22:69–91

Frankel AN (1950) Pregnancy complicated by diabetes. N Y St J Med 50:1233–1236

Franks PW, Looker HC, Kobes S et al (2006) Gestational glucose tolerance and risk of type 2 diabetes in young Pima Indians. Diabetes 55:460–465

Fraser FC (1960) Discussion. In: Wolstenholme GE, O'Connor CM (eds) Ciba Foundation symposium on congenital malformations. Little Brown, Boston, p 236

Fraser FC (1976) The multifactorial/threshold concept–uses and misuses. Teratology 14:267–280

Fraser R (1994) Diabetes in pregnancy. Arch Dis Child 71:F224–F230

Fredrikson H, Hagbard L, Olow I et al (1957) Follow-up investigation of children of diabetic mothers. Nord Med 57:669–671

Freinkel N (1989) The metabolic basis for birth defects in pregnancies complicated by diabetes mellitus. In: Sutherland HW et al (eds) Carbohydrate metabolism in pregnancy and the newborn. IV. Springer, New York, pp 39–49

Freinkel N, Gabbe SG, Hadden DR et al (1985) Summary and recommendations of the Second International Workshop-Conference on Gestational Diabetes Mellitus. Diabetes 34:123–126

Freinkel N, Metzger BE, Phelps RL et al (1986) Gestational diabetes mellitus: a syndrome with phenotypic and genotypic heterogeneity. Horm Metab Res 18:427–430

Frézal J, Kelley J, Guillemot ML et al (1964) Anencephaly in France. Am J Hum Genet 16:336–350

Friedman JM, Fialkow PJ (1980) The genetics of diabetes mellitus. Prog Med Genet 4:199–232

Fritz H, Hess R (1970) Ossification of the rat and mouse skeleton in the perinatal period. Teratology 3:331–338

Froehlich LA, Fujikura T (1969) Congenital malformations in perinatal, infant and child deaths. In: Nishimura H, Miller JR (eds) Methods for teratological studies in experimental animals and man. Igaku Shoin, Tokyo, pp 167–194

Froewis J, Rogovits N (1969) Diabetische Schwangerschaft und Geburt. Wien Klin Wochensch 81:129–135

Fuhrmann K (1982) Diabetic control and outcome in the pregnant patient. In: Peterson CM (ed) Diabetes management in the '80s. Praeger, New York, pp 66–79

Fuhrmann K, Reiher H, Semmler K et al (1983) Prevention of congenital malformations in infants of insulin-dependent diabetic mothers. Diabetes Care 6:219–223

Fuhrmann K, Reiher H, Semmler K et al (1984) The effect of intensified conventional insulin therapy before and during pregnancy on the malformtion rate in offspring of diabetic mothers. Exp Clin Endocrinol 83:173–177

Fuhrmann K, Reiher H, Semmler K et al (1986) Congenital anomalies: etiology, prevention, and prenatal diagnosis. In: Jovanovic L et al (eds) Diabetes and pregnancy: teratology, toxicology and treatment. Praeger, New York, pp 168–184

Funaki K, Mikamo K (1983) Developmental-stage-dependent teratogenic effects in the Chinese hamster. Diabetes 32:637–643

Futcher PH, Long NW (1954) Hospital data on the birth of large infants to "prediabetic" women. Bull Johns Hopkins Hosp 94:128–138

Gabbe SG (1977) Congenital malformations in infants of diabetic mothers. Obstet Gynecol Surv 32:125–132

Gabbe SG (1986) Diabetes mellitus. In: Danforth DN, Scott JR (eds) Obstetrics and gynecology. Lippincott, Philadelphia, pp 546–551

Gabbe SG, Landon MB (1989) Management of diabetes mellitus in pregnancy: survey of maternal-fetal medicine subspecialists in the United States. In: Sutherland HW et al (eds) Carbohydrate metabolism in pregnancy and the newborn. IV. Springer, London, pp 309–317

Gabbe SG, Lowensohn RI, Wu PY et al (1978) Current patterns of neonatal morbidity and mortality in infants of diabetic mothers. Diabetes Care 1:335–339

Gabbe SG, Mestman JG, Freeman RK, Anderson GV, Lowensohn RI (1977) Management and outcome of class A diabetes mellitus. Am J Obstet Gynecol 127(5):465–469

Gale EA (2002) The rise of childhood type 1 diabetes in the 20th century. Diabetes 51:3353–3361

Galindo A, Burguillo AG, Azriel S et al (2006) Outcome of fetuses in women with pregestational diabetes melitus. J Perinat Med 34:323–331

Gamsu HR (1978) Neonatal morbidity in infants of diabetic mothers. J Roy Soc Med 71:211–222

Gandhi JA, Zhang XY, Maidman JE (1995) Fetal cardiac hypertrophy and cardiac function in diabetic pregnancies. Am J Obstet Gynecol 173:1132–1136

Garcia-Patterson A, Corcoy R, Rigla M et al (1997) Does preconceptional counseling in diabetic women influence perinatal outcome? Ann Ist Super Sanita 33:333–336

Gardner RJ, Veale AM, Parslow MI, Becroft DM, Shaw RL, Fitzgerald PH, Hutchings HE, McCreanor HR, Wong J, Eiby JR, Howarth DA, Whyte SE (1973) A survey of 972 cytogenetically examined cases of Down's syndrome. N Z Med J 78(502):403–409

Garner P (1995) Type I diabetes mellitus and pregnancy. Lancet 346:157–161

Garner P, Okun N, Keely E et al (1997) A randomized control trial of strict glycemic control and tertiary level obstetric care versus routine obstetric care in the management of gestational diabetes: a pilot study. Am J Obstet Gynecol 177:190–195

Garner PR, D'Alton ME, Dudley DK et al (1990) Preeclamplsia in diabetic pregnancies. Am J Obstet Gynecol 163:505–508

Gaspar JL (1945) Diabetes mellitus and pregnancy: a survey of 49 deliveries. West J Surg 53:21–27

Gaspart E (1985) Glucose. In: Siest G, Henny J, Schiele F et al (eds) Interpretation of clinical laboratory tests. Biomedical Publications, Foster City, pp 253–269

Gellis SS, Hsia DY (1959) The infant of the diabetic mother. Am J Dis Child 97:1–41

Gendell M, Hellegers AE (1973) The influence of the changes in maternal age, birth order, and color on the changing perinatal death, Baltimore, 1961–1966. Health Serv Rep 88:733–742

Gens E, Michaelis D (1990) The frequency of disturbances of somatic development in young people with type I diabetes in dependence on duration and age at onset of the disease. Exp Clin Endocrinol 95:97–104

Gerritsen GC, Johnson MA, Soret MG et al (1974) Epidemiology of Chinese hamsters and preliminary evidence for genetic heterogeneity of diabetes. Diabetologia 10:581–588

Giavini E, Airoldi L, Broccia ML et al (1993) Effect of diets with different content in protein and fiber on embryotoxicity induced by experimental diabetes in rats. Biol Neonat 63:353–359

Giavini E, Broccia ML, Prati M et al (1986) Effects of streptozotocin-induced diabetes on fetal development of the rat. Teratology 34:81–88

Giavini E, Broccia ML, Pratti M et al (1991) Diet composition modifies embryotoxic effects induced by experimental diabetes in rats. Biol Neonat 59:278–286

Giavini E, Pratti M (1990) Morphogenesis of diabetes-induced congenital cataract in the rat. Acta Anat 137:132–136

Giavini E, Prati M, Roversi G (1990) Congenital malformations in offspring of diabetic rats: experimental study on the influence of the diet composition and magnesium intake. Biol Neonat 57:207–217

Gilbert JA (1949) The association of maternal obesity, large babies, and diabetes. BMJ 1:702–704

Gilbert JA, Dunlop DM (1949) Diabetic fertility, maternal mortality, and foetal loss rate. BMJ 1:48–51

Gillman J, Gilbert C, Gillman T et al (1948) A preliminary report on hydrocephalus, spina bifida, and other congenital anomalies in the rat produced by trypan blue. S Afr J Med Sci 13: 47–90

Gillmer MD, Oakley NW, Beard RW, Nithyananthan R, Cawston M (1980) Screening for diabetes during pregnancy. Br J Obstet Gynaecol 87(5):377–382

Gillmer MD, Holmes SM, Moore MP et al (1984) Diabetes in pregnancy: obstetric management 1983. In: Sutherland HW et al (eds) Carbohydrate metabolism in pregnancy and the newborn. Churchill, London, pp 102–118

Gittelsohn AM, Milham S (1965) Vital record incidence of congenital malformations in New York State. In: Neel JV et al (eds) Genetics and epidemiology of chronic disease. U.S. Department of Health, Education and Welfare, Washington pp 305–320

Given WP, Douglas RG, Tolstoi E (1951) Pregnancy and diabetes. Med Clin N Am 35:659–665

Given WP, Tolstoi E (1957) Present day management of the pregnant diabetic: success or failure? Surg Clin N Am 37:369–378

Given WP, Douglas RG, Tolstoi E (1950) Pregnancy and diabetes. Am J Obstet Gynecol 59:729–747

Gladman G, McCrindle BW, Boutin C et al (1997) Fetal echocardiographic screening of diabetic pregnancies for congenital heart disease. Am J Perinatol 14:59–62

Glasgow AC, Harley JM, Montgomery DA (1979) Congenital malformations in infants of diabetic mothers. Ulster Med J 48:109–117

Glenister TW (1964) Fantasies, facts and foetuses: the interplay of fancy and reason in teratology. Med Hist 8:18–30

Goldenberg RL, Humphrey JL, Hal CB et al (1983) Lethal congenital anomalies as a cause of birthweight-specific neonatal mortality. JAMA 250:513–515

Golde SH, Montoro M, Good-Anderson B, Broussard P, Jacobs N, Loesser C, Trujillo M, Walla C, Phelan J, Platt LD (1984) The role of nonstress tests, fetal biophysical profile, and contraction stress tests in the outpatient management of insulin-requiring diabetic pregnancies. Am J Obstet Gynecol 148(3):269–273

Golding J (1987) Epidemiology of fetal and neonatal death. In: Keeling JW (ed) Fetal and neonatal pathology. Springer, London, pp 151–165

Golding J (1991) The epidemiology of perinatal death. In: Kiely M (ed) Reproductive and perinatal epidemiology. CRC, Boca Raton, pp 401–436

Goldman JA (1976) Glucose tolerance in mothers of offspring with congenital malformations. Isr J Med Sci 10:1434–1437

Goldman JA, Dicker D, Feldberg D et al (1986) Pregnancy outcome in patients with insulin-dependent diabetes mellitus with preconceptional control: a comparative study. Am J Obstet Gynecol 155:293–297

Goldstein AI, Cronk DA, Garite T et al (1978) Perinatal outcome in the diabetic pregnancy: a retrospecive analysis. J Reprod Med 20:61–66

Goldstein E, Porter B, Galil A (1991) Neurodevelopmental outcome of offspring of the diabetic mother: need for further research. Am J Dis Child 145:602–603

Goldstein L, Murphy D (1929) Microcephalic idiocy following radium therapy for uterine cancer during pregnancy. Am J Obstet Gynecol 18:189–195

Golob EK, Rishi S, Becker KL et al (1970) Streptozotocin diabetes in pregnant and nonpregnant rats. Metabolism 19:1014–1019

Gomez KJ, Dowdy K, Allen G et al (1988) Evaluation of ultrasound diagnosis of fetal anomalies in women with pregestational diabetes: University of Florida experience. Am J Obstet Gynecol 159:584–586

Goodman MJ (1976) Maternal diabetes and congenital malformations among live births in Hawaii. Acta Diab Lat 13:99–106

Goto MP, Goldman AS (1994) Diabetic embryopathy. Curr Opin Pediat 6:486–491

Goudé H, Cozic A, Franck JB et al (1975) La grossesse chez la femme diabétique: à propos de neuf grossesses: conduite à tenir. J Gynecol Obstet Biol Reprod 4:541–550

Graefe (1898) Über die Einwirkung des Diabetes mellitus auf die weiblichen Sexualorgane und ihre Functionen. Munch Med Wochensch 14:127–128

Graham BD, Lowrey GH (1953) Chemical findings in infants born of diabetic mothers: a preliminary report. Univ Mich Med Bull 19:267–272

Graham G (1924) Pregnancy complicating diabetes treated with insulin. Lancet 206:953

Graham TP Jr, Gutgesell HP (1995) Ventricular septal defects. In: Emmanouilides GC et al (eds) Moss and Adams heart disease in children and adolescents including the fetus and young adult, 5th edn. Williams and Wilkins, Baltimore, pp 724–746

Granat M, Sharf M, Cooper A (1979) Glucose intolerance during pregnancy. Obstet Gynecol 53:157–161

Granroth G (1978) Defects of the central nervous system in Finland. III. Diseases and drugs in pregnancy. Early Hum Dev 2:147–162

Granroth G, Hakama M, Saxén L (1977) Defects of the central nervous system in Finland. I. Variations in time and space, sex distribution, and parental age. Br J Prev Soc Med 31:164–170

Graves WK, Neff R, Mark P (1967) Altered glucose metabolism in pregnancy: its determination and fetal outcome. Am J Obstet Gynecol 98:602–608

Graviss ER, Monteleone PA, Wampler LR et al (1980) Proximal femoral focal deficiency associated with the Robin anomalad. J Med Genet 17:390–392

Gray SH, Feemster LC (1926) Compensatory hypertrophy and hyperplasia of the islands of Langerhans in the pancreas of a child born of a diabetic mother. Arch Path Lab Med 1:348–355

Greb AE, Pauli RM, Kirby RS (1987) Accuracy of fetal death reports: comparison with data from an independent stillbirth assessment program. Am J Public Health 77:1202–1206

Greco P, Loverro G, Selvaggi L (1994) Does gestational diabetes represent an obstetrical risk? Gyn Obst Invest 37:242–245

Greene MF (1989) Congenital malformations. In: Hare JW (ed) Diabetes complicating pregnancy: the Joslin Clinic method. Liss, New York, pp 147–161

Greene MF, Allred EN, Leviton A (1995) Maternal metabolic control and risk of microcephaly among infants of diabetic mothers. Diabetes Care 18:166–169

Greene MF, Benacerraf BR (1991) Prenatal diagnosis in diabetic gravidas: utility of ultrasound and maternal serum alpha-fetoprotein screening. Obstet Gynecol 77:520–524

Greene MF, Hare JW, Cloherty JP et al (1989) First-trimester hemoglobin A_1 and risk for major malformation and spontaneous abortion in diabetic pregnancy. Teratology 39:225–231

Gregg MB (1979) Temporal trends in the incidence of birth defects–United States. MMWP 28:401–403

Gregg NM (1941) Congenital cataract following German measles in the mother. Trans Ophth Soc Aust 3:35–46

Gregory R, Scott AR, Mohajer M et al (1992) Diabetic pregnancy 1977–1990: have we reached a plateau? J Roy Coll Phys 26:162–166

Grenet P, Paillerets FD, Badoual J et al (1972) Le nouveau-né de mère diabétique. Arch Fr Pediatr 29:925–933

Grill V, Johansson B, Jalkanen P (1991) Influence of severe diabetes-mellitus early in pregnancy in the rat: effects of insulin sensitivity and insulin secretion in the offspring. Diabetologia 34:373–378

Grimaldi RD (1968) Significance and management of abnormal oral glucose tolerance tests during pregnancy. Obstet Gynecol 32:713–720

Gruenwald P (1947) Mechanisms of abnormal development. I. Causes of abnormal development in the embryo. II. Embryonic development of malformations. Arch Path 44:398–436, 495–559

Gruenwald P (1966) Growth of the human fetus. II. Abnormal growth in twins and infants of mothers with diabetes, hypertension or isoimmunization. Am J Obstet Gynecol 94:1120–1132

Grüneberg H (1963) The pathology of animals: a study of inherited skeletal disorders in animals. Wiley, New York

Gugliucci CL, O'Sullivan MJ, Opperman W et al (1976) Intensive care of the pregnant diabetic. Am J Obstet Gynecol 125:435–441

Gunton JE, McElduff A, Sulway M et al (2000) Outcome of pregnancies complicated by pregestational diabetes mellitus. Aust N Z Obstet Gynaecol 40:38–43

Gürakan B, Karaaslan E, Balci S (1996) Sirenomelia in an infant of a diabetic mother. Turk J Pediatr 38:393–397

Hadden DR (1975) Glucose tolerance tests in pregnancy. In: Sutherland HW, Stowers JM (eds) Carbohydrate metabolism in pregnancy and the newborn. Livingstone, Edinburgh, pp 19–41

Hadden DR (1979) Asymptomatic diabetes in pregnancy. In: Sutherland HW, Stowers JM (eds) Carbohydrate metabolism in pregnancy and the newborn 1978. Springer, Berlin, pp 407–424

Hadden DR (1980) Screening for abnormalities of carbohydrate metabolism in pregnancy 1966–1977: the Belfast experience. Diabetes Care 3(3):440–446
Hadden DR (1985) Geographic, ethnic, and racial variations in the incidence of gestational diabetes mellitus. Diabetes 34(2):8–12
Hadden DR (1986) Diabetes in pregnancy 1985. Diabetologia 29:1–9
Hadden DR (1989) The development of diabetes and its relation to pregnancy: the long-term and short-term historical viewpoint. In: Sutherland HW et al (eds) Carbohydrate metabolism in pregnancy and the newborn. V. Springer, New York, pp 1–8
Hadden DR, Alexander A, McCance DR et al (2001) Obstetric and diabetic care for pregnancy in diabetic women: 10 years outcome analysis, 1985–1995. Diabet Med 18:546–553
Hadden DR, Byrne E, Trotter I et al (1984) Physical and psychological health of children of Type 1 (insulin-dependent) diabetic mothers. Diabetologia 26:250–254
Hadden DR, Harley JM (1967) Potential diabetes and the foetus: a prospective study of the relation between maternal oral glucose tolerance and the foetal result. J Obstet Gynecol Br Comm 74:669–674
Hadden DR, Hillebrand B (1989) The first recorded case of diabetic pregnancy (Bennewitz HG, 1824, Univ of Berlin). Diabetologia 32:625
Hadden DR, Traub, AI, Harley JM (1988) Diabetes-related perinatal death and congenital fetal abnormality: a problem of audit. Diabet Med 5:321–323
Hagay ZJ, Weiss Y, Zusman I et al (1995) Prevention of diabetes-associated embryopathy by overexpression of the free radical scavenger copper zinc superoxide dismutase in transgenic mouse embryos. Am J Obstet Gynecol 173:1036–1041
Hagbard L (1956) Pregnancy and diabetes mellitus: a clinical study. Acta Obstet Gynecol Scand 35(1):1–180
Hagbard L (1958) The "pre-diabetic" period from an obstetric point of view. Acta Obstet Gynecol Scand 37:497–518
Hagbard L (1961) Pregnancy and diabetes mellitus. Thomas, Springfield, Ill
Hagbard L, Olow I, Reinand T (1959) A follow-up study of 514 children of diabetic mothers. Acta Paediatr 48:184–197
Hagbard L, Svanborg A (1960) Prognosis of diabetes mellitus with onset during pregnancy. A clinical study of seventy-one cases. Diabetes 9:296–302
Hakosalo JK (1973) Cumulative detection rates of congenital malformations in a ten-year follow-up study. Acta Path Microbiol Scand Sec A Suppl 242:7–58
Hall RE, Tillman AJ (1951) Diabetes in pregnancy. Am J Obstet Gynecol 61:1107–1115
Hamanishi C (1980) Congenital short femur: clinical, genetic and epidemiological comparison of the naturally occurring condition with that caused by thalidomide. J Bone Jt Surg 62B:307–320
Hamburger V (1988) The heritage of experimental embryology: Hans Spemann and the organizer. Oxford Univ, New York
Hamman L, Hirschman II (1917) Studies on blood sugar. Arch Int Med 20:761–808
Hanson U, Persson B (1993) Outcome of pregnancies complicated by type 1 insulin-dependent diabetes in Sweden: acute pregnancy complications, neonatal mortality and morbidity. Am J Perinat 10:330–333
Hanson U, Persson B, Enochsson E et al (1984) Self-monitoring of blood glucose by diabetic women during the third trimester of pregnancy. Am J Obstet Gynecol 150:817–821
Hanson U, Persson B, Thunell S (1990) Relationship between haemoglobin A_{1c} in early type 1 (insulin-dependent) diabetic pregnancy and the occurrence of spontaneous abortion and fetal malformation in Sweden. Diabetologia 33:100–104
Hansen JP (1986) Older maternal age and pregnancy outcome: a review of the literature. Obstet Gynecol Surv 41(11):726–742 (Review)
Hardy JB, Drage JS, Jackson EC (1979) The first year of life. Johns Hopkins Univ, Baltimore
Hare JW (1989) Medical management. In: Hare JW (ed) Diabetes complicating pregnancy: the Joslin Clinic method. Liss, New York, pp 3–51
Hare JW (1991) Insulin management of type I and type II diabetes in pregnancy. Clin Obstet Gynecol 34:494–506

Hare JW (1994) Diabetic complications of diabetic pregnancies. Semin Perinatol 18(5):451–458
Hare JW, White P (1980) Gestational diabetes and the White classification. Diabetes Care 3:394
Harjutsalo V, Sjöberg L, Tuomilehto J (2008) Time trends in the incidence of type 1 diabetes in Finnish childen: a cohort study. Lancet 371:1777–1782
Harlap S, Shiono PH, Ramcharan S (1980) A life table of spontaneous abortions and the effects of age, parity, and other variables. In: Porter IH, Hook EB (eds) Human embryonic and fetal death. Academic, New York, pp 145–158
Harlass FE, Brady K, Read JA (1991) Reproducibility of the oral glucose tolerance test in pregnancy. Am J Obstet Gynecol 164:564–568
Harley JM, Montgomery DA (1965) Management of pregnancy complicated by diabetes. BMJ 1:14–18
Harris EL (1990) Genetic epidemiology of hypospadias. Epidemiol Rev 12:29–40
Harris, JS, Woomer DF, Bruggers L (1963) Diabetes in pregnancy: experience in three general hospitals in Saginaw. J Mich Med Soc 62:769–774
Harris MI (1988) Gestational diabetes may represent discovery of preexisting glucose intolerance. Diabetes Care 11:403–411
Harris MI, Hadden, WC, Knowler WC et al (1987) Prevalence of diabetes and impaired glucose tolerance and plasma glucose levels in U.S. population aged 20–74 years. Diabetes 36:523–534
Hass J (1951) Congenital dislocation of the hip. Thomas, Springfield, Ill
Haust MD (1981) Maternal diabetes mellitus–effects on the fetus and placenta. In: Naeye RL et al (eds) Perinatal diseases. Williams and Wilkins, Baltimore, pp 201–285
Haworth JC, McRae KN, Dilling LA (1976) Prognosis of infants of diabetic mothers to neonatal hypoglycaemia. Dev Med Child Neurol 18:471–479
Hawthorne G, Robson S, Ryall EA et al (1997) Prospective population based survey of outcome of pregnancy in diabetic women: results of the Northern Diabetic Audit, 1994. BMJ 315:279–281
Hegge FN, Franklin RW, Watson PT et al (1990) Fetal malformations commonly detectable on obstetric ultrasound. J Reprod Med 35:391–398
Heinonen OP, Slone D, Shapiro S (1977) Birth defects and drugs in pregnancy. Publishing Sciences Group, Littleton, Mass
Heinze E, Vetter U (1987) Skeletal growth of fetuses from streptozotocin diabetic rat mothers: in vivo and in vitro studies. Diabetologia 30:100–103
Heisig N, Schall J (1971) Untersuchungen über die Gravidität und Nachkommenschaft des spontandiabetischen chinesischen Zwerghamsters. Arch Gynäkol 210:2–28
Heller SR, Lowe JM, Johnson IR et al (1984) Seven years experience of home management in pregnancy in women with insulin-dependent diabetes. Diabet Med 1:199–204
Henley WE (1947) Diabetes and pregnancy. N Z Med J 46:386–391
Henriques CU, Damm P, Tabor A et al (1991) Incidence of fetal chromosome abnormalities in insulin dependent diabetic women. Acta Obstet Gynecol Scand 70:295–297
Henriques CU, Damm P, Tabor A et al (1993) Decreased alpha-fetoprotein in amniotic fluid and maternal serum in diabetic pregnancy. Obstet Gynecol 82:960–964
Herman GH (1902) Diabetes and pregnancy. Edinb Med J 11:119–123
Herre HD, Horky Z (1964) The incidence of abnormalities in children of diabetic mothers. Zentralbl Gynakol 86:758–768 (Article in German)
Herrick WW, Tillman AJ (1938) Diabetes and pregnancy. Surg Gynecol Obstet 66:37–43
Hertz-Picciotto I, Samuels SJ (1988) Incidence of early loss of pregnancy. N Engl J Med 319:1483–1484
Herzstein J, Dolger H (1946) The fetal mortality in women during the prediabetic period. Am J Obstet Gynecol 51:420–422
Hexter AC, Harris JA (1991) Bias in congenital malformations information from the birth certificate. Teratology 44:177–180
Hiekkala H, Koskenoja M (1961) A follow-up study of children of diabetic mothers. I. General findings. Ann Paediat Fenn 7:17–31
Hiéronimus S, Cupelli C, Durand-Réville M et al (2004) Pregnancy and type 2 diabetes: which fetal prognosis? Gynecol Obstet Fertil 32:23–27

Hirst KM, Butler NR, Dawkins MJ (1968) Infant and perinatal death in England and Wales. PHS Publ. No. 1000, Ser. 3, No. 12. U.S. Government Printing Office, Washington

Hitti IF, Glasberg SS, Huggins-Jones D et al (1994) Bilateral femoral hypoplasia and maternal diabetes: case report and review of the literature. Pediatr Path 14:567–574

Hod M, Merlob P, Friedman S et al (1992) Prevalence of minor congenital anomalies in newborns of diabetic mothers. Eur J Obstet Gynecol Reprod Biol 44:111–116

Hod M, Rabinerson D, Kaplan B et al (1996) Perinatal complications following gestational diabetes mellitus: how 'sweet' is ill? Acta Obstet Gynecol Scand 75:809–815

Hod M, Damm P, Kaaja R et al (2008) Fetal and perinatal outcomes in type 1 diabetes pregnancy: a randomized study comparing insulin aspart with human insulin in 322 subjects. Am J Obstet Gynecol 198:186.e1–186.e7

Hoet JJ (1954) Carbohydrate metabolism during pregnancy. Diabetes 3:1–12

Hoet JJ, Geneesk BT (1958) Pregnancy & diabetes.14(1):17–24. (Dutch No abstract available)

Hoet JP, Gommers A, Hoet JJ (1960) Causes of congenital malformations. Wolstenholme GE, O'Connor CM (eds) CIBA Foundation Symposium on congenital malformations. Little Brown, Boston, pp 219–235

Hoffman JI (1968) Natural history of congenital heart disease: problems in its assessment with special reference to ventricular septal defects. Circulation 37:97–105

Hoffman JI (1987) Incidence, mortality and natural history. In: Anderson RH et al (eds) Paediatric cardiology. Churchill Livingstone, Edinburgh, pp 3–14

Hoffman JI (1990) Congenital heart disease: incidence and inheritance. Pediatr Clin N Am 37:25–43

Hoffman JI, Christianson R (1978) Congenital heart disease in a cohort of 19,502 births with long-term follow-up. Am J Cardiol 42:641–647

Holing EV, Brown ZZ, Beyer CS et al (1998) Why don't women with diabetes plan their pregnancies? Diabetes Care 21:889–895

Hollingsworth DR, Moore TR (1987) Postprandial walking exercise in pregnant insulin-dependent (type I) diabetic women: reduction of plasma lipid levels but absence of a significant effect on glycemic control. Am J Obstet Gynecol 157:1359–1363

Hollingsworth DR, Vaucher Y, Yamamoto TR (1991) Diabetes in pregnancy in Mexican Americans. Diabetes Care 14(3):695–705

Holmes LB (1976) Current concepts in genetics: congenital malformations. N Engl J Med 295:204–207

Holmes LB (1992) Fetal environmental toxins. Pediatr Rev 13:364–363

Holmes LB (1994) Spina bifida: anticonvulsants and other maternal influences. In: Bock G, Marsh J (eds) Neural tube defects. Wiley, Chichester, pp 232–239

Holmes LB, Cann, C, Cook C (1985) Examination of infants for both minor and major malformations to evaluate for possible teratogenic exposures. Prog Clin Biol Res 163B:59–63

Holmes LB, Driscoll SG, Atkins L (1976) Etiologic heterogeneity of neural-tube defects. N Engl J Med 294:365–369

Holmes LB, Kleiner, BC, Leppig KA et al (1987) Predictive value of minor anomalies. III. Use in cohort studies to identify teratogens. Teratology 36:291–298

Holthusen W (1972) The Pierre Robin syndrome: unusual associated developmental defects. Ann Radiol 15:253–262

Holu S, Carter B, Watson PD et al (2004) Increasing prevalence of type 2 diabetes in adolescents. J Paediatr Child Health 40:201–204

Hook EB, Porter IH (1980) Terminological conventions, methodological considerations, temporal trends, specific genes, environmental hazards, and some other factors pertaining to embryonic and fetal death. In: Porter IH, Hook EB (eds) Human embryonic and fetal death. Academic, New York, pp 1–18

Horii K, Watanabe G, Ingalls TH (1966) Experimental diabetes in pregnant mice: prevention of congenital malformations in offspring by insulin. Diabetes 15:194–204

Hosemann H (1950) Critical examination of prolonged pregnancies; reply to an article of like title by K. Freudenberg. Arch Gynakol 177(6):751–762 (Undetermined Language)

Höst HF (1925) Carbohydrate tolerance in pregnancy. Lancet 1:1022–1025

Hreidarsson AB, Geirsson RT, Helgason T (1993) Diabetes mellitus in Iceland: prevalence, organization of services, pregnancy outcome and long-term complications. Diabet Nutr Metab 6:333–334

Hsia DY, Gellis SS (1957) Birth weight in infants of diabetic mothers. Ann Hum Genet 22:80–92

Hubbell JP, Drorbaugh JE (1965) Infants of diabetic mothers: neonatal problems and their management. Diabetes 14:157–161

Hubbell JP, Muirhead DH, Drorbaugh JE (1965) The newborn infant of the diabetic mother. Med Clin N Am 49:1035–1052

Huber J, Reinold E (1985) Die perinatal verstorbenen Kinder in der I. Universitäts-Frauenklinik Wien zwischen 1981 und 1983. Wien Med Wochensch 135:197–200

Hultquist GT (1950) Diabetes and pregnancy: an animal study. Acta Path Microbiol Scand 27:695–719

Hurley LS (1977) Nutritional deficiencies and excesses. In: Wilson JG, Fraser FC (eds) Handbook of teratology, vol 1. Plenum, New York, pp 261–308

Hunter DJ, Burrows RF, Mohide PT, Whyte RK (1993) Influence of maternal insulin-dependent diabetes mellitus on neonatal morbidity. CMAJ 149(1):47–52

Hurst D, Johnson DF (1980) Brief clinical report: femoral hypoplasia-unusual facies syndrome. Am J Med Genet 5:255–258

Hurwitz D, Higano N (1952) Diabetes and pregnancy. N Engl J Med 247:305–309

Hurwitz D, Irving FC (1937) Diabetes and pregnancy. Am J Med Sci 194:85–92

Hurwitz D, Jensen D (1946) Carbohydrate metabolism in normal pregnancy. N Engl J Med 234:327–329

Hyett JA, Moscoso G, Nicolaides KH (1995) First-trimester nuchal translucency and cardiac septal defects in fetuses with trisomy 21. Am J Obstet Gynecol 172:1411–1413

Hyett JA, Perdu M, Sharland G et al (1999) Using fetal nuchal translucency to screen for major congenital cardiac defects at 10–14 weeks of gestation: population based cohort study. BMJ 318:81–85

Imerslund O (1948) Den føtale og neonatale dødelighet og fødselsvekten hos barn født av prediabetiske mødre. Sartryck Nord Med 40:1880–1882

Incerpi MH, Miller DA, Samadi R et al (1998) Stillbirth evaluation: what tests are needed? Am J Obstet Gynecol 178:1121–1125

Irsigler K, Leodolter S, Rosenkranz A et al (1986) Different approaches toward normoglycemia in pregnancy: the Vienna experience. In: Jovanovic L et al (eds) Diabetes and pregnancy: teratology, toxicology and treatment. Praeger, New York, pp 263–290

Ivy RH (1968) Congenital deformities recorded on birth certificates in Pennsylvania, 1961–1965. Plast Reconstr Surg 41(1):50–53

Jackson WP (1952) Studies in pre-diabetes. BMJ 2:690–696

Jackson WP (1959) Prediabetes: a synthesis. Postgrad Med J 35:287–296

Jackson WP (1961) Is pregnancy diabetogenic? Lancet 2:1369–1372

Jacobs HR (1937) Hypoglycemic action of alloxan. Proc Soc Exp Biol Med 37:407–409

Jacobson JD, Cousins L (1989) A population-based study of maternal and perinatal outcome in patients with gestational diabetes. Am J Obstet Gynecol 161:981–986

Jährig D, Stiete S, Jonas C (1993) Offspring of diabetic mothers: problems of morbidity. Diabet Metab 19:207–212

Janerich DT, Polednak AP (1983) Epidemiology of birth defects. Epidemiol Rev 5:16–37

Jankowski MA, Uriu-Hare JY, Rucker RB et al (1993) Effect of maternal diabetes and dietary copper on fetal development in rats. Reprod Toxic 7:589–598

Jansen RP (1982) Spontaneous abortion incidence in the treatment of infertility. Am J Obstet Gynecol 143:451–473

Janssen PA, Rothman I, Schwartz SM (1996) Congenital malformations in newborns of women with established and gestational diabetes in Washington State, 1984–1991. Paediatr Perinat Epidemiol 10:52–63

Janz D (1982) On major malformations and minor anomalies in the offspring of parents with epilepsy. In: Janz D et al (eds) Epilepsy, pregnancy, and the child. Raven, New York, pp 211–222
Jarrett RJ (1981) Reflections on gestational diabetes mellitus. Lancet 2:1220–1222
Jarrett RJ (1993) Gestational diabetes: a non-entity? BMJ 306:37–38
Jarrett RJ (1997) Should we screen for gestational diabetes? BMJ 315:736–739
Jawerbaum A, White V (2010) Animal models in diabetes and pregnancy. Endocr Rev 31:680–701
Jensen DM, Damm P, Moelsted-Pedersen L et al (2004) Outcomes in type 1 diabetic pregnancies: a nationwide, population-based study. Diabetes Care 27:2819–2823
Jensen DM, Korsholm L, Ovesen P et al (2009) Peri-conceptional A_{1C} and risk of serious adverse pregnancy outcome in 933 women with type 1 diabetes. Diabetes Care 32:1046–1048
Jervell J, Bjerkedal T, Moe N (1980) Outcome of pregnancies in diabetic mothers in Norway, 1967–1976. Diabetologia 18:131–134
Jervell J, Moe N, Skjaeraasen J et al (1979) Diabetes mellitus and pregnancy–management and results at Rikshospitalet, Oslo, 1970–1977. Diabetologia 16:151–155
Johnson JM, Lange IR, Harman CR et al (1988) Biophysical profile scoring in the management of the diabetic pregnancy. Obstet Gynecol 72:841–846
Johnson JP, Carey JC, Gooch WM et al (1983) Femoral hypoplasia-unusual facies syndrome in infants of diabetic mothers. J Pediatr 102:866–872
Johnstone FD, Lindsay RS, Steel J (2006) Type 1 diabetes and pregnancy: trends in birth weight over 40 years at a single clinic. Obstet Gynecol 107:1297–1302
Jokipii SG (1955) Diabetes and pregnancy. Ann Med Int Fenn 44:185–205
Jonasson JM, Brismar K, Sparén P et al (2007) Fertility in women with type 1 diabetes: a population-based cohort study in Sweden. Diabetes Care 30:2271–2276
Jones KL (ed) (1988) Smith's recognizable patterns of human malformations. Saunders, Philadelphia
Jones WS (1952) Diabetes in pregnancy: a preliminary report. Rhode Isl Med J 35:662–664, 666, 668
Jones WS (1953) Diabetes in pregnancy. Am J Obstet Gynecol 66:322–334
Jones WS (1956) The severity of diabetes in pregnancy. Am J Obstet Gynecol 71:319–325
Jones WS (1958) Management of the pregnant diabetic. Diabetes 7:439–445
Joslin EP (1915) Pregnancy and diabetes mellitus. Bost Med Surg J 23:841–849
Joslin EP (1923) Pregnancy and diabetes. In: Joslin EP (ed) The treatment of diabetes mellitus. Lea & Febiger, Philadelphia, pp 649–665
Jovanovic L, Druzin M, Peterson CM (1981) Effect of euglycemia on the outcome of pregnancy in insulin-dependent women as compared with normal control subjects. Am J Med 71:921–927
Jovanovic L, Peterson CM (1985) Screening for gestational diabetes: optimum timing and criteria for retesting. Diabetes 34(2):21–23
Joyce J (1986) Ulysses (corrected text). Vintage, New York
Julian-Reynier C, Philip N, Scheiner C et al (1994) Impact of prenatal diagnosis by ultrasound on the prevalence of congenital anomalies at birth in southern France. J Epidemiol Community Health 48:290–296
Junod A, Lambert AE, Orci L et al (1967) Studies of the diabetogenic action of streptozotocin. Proc Soc Exp Biol Med 126:201–205
Kaaja R, Rönnemaa T (2008) Gestational diabetes: pathogenesis and consequences to mother and offspring. Rev Diabetic Stud 5:194–202
Kade H, Dietel H (1952) Die Prognose der Schwangerschaft bei prädiabetischen und diabetischen Frauen. Dtsch Med Wochensch 77:673–675
Kaku K, McGill J, Province M et al (1989) A single major gene controls most of the difference in susceptibility to streptozotocin-induced diabetes between C57BL/6 J and C3H/HeJ mice. Diabetologia 32:716–723
Kalamchi A, Cowell GH, Kim KI (1985) Congenital deficiency of the femur. J Pediat Orthop 5:129–134
Kalitzki M (1965) Congenital malformations and diabetes. Lancet 2:641–642

Kalkhoff RK (1985) Therapeutic results of insulin therapy in gestational diabetes mellitus. Diabetes 34(Suppl 2):97–100 (Review)

Källén B (1985) Analysis of deliveries among diabetic women in Sweden: 1978–1981. Personal communication

Källén B (1987a) Search for teratogenic risks with the aid of malformation registries. Teratology 35:47–52

Källén B (1987b) Caudal aplasia. In: Vinker PJ et al (eds) Handbook of clinical neurology. Malformations, vol 50. Elsevier, Amsterdam, pp 509–518

Källén B (1989a) Population surveillance of congenital malformations: possibilities and limitations. Acta Paediatr Scand 78:657–663

Källén B (1989b) A prospective study of some aetiological factors in limb reduction defects in Sweden. J Epidemiol Comm Health 43:86–96

Källén B, Castilla EE, Lancaster PA et al (1992) The cyclops and the mermaid: an epidemiological study of two types of rare malformation. J Med Genet 29:30–35

Källén B, Hay S, Klingberg M (1984) Birth defects monitoring systems: accomplishments and goals. In: Kalter H (ed) Issues and reviews in teratology, vol 2. Plenum, New York, pp 1–22

Källén B, Winberg J (1968) A Swedish register of congenital malformations: experience with continuous registration during 2 years with special reference to multiple malformations. Pediatrics 41:765–776

Källén B, Winberg J (1974) Caudal mesoderm pattern of anomalies: from renal agenesis to sirenomelia. Teratology 9:99–111

Kalter H (1954) The inheritance of susceptibility to the teratogenic effects of cortisone in mice. Genetics 39:185–196

Kalter H (1968) Teratology of the central nervous system: induced and spontaneous malformations of laboratory, agricultural, and domestic animals. Univ of Chicago, Chicago

Kalter H (1980) The relation between congenital malformations and prenatal mortality in experimental animals. In: Porter IH, Hook EB (eds) Human embryonic and fetal death. Academic, New York, pp 29–44

Kalter H (1987) Diabetes and spontaneous abortion: a historical review. Am J Obstet Gynecol 156:1243–1253

Kalter H (1990) Perinatal death and congenital malformations in infants born to women with insulin-dependent diabetes mellitus–United States, Canada, and Europe, 1940–1988. MMWP 39:363–365

Kalter H (1991) Five-decade international trends in the relation of perinatal death and congenital malformations: stillbirth and neonatal death compared. Int J Epidemiol 20:173–179

Kalter H (1993) Case reports of malformations associated with maternal diabetes: history and critique. Clin Genet 43:174–179

Kalter H (1997) Flawed study alleging prevention of diabetic embryopathy. Am J Obstet Gynecol 177:1273 (letter)

Kalter H (1998) The non-teratogenicity of gestational diabetes. Paediat Perinat Epidemiol 12:456–458

Kalter H (2000) Of diabetic mothers and their babies. Harwood Academic Publishers, Amsterdam

Kalter H (2007) Mortality and maldevelopment. Part 1: congenital cardiovascular malformations. The Netherlands, Springer

Kalter H (2009) Mortality and maldevelopment. Part 2: the saga of neural tube defects. The Netherlands, Springer

Kalter H (2010) Teratology in the twentieth century plus ten. Springer, Amsterdam

Kalter H, Warkany J (1961) Experimental production of congenital malformations in strains of inbred mice by maternal treatment with hypervitaminosis A. Am J Path 38:1–20

Kalter H, Warkany J (1983) Congenital malformations: etiologic factors and their role in prevention. N Engl J Med 308:424–431, 491–497

Kampmeier OF (1927) On sireniform monsters, with a consideration of the causation and the predominance of the male sex among them. Anat Rec 34:365–389

Kaneko S, Kondo T (1995) Antiepileptic drugs and birth defects: incidence, mechanisms and prevention. CNS Drug 3:41–55

Kangas T (1949) Über die perinatale Mortalität bei ausgetragenen Kindern. Acta Obstet Gynecol Scand 29(2):1–128

Kaplan S (1979) A mechanistic approach to teratogenesis: analysis of caudal dysplasia syndrome (sacral agenesis). In: Persaud T (ed) Advances in the study of birth defects, vol 1. MTP Press, Lancaster, PA, pp 177–197

Karlsson K, Kjellmer I (1972) The outcome of diabetic pregnancies in relation to the mother's blood sugar level. Am J Obstet Gynecol 112:213–220

Kawaguchi M, Tanigawa K, Tanaka O et al (1994) Embryonic growth impaired by maternal hypoglycemia during early organogenesis in normal and diabetic rats. Acta Diabet 31:141–146

Keeling, JW (1987) Macerated stillbirth. In: Keeling JW (ed) Fetal and neonatal pathoogy. Springer, London, pp 167–177

Keen H (1991) Gestational diabetes: can epidemiology help? Diabetes 40:3–7

Kenna AP, Smithells RW, Fielding DW (1975) Congenital heart disease in Liverpool: 1960–1969. QJM 44:17–44

Kennedy WP (1967) Epidemiologic aspects of the problem of congenital malformations. Birth Defects 3:1–18

Kerunanayake EH, Hearse DJ, Mellows G (1976) Streptozotocin: its excretion and metabolism in the rat. Diabetologia 12:483–488

Kervran A, Guillaume M, Jost A (1978) The endocrine pancreas of the fetus from diabetic pregnant rat. Diabetologia 15:387–394

Key TC, Giuffrida R, Moore TR (1987) Predictive value of early pregnancy glycohemoglobin in the insulin-treated diabetic patient. Am J Obstet Gynecol 156:1096–1100

Khera KS (1984) Maternal toxicity: a possible etiological factor in embryo-fetal deaths and fetal malformations of rodent-rabbit species. Teratology 31:129–153

Khoury MJ (1989) Epidemiology of birth defects. Epidemiol Rev 11:244–248

Khoury MJ, Becerra, JE, Cordero J et al (1989) Clinical-epidemiological assessment of patterns of birth defects associated with human teratogens: application to diabetic embryopathy. Pediatrics 84:658–665

Kiely JL. (1991) Some conceptual problems in multivariable analyses of perinatal mortality. Paediatr Perinat Epidemiol 5(3):243–257

Kilpatrick ES, Rumley AG, Dominiczak MH et al (1994) Glycated haemoglobin values: problems in assessing blood glucose control in diabetes mellitus. BMJ 309:983–985

Kim C, Newton KM, Knopp RH (2002) Gestational diabetes and the incidence of type 2 diabetes: a systematic review. Diabetes Care 25:1862–1868

Kimmerle R, Heinemann L, Delecki A et al (1992) Severe hypoglycemia incidence and predisposing factors in 85 pregnancies of type I diabetic women. Diabetes Care 15:1034–1037

Kimmerle R, Zass RP, Cupisti S et al (1995) Pregnancies in women with diabetic nephropathy: long-term outcome for mother and child. Diabetologia 38:227–235

Kirk JS, Comstock H, Lee W et al (1997) Sonographic screening to detect fetal cardiac anomalies: a 5-year experience with 111 abnormal cases. Obstet Gynecol 89:227–232

Kirk RL, Serjeantson SW, King H et al (1985) The genetic epidemiology of diabetes mellitus. In: Chakraborty R, Szathmary EJ (eds) Diseases of complex etiology in small populations. Liss, New York, pp 119–146

Kiss AC, Lima PH, Sinzato YK et al (2009) Animal models for clinical and gestational diabetes: maternal and fetal outcomes. Diabetol Metab Syndr 1:21

Kitzmiller JL (1986) Macrosomia in infants of diabetic mothers: characteristics, causes, prevention. In: Jovanovic L et al (eds) Diabetes and pregnancy: teratology, toxicology and treatment. Praeger, New York, pp 85–119

Kitzmiller JL (1993) Sweet success with diabetes: the development of insulin therapy and glycemic control for pregnancy. Diabetes Care 16:107–121

Kitzmiller JL, Aiello LM, Kaldany A et al (1981) Diabetic vascular disease complicating pregnancy. Clin Obstet Gynecol 24:107–123

Kitzmiller JL, Buchanan TA, Kjos S et al (1996) Pre-conception care of diabetes, congenital malformations, and spontaneous abortions. Diabetes Care 19:514–541

Kitzmiller JL, Cloherty JP, Graham CA (1982) Management of diabetes and pregnancy. In: Kozak GP (ed) Clinical diabetes mellitus. Saunders, Philadelphia, pp 203–214

Kitzmiller JL, Cloherty JP, Younger MD et al (1978) Diabetic pregnancy and perinatal morbidity. Am J Obstet Gynecol 131:560–580

Kitzmiller JL, Combs CA (1993) Maternal and perinatal implications of diabetic nephropathy. Clin Perinat 20:561–570

Kitzmiller JL, Gavin LA, Gin GD et al (1991) Preconception care of diabetes: glycemic control prevents congenital anomalies. JAMA 265:731–736

Kitzmiller JL, Hoedt LA, Gunderson EP et al (1988) Macrosomia and birth trauma in infants of diet treated gestational diabetic women. In: Weiss PA, Coustan DR (eds) Gestational diabetes. Springer, New York, pp 160–166

Kitzmiller JL, Wallerstein R, Correa A et al (2010) Preconception care for women with diabetes and prevention of major congenital malformations. Birth Defects Res A 88:791–803

Kjaer K, Hagen C, Sandø SH et al (1992a) Epidemiology of menarche and menstrual disturbances in an unselected group of women with insulin-dependent diabetes mellitus compared to controls. J Clin Endocr Metab 75:524–529

Kjaer K, Hagen C, Sandø SH et al (1992b) Inferility and pregnancy outcome in an unselected group of women with insulin-dependent diabetes mellitus. Am J Obstet Gynecol 166:1412–1418

Klebe JG, Espersen T, Allen J (1986) Diabetes mellitus and pregnancy: a seven-year material of pregnant diabetics, where control during pregnancy was based on a centralized ambulant regime. Acta Obstet Gynecol Scand 65:235–240

Klemetti A (1978) Congenital defects in a cohort followed for seven years. Acta Paediat Scand 67:601–606

Klingberg MA, Papier CM (1979) Teratoepidemiology. J Biosoc Sci 11:233–258

Knight G, Worth RC, Ward JD (1983) Macrosomy despite a well-controlled diabetic pregnancy. Lancet 2:1431

Knowler WC, Bennett PH, Hamman RF et al (1978) Diabetes incidence and prevalence in Pima Indians: a 19-fold greater difference than in Rochester, Minnesota. Am J Epidemiol 108:497–505

Knowler WC, Pettitt DJ, Bennett PH et al (1983) Diabetes mellitus in the Pima Indians: genetic and evolutionary considerations. Am J Phys Anthropol 62:107–114

Knox EG, Armstrong, EH, Lancashire R (1984) The quality of notification of congenital malformations. J Epidemiol Community Health 38:296–305

Koch R, Levy HL, Matalon R et al (1994) The international collaborative study of maternal phenylketonuria: status report 1994. Acta Paediatr Suppl 407:111–119

Koch S, Lösche G, Jager-Röman E et al (1992) Major and minor birth malformations and antiepileptic drugs. Neurology 42:83–88

Koenig RJ, Peterson CM, Jones RL et al (1976a) Correlation of glucose regulation and hemoglobin A_{1c} in diabetes mellitus. N Engl J Med 295:417–420

Koenig RJ, Peterson CM, Kilo C et al (1976b) Hemoglobin A_{1c} as an indicator of the degree of glucose intolerance in diabetes. Diabetes 25:230–232

Koller O (1953) Diabetes and pregnancy. Acta Obstet Gynecol Scand 32:80–103

Koman LA, Meyer LC, Warren FH (1982) Proximal femoral focal deficiency: a 50-year experience. Dev Med Child Neurol 24:344–355

Komrower GM, Langley FA (1961) The fate of the diabetic woman's child. Manchester Med Gaz 40:166–171

Koskenoja M (1961) Alloxan diabetes in the pregnant mouse. Acta Ophth Suppl 68:1–92

Kotzot D, Weigi J, Huk W et al (1993) Hydantoin syndrome with holoprosencephaly: a possible rare teratogenic effect. Teratology 48:15–19

Kousseff BG, Diamond T (1991) Class A diabetes mellitus as a human teratogen. Teratology 43:424

Krall LP (1965) When is diabetes? Med Clin North Am 49:893–904

Kramer W (1936) Diabetes and pregnancy: a survey of 665 cases. Penn Med 39:702–707

Kreipe U (1967) Missbildungen innerer Organe bei Thalidomidembryopathie. Ein Beitrag zur Bestimmung der sensiblen Phase bei Thalidomideinnahme in der Frühschwangerschaft. Arch Kinderheilk 176:33–61

Kreshover SJ, Clough OW, Bear DM (1953) Prenatal influences on tooth development. I. Alloxan diabetes in rats. J Dent Res 32:246–261

Kriss JP, Futcher PH (1948) The relation between infant birthweight and subsequent development of maternal diabetes mellitus. J Clin Endocr 8:380–389

Kubryk N, Schmatko M, Borde M et al (1981) Le syndrome de régression caudale: à propos d'une observation. Ann Pediat 28:597–600

Kučera J (1971a) Rate and type of congenital anomalies among offspring of diabetic women. J Reprod Med 7:61–70

Kučera J (1971b) Movement of the frequencies of congenital malformations in time and space. Soc Biol 18:422–430

Kučera J, Lenz W (1967) Caudale Regression mit Oesophagusatresie und Nierenagenesie–ein Syndrom. Z Kinderheilk 98:326–329

Kučera J, Lenz W, Maier W (1965) Missbildungen der Beine und der kaudalen Wirbelsäule bei Kindern diabetischer Mutter. Dtsch Med Wochensch 90:901–905

Kühl C, Møller-Jensen B (1989) Intensified insulin treatment in diabetic pregnancy. In: Sutherland HW et al (eds) Carbohydrate metabolism in pregnancy and the newborn. IV. Springer, London, pp 161–171

Kühne H, Steinbach C, Gstöttner H (1984) Das neonatale Risiko bei frühmanifestiertem mütterlichem Diabetes. Zentralbl Gynakol Gyn 106:500–505

Kyle GC (1963) Diabetes and pregnancy. Ann Int Med 59:1–82

Labarrere CA, Faulk WP (1991) Diabetic placentae: studies of the battlefield after the war. Diabetes Metab Rev 7(4):253–263

Labate JS (1947) A study of the causes of fetal and neonatal mortality on the obstetric service of Bellevue Hospital. Am J Obstet Gynecol 54:188–200

Lage JM, Driscoll SG, Bieber FR (1987) Transposition of the external genitalia associated with caudal regression. J Urol 138:387–389

Lambie CG (1926) Diabetes and pregnancy. J Obstet Gynecol 33:563–606

Lammer EJ, Opitz JM (1986) The DiGeorge anomaly as a developmental field defect. Am J Med Genet Suppl 2:113–127

Lancaster P, Hurst T (2001) Trends in neural tube defects in Australia. Australian Food and Nutrition Monitoring and Surveillance Project

Landon MB, Gabbe SG (1985) Antepartum fetal surveillance in gestational diabetes mellitus. Diabetes 34(2):50–54

Landon MB, Gabbe SG (1995) Diabetes mellitus. In: Barron WM, Lindheimer MD, Davison JM (eds) Medical disorders during pregnancy, 2nd edn. Mosby, St. Louis, pp 63–88

Landon MB, Gabbe SG, Piana R et al (1987) Neonatal morbidity in pregnancy complicated by diabetes mellitus: predictive value of maternal glycemic profiles. Am J Obstet Gynecol 156:1089–1095

Landon MB, Mintz MC, Gabbe SG (1989) Sonographic evaluation of fetal abdominal growth: predictor of the large-for-gestational-age infant in pregnancies complicated by diabetes mellitus. Am J Obstet Gynecol 160:115–121

Lang U, Künzel W (1989) Diabetes mellitus in pregnancy. Management and outcome of diabetic pregnancies in the state of Hesse, F.R.G.; a five-year-survey. Eur J Obstet Gynecol Reprod Biol 33(2):115–129

Langer O (2010) Changing the diagnosis criteria of type 2 diabetes in pregnancy: do the ends justify the means? J Mat Fet Neonat Med 23:234–238

Langer O, Mazze R (1988) The relationship between large-for-gestational-age infants and glycemic control in women with gestational diabetes. Am J Obstet Gynecol 159:1478–1483

Langer O, Rodriguez DA, Xenakis EM et al (1994) Intensified versus conventional management of gestational diabetes. Am J Obstet Gynecol 170:1036–1047

Larsson G, Spjuth J, Ranstam J et al (1986) Prognostic significance of birth of large infant for subsequent development of maternal non-insulin-dependent diabetes mellitus: a prospective study over 20–27 years. Diabetes Care 9:359–364

Laurence KM, Carter CO, David PA (1967) Major central nervous system malformations in South Wales. I. Incidence, local variations and geographical factors. Br J Prev Soc Med 21:146–160

Laursen HB (1980) Some epidemiological aspects of congenital heart disease in Denmark. Acta Paediat Scand 69:619–624

Lavietes PH, Leary DC, Winkler AW et al (1943) Diabetes mellitus and pregnancy. Yale J Biol Med 16:151–166

Lavin JP, Lovelace DR, Miodovnik M et al (1983) Clinical experience with one hundred seven diabetic pregnancies. Am J Obstet Gynecol 147:742–751

Law SW, Gibbons, W, Poindexter AN (1980) Patient cooperation: a determinant of perinatal outcome in the pregnant diabetic. J Reprod Med 24:197–201

Lawrence AM, Contopoulos AN (1960) Reproductive performance in the alloxan diabetic rat. Acta Endocr 33:175–184

Lawrence RD, Oakley W (1942) Pregnancy and diabetes. QJM 11:45–75

Layde PM, Dooley K, Erickson JD et al (1980) Is there an epidemic of ventricular septal defects in the U.S.A.? Lancet 1:407–408

Lazarow A, Heggestad CB (1970) Offspring of animals with experimental diabetes. In: Camerini-Davalos RA, Cole HS (eds) Early diabetes. Academic, New York, pp 229–237

Leck I (1972) The etiology of human malformations: insights from epidemiology. Teratology 5(3):303–3614

Leck I (1984) Fetal malformations. In: Barron SL, Thomson AM (eds) Obstetrical epidemiology. Academic, London, pp 263–317

Leck I (1993) The contribution of epidemiologic studies to understanding human malformations. In: Stevenson RE, Hall JG, Goodan RM (eds) Human malformations and related anomalies. Oxford Univ, New York, pp 65–93

Leck I, Record RG, McKeown T et al (1968) The incidence of malformations in Birmingham, England, 1950–1959. Teratology 1:263–280

Lecorché E (1885) Du diabète: dans ses rapports avec la vie utérine la menstruation et la grossesse. Ann Gynecol 24:257–273

Leikin E, Jenkins JH, Graves WL (1987) Prophylactic insulin in gestational diabetes. Obstet Gynecol 70:587–592

Leinonen PJ, Hiilesmaa VK, Kaaja RJ et al (2001) Maternal mortality in type 1 diabetes. Diabetes Care 24:1501–1502

Leiter EH, Prochazka M, Coleman DL (1987) Animal model of human disease: the non-obese diabetic (NOD) mouse. Am J Path 128:380–383

Leiva A (1996) Frontiers of clinical research in type 1 diabetes. Horm Res 45 (Suppl) 1:32–5

Lejeune J, Turpin R, Goutier M (1959) Le mongolisme: premier example d'aberration autosomique humaine. Ann Génét 1:s41–s49

Lemire RJ, Beckwith JB, Warkany J (1978) Anencephaly. Raven, New York

Lemons JA, Vargas P, Delaney JJ (1981) Infants of the diabetic mother: a review of 225 cases. Obstet Gynecol 57:187–192

Leng-Lévy J, Aubertin J, Le Gall F et al (1972) Pronostic de la grossesse chez les diabétiques en fonction de la correction du diabète pendant la gestation. Bord Med 5:887–896

Lenz W (1961) Discussionsbemerkung zu dem Vortrag von R.A. Pfeiffer und K. Kosenow: Zur Frage der exogenen Entstehung schwerer Extremitätenmissbildungen. In: Tagung der Rheinisch-Westfälischen Kinderärztevereinigung in Düsseldorf 19.11

Lenz W, Knapp K (1962) Thalidomide embryopathy. Arch Environ Health 5:100–105

Lenz W, Kučera J (1967) L'étiologie de la régression caudale (agénésie du sacrum). Med Hyg 25:241–243

Lenz W, Maier W (1964) Congenital malformations and maternal diabetes. Lancet 2:1124–1125

Lenz W, Passarge E (1965) Syndrome of caudal regression in infants of diabetic mothers. Abstracts of the 5th Annual Meeting of the Teratology Society, San Francisco, May 26–28, p 16

Leonhardt T, Samuelson G, Spetz S (1978) Erfarenheter av skötsel av gravida diabetiker vid ett länssjukhus. Lakartidningen 75:2709–2711

Lepercq J, Jacqueminet S, Hiéronimus S et al (2010) Use of insulin glargine throughout pregnancy in 102 women with type 1 diabetes. Diabetes Med 36:209–212

Leppig KA, Werler MM, Cann CI et al (1987) Predictive value of minor anomalies. 1. Association with major malformations. J Pediat 110:531–537

Leridon H (1976) Facts and artifacts in the study of intrauterine mortality: a reconsideration from pregnancy histories. Popul Stud 30:319–336

Leridon H (1977) Human fertility: the basic components. Univ of Chicago, Chicago

Leroy JL, May JP, Codaccioni X et al (1974) La surveillance de la diabétique enceinte: une expériebce de 12 années: 1962–1973 (201 observations). J Gynecol Obstet Biol Reprod 3:813–820

Leslie RDG, Pyke DA, John PN, White JM (1978) Haemoglobin A_1 in diabetic pregnancy. Lancet 2:958–959

Leveno KL, Jauth JC, Gilstrap LC et al (1979) Appraisal of "rigid" blood glucose during pregnancy of the overtly diabetic woman. Am J Obstet Gynecol 135:853–859

Levy-Marchal C, Czernichow P (eds) (1992) Epidemiology and etiology of insulin-dependent diabetes in the young. Karger, Basel

Limb CJ, Holmes LB (1994) Anencephaly: changes in prenatal detection and birth status, 1972–1990. Am J Obstet Gynecol 170:1333–1338

Lin Y, Lee M, Leichter J (1995) Interactive effects of alcohol and diabetes during pregnancy on the rat fetus. Teratogen Carcinogen Mutagen 15:147–153

Lind T (1984) Reflections on the 1983 workshop on gestational diabetes. In: Sutherland HW, Stowers JM (eds) Carbohydrate metabolism in pregnancy and the newborn. Livingstone, Edinburgh, pp 220–225

Lind T, Phillips PR, The Diabetic Pregnancy Study Group of the European Association for the Study of diabetes. (1991) Influence of pregnancy on the 75-g OTGT: a prospective multicenter study. Diabetes 40:8–13

Linn T, Lowek E, Schneider K et al (1993) Spontaneous glucose intolerance in the progeny of low dose streptozotocin-induced diabetic mice. Diabetologia 36:1245–1251

Lisowski LA, Verheijen PM, Copel JA et al (2010) Congenital heart disease in pregnancies complicated by maternal diabetes mellitus: an international clinical collaboration, literature review, and meta-analysis. Herz 35:19–26

Little DJ, Stubbs SM, Brudenell M et al (1979) Early growth retardation in diabetic pregnancy. BMJ 1:488

Little J, Carr-Hill RA (1984) Problems of ascertainment of congenital anomalies. Acta Genet Med Gemell 33:97–105

Little J, Elwood JM (1991) Epidemiology of neural tube defects. In: Kiely M (ed) Reproductive and perinatal epidemiology. CRC, Boca Raton, Fla, pp 251–336

Little RR, McKenzie EM, Shyken JM et al (1990) Lack of relationship between glucose tolerance and complications of pregnancy in nondiabetic women. Diabetes Care 13:483–487

Livshits A, Seidman DS (2009) Fertility issues in women with diabetes. Womens Health (Lond Engl) 5:701–707

Lizan G, Lucas P, Muller G (1985) Diabète et grossesse: notre expérience de la pompe à insuline. Rev Fr Gynecol Obstet 80:451–457

Lloyd DJ, Duffty P (1984) Management of the infant of the diabetic mother: recent experience. In: Sutherland HW, Stowers JM (eds) Carbohydrate metabolism in pregnancy and the newborn. Churchill, Edinburgh, pp 144–149

Loh KJ (1988) Diabetes und Schwangerschaft: gynäkologische Aspekte. Arch Gynecol Obstet 245:266–272

Long WN, Hartmann WL, Futcher PH et al (1954) Diabetes mellitus and pregnancy. Obstet Gynecol 3:160–168

López-Quijada C, Carrion LC (1974) Maternal disorders of carbohydrate metabolism in cases of cardiac embryopathy. Acta Diabet Lat 11:140–148

Lord J, Beighton P (1981) The femoral hypoplasia-unusual facies syndrome: a genetic entity? Clin Genet 20:267–275

Lowy C, Beard RW, Goldschmidt J (1986a) Congenital malformations in babies of diabetic mothers. Diabetes Med 3:458–462

Lowy C, Beard RW, Goldschmidt J (1986b) The UK diabetic pregnancy survey. Acta Endocr Suppl 277:86–89

Lubetzki J, Duprey J, Sambourg C (1973) Influence of mother's age, parity, obesity, and diabetes upon birth weight. Diabetologia 9:79

Lübken W (1970) Schwangerschaft und Diabetes mellitus. Munch Med Wochensch 112:684–689

Lucas MJ, Leveno, KJ, Williams ML et al (1989) Early pregnancy glycosylated hemoglobin, severity of diabetes, and fetal malformations. Am J Obstet Gynecol 161:426–431

Lufkin EG, Nelson RL, Hill LM et al (1984) An analysis of diabetic pregnancies at Mayo Clinic, 1950–1979. Diabetes Care 7:539–547

Lukens FD (1948) Alloxan diabetes. Physiol Rev 28:304–330

Lund CJ, Weese WH (1953) Glucose tolerance and excessively large babies in nondiabetic mothers. Am J Obstet Gynecol 65(4):815–832

Lundbaek K (1962) Intravenous glucose tolerance as a tool in definition and diagnosis of diabetes mellitus. BMJ 1:1507–1513

Lurie S, Matzkel A, Weissman A, Gotlibe Z, Friedman A (1992) Outcome of pregnancy in class A1 and A2 gestational diabetic patients delivered beyond 40 weeks' gestation. Am J Perinatol 9(5–6):484–488

Macafee CA, Beischer NA (1974) The relative value of the standard indications for performing a glucose tolerance test in pregnancy. Med J Aust 1:911–914

MacDorman MF, Kirmeyer S (2009) Fetal and perinatal death, United States. Nat Vit Stat Rep 57(8). Hyattsville, MD, National Center for Health Statistics

Macintosh MC, Fleming KM, Bailey JA et al (2006) Perinatal mortalityea and congenital anomalies in babies of women with type 1 or type 2 diabetes in England, Wales, and Northbern Ireland: population based study. BMJ 333:177 Epub 2006 Jun 16

Mackeprang M, Hay S, Lunde S (1972) Completeness and accuracy of reporting of malformations on birth certificates. HSMHA Health Rep 87:43–49

Magnus R, Rogers JG, Haan EA (1983) Does sacral agenesis predispose to spina bifida? J Med Genet 20:313

Maher JE, Colvin, EV, Samdarshi TE et al (1994) Fetal echocardiography in gravidas with historic risk factors for congenital heart diaeasse. Am J Perinat 11:334–336

Maisels DO, Stilwell JH (1980) The Pierre Robin syndrome associated with femoral dysgenesis. Br J Plast Surg 33:237–241

Majewski A (1953) Beobachtungen an Neugeborenen diabetischer Mütter. Geburts Frauenheilk 13:25–34

Majewski F, Nothjunge J, Bierich JR (1979) Alcohol embryopathy and diabetic fetopathy in the same newborn. Helv Paediat Acta 34:135–140

Makhoul IR, Aviram-Goldring A, Paperna T et al (2001) Caudal dysplasia sequence with penile enlargement: case report and a potential pathogenic hypothesis. Am J Med Genet 99:54–58

Makino S, Kunimoto K, Muraoka Y et al (1980) Breeding of a non-obese, diabetic strain of mice. Exp Anim 29:1–13

Malins JM (1968) Clinical diabetes mellitus. Eyre & Spottiswoode, London

Malins JM (1978) Congenital malformations and fetal mortality in diabetic pregnancy. J Roy Soc Med 71:205–207

Malins JM (1979) Fetal anomalies related to carbohydrate metabolism: the epidemiological approach. In: Sutherland HW, Stowers JM (eds) Carbohydrate metabolism in pregnancy and the newborn. Springer, Berlin, pp 229–246

Malins JM, FitzGerald MG (1965) Childbearing prior to recognition of diabetes: recollected birth weights and stillbirth rate in babies born to parents who developed diabetes. Diabetes 14:175–178

Mall FR (1908) A study of the causes underlying the origin of human monsters. Wistar, Philadelphia

Malpas P (1937) The incidence of human malformations and the significance of changes in the environment in their causation. J Obstet Gynecol Br Emp 44:434–454

Manning FA, Morrison I, Lange IR et al (1985) Fetal assessment based on fetal biophysical profile scoring:experince in 12,620 referred high-risk pregnancies. I. Perinatal death by frequency and etiology. Am J Obstet Gynecol 151:343–350

Manzke H, Cromme E, Gutezeit G (1977) Entwicklung von Kindern diabetischer Mütter. Med Welt 28:1409–1414

Marble, A (1985) Insulin in the treatment of diabetes. In: Marble A, Krall LP, Bradley RF et al (eds) Joslin's diabetes mellitus. Lea & Febiger, Philadelphia, pp 380–405

Marden PM, Smith DW, McDonald J (1964) Congenital anomalies in the newborn infant, including minor variations. J Pediatr 64:357–371

Maresh M, Beard RW, Bray CS et al (1989) Factors predisposing to and outcome of gestational diabetes. Obstet Gynecol 74:324–326

Mariani AJ, Stern J, Khan AU et al (1979) Sacral agenesis: an analysis of 11 cases and review of the literature. J Urol 122:684–686

Marks HH, Krall LP, White P (1971) Epidemiology and detection of diabetes. In: Marble A et al (eds) Joslin's diabetes mellitus. Lea & Febiger, Philadelphia, pp 10–34

Marliss EB, Nakhooda AF, Poussier P et al (1982) The diabetic syndrome of the "BB" Wistar rat: possible relevance to type 1 (insulin-dependent) diabetes in man. Diabetologia 22: 225–232

Marquardsen G (1952) Fertilitäts- und Graviditätskatamnese von 100 Diabetikerinnen. Arzt Wochensch 7:700–704

Marquette GP, Klein VR, Niebyl JR (1985) Efficacy of screening for gestational diabetes. Am J Perinatol 2:7–9

Martin E (1880) Histoire des monstres depuis l'antiquité jusqu'a nos jours. Reinwald, Paris

Martin GR, Perry LW, Ferencz C (1989) Increased prevalence of ventricular septal defects: epidemic or improved diagnosis. Pediatrics 83:200–203

Martin AA, Barrio AM, Guerrero GC (1990) Sirenomelia: presentacion de tres casos. An Esp Pediatr 33:87–89

Martin RA, Fineman RM, Jorde LB (1983) Phenotypic heterogeneity in neural tube defects: a clue to causal heterogeneity. Am J Med Genet 16:519–526

Martin TR, Allen AC, Stinson D (1979) Overt diabetes in pregnancy. Am J Obstet Gynecol 133:275–280

Martinez C, Grande F, Bittner JJ (1954) Alloxan diabetes in different strain of mice. Proc Soc Exp Biol Med 87:236–237

Martínez-Frías ML (1994) Epidemiological analysis of outcomes of pregnancy in diabetic mothers: identification of the most characteristic and most frequent congenital anomalies. Am J Med Genet 51:108–113

Martínez-Frías ML, Bermejo E, Cereijo A (1992) Preaxial polydactyly of feet in infants of diabetic mothers: epidemiological test of a clinical hypothesis. Am J Med Genet 42:643–646

Martínez-Frías ML, Bermejo E, García A et al (1994) Holoprosencephaly associated with caudal dysgenesis: a clincal epidemiological analysis. Am J Med Genet 53:46–51

Martínez-Frías ML, Bermejo E, Rodriguez-Pinilla L et al (1998) Epidemiological analysis of outcomes of pregnancy in gestational diabetic mothers. Am J Med Genet 78:140–145

Martínez-Frías ML, Frías JL, Salvador J (1989) Clinical/epidemiological analysis of malformations. Am J Med Genet 35:121–125

Mather HM, Keen H (10985) The Southall Diabetes Survey: prevalence of known diabetes in Asians and Europians. BMJ 291:1081–1085

Mathers CD, Field B (1983) Some international trends in the incidence of neural tube defects. Community Health Stud 7:60–66

Matsunaga E, Shiota K (1977) Holoprosencephaly in human embryos: epidemiologic studies of 150 cases. Teratology 16:261–272

Matsunaga E, Shiota K (1980) Search for maternal factors associated with malformed human embryos: a prospective study. Teratology 21:323–331

Mayer JB (1964) Der Einfluss des mütterlichen Diabetes auf das werdende Kind: die diabetogenen Embryopathien. Bull Schweiz Akad Med Wiss 20:470–486

Mayer JP (1952) Die Embryopathia diabetica. Z Kinderheilk 71:183–201

Mayer TK, Freedman ZR (1983) Protein glycosylation in diabetes mellitus: a review of laboratory measurements and of their clinical utility. Clin Chim Acta 127:147–184

Mazze RS, Krogh CL (1992) Gestational diabetes mellitus: now is the time for detection and treatment. Mayo Clin Proc 67(10):995–1002

McBride WG (1961) Thalidomide and congenital abnormalities. Lancet 2:1358

McCain JR, Lester WM (1950) Diabetes in pregnancy. J Med Ass Ga 39:57–63

McCarter RJ, Kessler II, Comstock GW (1987) Is diabetes mellitus a teratogen or a coteratogen? Am J Epidemiol 125:195–205

McCracken JS (1965) Absence of foetal femur and maternal prediabetes. Lancet 1:1274–1275

McDermott RA, Li M, Campbell SK (2010) Incidence of type 2 diabetes in two indigenous Australian populations: a 6-year follow-up study. Med J Aust 192:562–565

McDonald AD (1961) Maternal health in early pregnancy and congenital defect: final report on a prospective inquiry. Br J Prev Soc Med 15:154–166

McDonald GW, Fisher GF, Burnham C (1965) Reproducibility of the oral glucose tolerance test. Diabetes 14:473–480

McElvy SS, Miodovnik M, Rosenn B et al (2000) A focused preconceptional and early pregnancy program in women with type 1 diabetes reduces perinatal death and malformation rates to population levels. J Matern Fetal Med 9:14–20

McFarland KF, Case CA (1985) The relationship of maternal age on gestational diabetes. Diabetes Care 8:598–600

McFarland KF, Hemaya E (1985) Neonatal mortality in infants of diabetic mothers. Diabetes Care 8:333–336

McFarland KF, Pai MS, Coleman JL (1981) Outcome of diabetic pregnancies. J S Carol Med Ass 77:485–488

McIntosh R, Merritt KK, Richards MR et al (1954) The incidence of congenital malformations: a study of 5,964 pregnancies. Pediatrics 14:505–521

McIntyre HD, Thomae MK, Wong SF et al (2009) Pregnancy in type 2 diabetes mellitus–problems & promises. Curr Diabetes Rev 5:190–2000

McKeown T (1988) The origins of human disease. Blackwell, London

McKeown T, Record RG (1960) Malformations in a population observed for five years after birth. In: Wolstenholme GE, O'Connor CM (eds) Ciba Foundation symposium on congenital malformations. Little Brown, Boston, pp 2–16

McKusick VA (ed) (1992) Mendelian inheritance in man: catalogs of autosomal dominant, autosomal recessive, and X-linked phenotypes. Johns Hopkins Univ, Baltimore

McLendon H, Bottomy JR (1960) A critical analysis of the management of pregnancy in diabetic women. Am J Obstet Gynecol 80:641–652

McNeil C (1943) The first month of life: general survey. Edinb Med J 50:491–499

Meberg A, Otterstad JE, Frøland G et al (1994) Increased incidence of ventricular septal defects caused by improved detection rate. Acta Paediatr 83:653–657

Medical Research Council (1955) The use of hormones in the management of pregnancy in diabetics. Lancet 2:833–836

Méhes K (1983) Minor malformations in the neonate. Akadémiai Kiadó, Budapest

Méhes K (1988) Informative morphogenetic variants in the newborm infant. Akadémiai Kiadó, Budapest

Meinert CL (1972) Standardization of the oral glucose tolerance test: criticisms and suggestions invited. Diabetes 21:1197–1198

Meirik O, Smedby B, Ericson A (1979) Impact of changing age and parity distributions of mothers on perinatal death in Sweden, 1953–1975. Int J Epidemiol 8:361–364

Melamed N, Hod M (2009) Perinatal death in pregestational diabetes. Int J Gynaecol Obstet 104(Suppl 1):S20–S24

Mellin GW (1963) The frequency of birth defects. In: Fishbein M (ed) Birth defects. Lippincott, Philadelphia, pp 1–17

Mello G, Parretti E, Mecacci P et al (1997) Livelli glicemici "soglia" e aborto spontaneo nel I trimestre nelle gestanti affette da diabete melito insulino-dipendente. Minerva Ginecol 49:365–370

Mengert WF, Laughlin KA (1939) Thirty-three pregnancies in diabetic women. Surg Gynecol Obstet 69:615–617

Merkatz IR, Duchon MA, Yamashita TS, Houser HB (1980) A pilot community-based screening program for gestational diabetes. Diabetes Care 3:453–457

Merlob P (1994) Mild errors of morphogenesis: one of the most controversial subjects in dysmorphology. In: Kalter H (ed) Issues and reviews in teratology, vol 7. Plenum, New York, pp 57–102

Merlob P, Papier CM, Klingberg MA et al (1985) Incidence of congenital malformations in the newborn, particularly minor abnormalities. In: Marois M (ed) Prevention of physical and mental congenital defects. Liss, New York, pp 51–56

Mestman JH (1980) Outcome of diabetes screening in pregnancy and perinatal morbidity in infants of mothers with mild impairment in glucose tolerance. Diabetes

Metzger B (1991) 1990 overview of GDM. Accomplishments of the last decade-challenges for the future. Diabetes 40(Suppl 2):1–2

Metzger BE, The Organizing Committee (1991) Summary and recommendations of the third international workshop-conference on gestational diabetes nellitus. Diabetes Care 40:197–201

Metzger BE, Buchanaan TA, Coustan DR et al (2007) Summary and recommendations of the fifth international workshop-conference on gestational diabetes mellitus. Diabetes Care 30(2):S251–S260

Meyer-Wittkopf M, Simpson JM, Sharland GK (1996) Incidence of congenital heart defects in fetuses of diabetic mothers: a retrospective study of 326 cases. Ultrasound Obstet Gynecol 8:8–10

Michelsson K, Tiisala R, Wist A (1968) Perinatal death in diabetic pregnancy. Ann Chir Gynecol Fenn 57:402–404

Miller E, Hare JW, Cloherty JP et al (1981) Elevated maternal hemoglobin A_{1c} in early pregnancy and major congenital anomalies in infants of diabetic mothers. N Engl J Med 304:1331–1334

Miller HC (1945) The effect of the prediabetic state on the survival of the fetus and the birth weight of the newborn infant. N Engl J Med 233:376–378

Miller HC (1947) The effect of pregnancy complicated by alloxan diabetes on the fetuses of dogs, rabbits and rats. Endocrinology 40:251–258

Miller HC (1956) Offspring of diabetic and prediabetic mothers. In: Levine SZ (ed) Advances in pediatrics, vol 8. Year Book, Chicago. pp 137–163

Miller HC, Hurwitz D, Kuder K (1944) Neonatal mortality in pregnancies complicated by diabetes mellitus. JAMA 124:271–275

Miller JM (1983) A reappraisal of "tight control" in diabetic pregnancies. Am J Obstet Gynecol 147:158–162

Miller M (1965) Diabetic pregnancy and foetal survival in a large metropolitan area. In: Leibel BS, Wrenshall GA (eds) On the nature and treatment of diabetes. Excerpta Medica, Amsterdam, pp 714–717

Miller RW, Blot WJ (1972) Small head size after in-utero exposure to atomic radiation. Lancet 2:784–787

Miller RW, Mulvihill JJ (1976) Small head size after atomic radiation. Teratology 16:355–357

Miller SF (1972) Transposition of the external genitalia associated with the syndrome of caudal regression. J Urol 108:818–822

Mills JL (1982) Malformations in infants of diabetic mothers. Teratology 25(3):385–394

Mills JL, Baker L, Goldman AS (1979) Malformations in infants of diabetic mothers occur before the seventh gestational week: implications for treatment. Diabetes 28:292–293

Mills JL, Fishl AR, Knopp RH et al (1983) Malformations in infants of diabetic mothers: problems in study design. Prev Med 12:274–286

Mills JL, Knopp RH, Simpson JL et al (1988b) Lack of relation of increased malformation rates in infants of diabetic mothers to glycemic control during organogenesis. N Engl J Med 318:671–676

Mills JL, Simpson JL, Driscoll SG et al (1988a) Incidence of spontaneous abortion among normal women and insulin-dependent diabetic women whose pregnancies were identified within 21 days of conception. N Engl J Med 319:1617–1623

Mills JL, Withiam MJ (1986) Diabetes, pregnancy, and malformations: an epidemiologic perspective. In: Jovanovic L et al (eds) Diabetes and pregnancy: teratology, toxicity and treatment. Praeger, New York, pp 3–14

Milunsky A, Alpert E, Kitzmiller JL et al (1982) Prenatal diagnosis of neural tube defects. VIII. The importance of serum alpha-fetoprotein screening in diabetic pregnant women. Am J Obstet Gynecol 142:1030–1032

Mimouni F, Miodovnik M, Rosenn B et al (1992) Birth trauma in insulin-dependent diabetic pregnancies. Am J Perinat 9:205–208

Mimouni F, Miodovnik M, Tsang RC et al (1987) Decreased maternal serum magnesium concentration and adverse fetal outcome in insulin-dependent diabetic women. Obstet Gynecol 70:85–88

Mimouni M (1972) Les malformations congénitales des enfants nés de mères diabétiques traitées par l'insuline. J Pediatr 53:579–585

Miodovnik M, Lavin JP, Knowles HC et al (1984) Spontaneous abortion among insulin-dependent diabetic women. Am J Obstet Gynecol 150:372–375

Miodovnik M, Mimouni F, Dignan PS et al (1988) Major malformations in infants of IDDM women: vasculopathy and early trimester poor glycemic control. Diabetes Care 11:713–718

Miodovnik M, Mimouni F, Tsang RC et al (1986) Glycemic control and spontaneous abortion in insulin-dependent diabetic women. Obstet Gynecol 68:366–369

Miodovnik M, Skillman C, Holroyde JC et al (1985) Elevated maternal glycohemoglobin in early pregnancy and spontaneous abortion among insulin-dependent diabetic women. Am J Obstet Gynecol 153:439–442

Misenheimer HR, Kaltreider DF (1969) Preterm delivery of patients with decreased glucose tolerance. Obstet Gynecol 33:642–646

Mitchell SC, Berendres HW, Clark WM Jr (1967) The normal closure of the ventricular septum. Am Heart J 83:334–338

Mitchell SC, Korones SB, Berendes HW (1971b) Congenital heart disease in 56,109 births: incidence and natural history. Circulation 43:323–332

Mitchell SC, Sellman AH, Westphal MC et al (1971a) Etiologic correlates in a study of congenital heart diaease in 56,109 births. Am J Cardiol 28:653–657

Modanlou HD, Dorchester WL, Thorosian A et al (1980) Macrosomia–maternal, fetal, and neonatal implications. Obstet Gynecol 55:420–424

Modvig J, Schmidt L, Damsgaard MT (1990) Measurement of total risk of spontaneous abortion: the virtue of conditional risk estimation. Am J Epidemiol 132:1021–1038

Moe DG, Guntheroth WG (1987) Spontaneous closure of uncomplicated ventricular septal defect. Am J Cardiol 60:674–678

Moe N, Paul P, Jervell J et al (1987) Diabetes mellitus og graviditet. T Norske Laegeforen 107:1746–1750

Moley KH, Vaughn WK, DeCherney AH et al (1991) Effect of diabetes mellitus on mouse preimplantation embryo development. J Reprod Fert 93:325–332

Möllerström J (1950) Graviditetsförloppet vid diabetes. Nord Med 44:1570–1571

Mølsted-Pedersen L (1980) Congenital malformations in the offspring of diabetic women. In: Waldhaüsl WK, ed. Diabetes 1979. Proceedings of the 10th Congress of IDF, Vienna, Austria. Excerpta Medica, Amsterdam, pp 758–762

Mølsted-Pedersen L (1984) Detection of gestational diabetes. In: Sutherland HW, Stowers M (eds) Carbohydrate metabolism in pregnancy and the newborn. Livingstone, Edinburgh, pp 209–214

Mølsted-Pedersen L, Pedersen J (1967) Causes of perinatal death in diabetic pregnancy: a clinico-pathological analysis. Acta Med Scand Suppl 476:175–181
Mølsted-Pedersen L, Pedersen J (1985) Congenital malformations in diabetic pregnancies. Acta Paediat Scand Suppl 320:79–84
Mølsted-Pedersen L, Tygstrup I, Pedersen J (1964) Congenital malformations in newborn infants of diabetic women: correlation with maternal diabetic vascular complications. Lancet 1:1124–1126
Monier D, Guimond P, Dandavino A (1981) Diabète et grossesse: mortalité et morbidité périnatales 1975–1980. Union Med Can 110:996–998, 1004
Moore WM (1991) Naegele's rule. Lancet 337:910
Moreau R, Deuil R, Hadjissotiriou G et al (1955) L'importance de la mortalité et la fréquence des gros enfants chez les diabétiques et les prédiabétiques. Sem Hôp 31:652–655
Morishima M, Ando M, Takao A (1991) Visceroatrial heterotaxy syndrome in the NOD mouse with particular reference to the atrial sinus. Teratology 44:91–100
Morison SE (1971) The European discovery of America: the northern voyages. AD 500–1600. Oxford Univ, New York
Morris JK, Wald NJ (2007) Prevalence of neural tube defect pregnancies in England and Wales from 1965 to 2004. J Med Screen 14:55–59
Morris MA, Grandis AS, Litton JC (1985) Glycosylated hemoglobin concentration in early gestation associated with neonatal outcome. Am J Obstet Gynecol 153:651–654
Morris NM, Udry JR, Chase CL (1975) Shifting age-parity distribution of births and the decrease in infant mortality. Am J Publ Health 65:359–362
Moss JM, Connor EJ (1965) Pregnancy complicated by diabetes: report of 102 pregnancies including eleven treated with oral hypoglycemic drugs. Med Ann DC 34:253–260
Moss JM, Mulholland HB (1951) Diabetes and pregnancy: with special reference to the prediabetic state. Ann Int Med 34:678–691
Moyer JH, Womack CR (1950) Glucose tolerance. I. A comparison of 4 types of diagnostic tests in 103 control subjects and 26 patients with diabetes. Am J Med Sci 219:161–173
Mufarrij IK, Kilejian VO (1963) Anencephaly. Obstet Gynecol 22:657–661
Müller F, O'Rahilly R (1989) Mediobasal prosencephalic defects, including holoprosencephaly and cyclopia, in relation to the development of the human forebrain. Am J Anat 185:391–414
Murphy DP (1929) Outcome of 625 pregnancies in women subjected to pelvic radium or roentgen irradiation. Am J Obstet Gynecol 18:179–187
Murphy DP (1933) Excretion of ovary stimulating hormone in urine during pregnancy: its relation to urinary output. Surg Gynecol Obstet 56:914–917
Murphy DP (1939) Congenital malformations: a study of parental characteristics with special reference to the reproductive process. Univ of Pennsylvania, Philadelphia
Murphy EA (1966) A scientific viewpoint on normalcy. Perspect Biol Med 9:333–348
Murphy J, Peters J, Morris P et al (1984) Conservative management of pregnancy in diabetic women. BMJ 288:1203–1205
Murphy NJ, Bulkow LR, Schraer CD et al (1993) Prevalence of diabetes mellitus in pregnancy among Yup'ik Eskimos, 1987–1988. Diabetes Care 16(Suppl 1):315–317
Muylder XD (1984) Perinatal complications of gestational diabetes: the influence of the timing of the diagnosis. Eur J Obstet Gynecol Reprod Biol 18:35–42
Mylvaganam R, Stowers JM, Steel JM et al (1983) Insulin immunogenicity in pregnancy: maternal and fetal studies. Diabetologia 24:19–25
Myrianthopoulos NC (1985) Malformations in children from one to seven years: a report from the Collaborative Perinatal Project. Liss, New York
Myrianthopoulos NC, Chung CS (1974) Congenital malformations in singletons: epidemiologic survey. Report from the Collaborative Perinatal project. Birth Defects Orig Artic Ser 10(11):1–58
Naeye RL (1978) The outcome of diabetic pregnancies: a prospective study. Ciba Found Symp (63):227–241 (Mar 30-Apr 1)
Naeye RL (1990) Maternal body weight and pregnancy outcome. Am J Clin Nutr 52(2):273–279

Naggan L, MacMahon B (1967) Ethnic differences in the prevalence of anencephaly and spina bifida in Boston, Massachusetts. N Engl J Med 277:1119–1123

Nakamoto T, Quinby GE Jr (1987) Effects of maternal dietary protein on the mandibular growth of fetuses from diabetic dams. Res Comm Path Pharmacol 56:273–276

Nakhooda AF, Like AA, Chappel CI et al (1976) The spontaneously diabetic Wistar rat: metabolic and morphologic studies. Diabetes 26:100–112

Naqshbandi M, Harris SB, Esler JG et al (2008) Global complication rates of type 2 diabetes in Indigenous peoples: a comprehensive review. Diabetes Res Clin Pract 82:1–17

Nathanson JN (1950) The excessively large fetus as an obstetric problem. Am J Obstet Gynecol 60:54–63

National Center for Health Statistics (1992) Annual summary of births, marriages, divorces, and deaths: United States, 1991. Mon Vit Stat Rep 40(13):1–28

National Center for Health Statistics (1998) Births, marriages, divorces, and deaths for October 1997. Mon Vit Stat Rep 46(10):1–20

National Diabetes Data Group (1979) Classification and diagnosis of diabetes mellitus and other categories of glucose intolerance. Diabetes 28:1039–1057

Nau H (1987) Species differences in pharmacokinetics, drug metabolism, and teratogenesis. In: Nau H, Scott WJ (eds) Pharmacokinetics in teratogenesis, vol 1. CRC, Boca Raton, Fla, pp 81–106

Navarrete VN, Torres IH, Rivera IR et al (1967) Maternal carbohydrate disorder and congenital malformations. Diabetes 16:127–129

Naylor AF (1974) Sequential aspects of spontaneous abortion: maternal age, parity, and pregnancy compensation artifact. Soc Biol 21:195–204

Naylor CD (1989) Diagnosing gestational diabetes mellitus: is the gold standard valid? Diabetes Care 12:565–572

Naylor CD, Sermer M, Chen E et al (1997) Selective screening for gestational diabetes mellitus. N Engl J Med 337:1591–1596

Neave C (1967) Congental malformations in offspring of diabetics. Doctor of Public Health Thesis, Harvard Univ, Boston

Neave C (1984) Congenital malformations in offspring of diabetics. Perspect Pediatr Path 8:213–222

Neel JV (1958) A study of major congenital defects in Japanese infants. Am J Hum Genet 10:398–445

Neilson DR, Bolton RN, Prins RP et al (1991) Glucose challenge testing in pregnancy. Am J Obstet Gynecol 164:1673–1679

Nelson HB, Gillespie L, White P (1953) Pregnancy complicated by diabetes mellitus. Obstet Gynecol 1:219–225

Nelson RL (1986) Diabetes and pregnancy: control can make a difference. Mayo Clin Proc 61:825–829

Nevinny H, Schretter G (1930) Zuckerkrankheit und Schwangerschaft. Arch Gynäk 140:397–427

Newman G (1906) Infant mortality: a social problem. London, Methuen

Newman TB (1985) Etiology of ventricular septal defects: an epidemiologic approach. Pediatrics 76:741–749

Newsholme A (1910) Report by the Medical Officer on Child Mortality. Supplement to the 30th Annual Report. Local Government Board, London

Nicolini U, Kustermann A, Gargiulo M et al (1986) Esiti perinatali nelle gravide diabetiche:1963–1975 e 1978–1983. Ann Ostet Ginecol 107:243–250

Nielsen GL, Hostrup P (1990) Malformations in 238 diabetic pregnancies: no correlation between HbA_{1c} and malformations. Diabetologia 33:A138

Nielsen GL, Møller M, Sørensen HT (2006a) HbA_{1c} in early diabetic pregnancy and pregnancy outcomes: a Danish population-based cohort study of 573 pregnancies in women with type 1 diabetes. Diabetes Care 29:2612–2616

Nielsen GL, Nielsen PH (1993) Outcome of 328 pregnancies in 205 women with insulin-dependent diabetes mellitus in the county of Northern Jutland from 1976 to 1990. Eur J Obstet Gynecol Reprod Biol 50:33–38

Nielsen GL, Nielsen PH (1994) Results of 312 pregnancies among White class B-F mothers in northern Jutland from 1976 to 1992. Dan Med Bull 41:115–118

Nielsen GL, Sørensen HT, Nielsen PH et al (1997) Glycosylated hemoglobin as predictor of adverse fetal oputcome in type I diabetic pregnancies. Acta Diabetol 34:217–222

Nielsen LR, Damm P, Mathiesen ER (2009) Improved pregnancy outcome in type 1 diabetic women with microalbuminuria or diabetic nephropathy: effect of intensified antihypertensive therapy? Diabetes Care 32:38–44

Nielsen LR Müller C, Damm P et al (2006b) Reduced prevalence of early preterm delivery in women with type 1 diabetes and microalbuminuria–possible effect of early antihypertensive treatment during pregnancy. Diabet Med 23:426–431

Nishimura H, Takano K, Tanimura T et al (1968) Normal and abnormal development of human embryos: first report of the analysis of 1,213 intact embryos. Teratology 1:281–290

Niswander KR, Gordon M (1972) The Women and their pregnancies. Saunders, Philadelphia

Nizard J, Ville Y (2009) The fetus of a diabetic mother: sonographic evaluation. Semin Fetal Neonatal Med 14:101–105

Nordström L, Spetz E, Wallström K et al (1998) Metabolic control and pregnancy outcome among women with insulin-dependent diabetes melitus. A twelve-year follow-up in the county of Jämtland, Sweden. Acta Obstet Gynecol Scand 77:284–289

Northern Regional Survey Steering Group (1992) Fetal abnormality: an audit of its recognition and management. Arch Dis Child 67:770–774

Nothmann M, Hermstein A (1932) Diabetes und Gravidität. I. Mitteilung. Arch Gynäk 150:287–301

Nowack E (1965) Die sensible phase bei der thalidomid-embryopathie. Humangenetik 1:516–536

O'Rahilly R, Müller F (1989) Interpretation of some median anomalies as illustrated by cyclopia and symmelia. Teratology 40:409–422

O'Shaughnessy R, Russ J, Zuspan FP (1979) Glycosylated hemoglobins and diabetes mellitus in pregnancy. Am J Obstet Gynecol 135:783–790

O'Sullivan JB (1961) Gestational diabetes: unsuspected, asymptomatic diabetes in pregnancy. N Engl J Med 264:1082–1085

O'Sullivan JB (1979) Gestational diabetes: factors influencing the rates of subsequent diabetes. In: Sutherland HW, Stowers JM (eds) Carbohydrate metabolism in pregnancy and the newborn 1978, Springer, Berlin, pp 425–434

O'Sullivan JB (1980) Establishing criteria for gestational diabetes. Diabetes Care 3:437–439

O'Sullivan JB, Gellis SS, Dandrow RV et al (1966) The potential diabetic and treatment in pregnancy. Obstet Gynecol 27:683–689

O'Sullivan JB, Mahan CM (1964) Criteria for the oral glucose tolerance test in pregnancy. Diabetes 13:278 -285 (May-June)

O'Sullivan JB, Mahan CM (1966) Glucose tolerance test: variability in pregnant and nonpregnant women. Am J Clin Nutr 19:345–351

O'Sullivan JB, Mahan CM (1980) Diabetes Care. 3(3):482–485

O'Sullivan JB, Mahan CM, Charles D, Dandrow RV (1973) Screening criteria for high-risk gestational diabetic patients. Am J Obstet Gynecol 116(7):895–900

O'Sullivan JB, Mahan CM, Charles D, Dandrow RV (1974a) Medical treatment of the gestational diabetic. Obstet Gynecol 43(6):817–821 (June)

O'Sullivan JB, Mahan CM, D'Agostino RB, Charles D (1974b) Glucose disposal rates and the glucose challenge in pregnant women. J Clin Endocrinol Metab 39(6):1067–1071

Oakley GP, Erickson JD, James LM et al (1994) Prevention of folic acid-preventable spina bifida and anencephaly. In: Bock G, Marsh J (eds) Neural tube defects. Wiley, Chichester, pp 212–231

Oakley W (1953) Prognosis in diabetic pregnancy. BMJ 1(4825):1413–1415
Oakley W (1965) The treatment of pregnancy in diabetes mellitus. In: Leibel BS, Wrenshall GA (eds) On the nature and treatment of diabetes mellitus. Excerpta Medica, Amsterdam, pp 673–678
Oats JN, Beischer NA (1986) Gestational diabetes. Aust N Z J Obstet Gynecol 26:2–10
Ober C, Simpson JL (1986) Diabetes mellitus: preventing anomalies through maternal metabolic intervention. Clin Obstet Gynecol 29:558–568
Oh W, Gelardi NL, Cha C-J (1988) Maternal hyperglycemia in pregnant rats: its effect on growth and carbohydrate metabolism in the offspring. Metabolism 37:1146–1151
Olofsson P, Liedholm H, Sartor G et al (1984a) Diabetes and pregnancy: a 21-year Swedish material. Acta Obstet Gynecol Scand Suppl 122:3–62
Olofsson P, Sjöberg NO, Solum T et al (1984b) Changing panorama of perinatal and infant mortality in diabetic pregnancy. Acta Obstet Gynecol Scand 63:467–472
Olsen CL, Hughes JP, Youngblood LG et al (1997) Epidemiology of holoprosencephaly and phenotypic characteristics of affected children: New York State, 1984–1989. Am J Med Genet 73:217–226
Ooshima Y, Shiota K (1991) Congenital malformations in genetically diabetic mice, yellow KK. Teratology 44:13B
Opitz JM (1994) Associations and syndromes: terminology in clinical genetics and birth defects epidemiology. Am J Med Genet 49:14–20
Orchard TJ, Dorman JS, LaPorte RE et al (1986) Host and environmental interactions in diabetes mellitus. J Chron Dis 39:979–1000
Ornoy A, Ratzo, N, Greenbaum C et al (1994) The development of children born to diabetic mothers at the age of 6–10 years. Teratology 50:25A
Orr SC (1888) Strange freak of nature. J Comp Med Surg 10:377–378
Osler W (1885) The Gulstonian Lectures, on malignant endocarditis. BMJ 1:467–470
Österlund K, Rantakallio P (1964) Perinatal death in diabetic pregnancies. Ann Paediatr Fenn 10:84–91
Otani H, Tanaka O, Tatekawi R et al (1991) Diabetic environment and genetic disposition as causes of congenital malformations in NOD mouse embryos. Diabetes 40:1245–1250
Ounsted M, Moar VA, Cockburn J, et al (1984) Factors associated with the intellectual ability of children born to women with high risk pregnancies. BMJ 228:1038–1041
Padmanabhan R, Al-Zuhair AG (1988) Congenital malformations and intrauterine growth retardation in streptozotocin induced diabetes during gestation in the rat. Reprod Toxic 1:117–125
Palacin M, Lasunción MA, Martin A et al (1985) Decreased uterine blood flow in the diabetic pregnant rat does not modify the augmented glucose transfer to the fetus. Biol Neonat 48:197–203
Pallardo LF, Grande C, Luna R et al (1990) Diabetes y embarazo: nuestra experiencia en diabetes gestacional (1977–1988). Med. Clin 95:406–410
Palmer LJ, Barnes RH (1945) Pregnancy in the diabetic. West J Surg Obstet Gynecol 53:195–202
Palumbo L (1954) Diabetes mellitus complicated by pregnancy. N Carol Med J 15:120–123
Pang D (1993) Sacral agenesis and caudal spinal cord malformations. Neurosurgery 32:755–778
Pang D, Hoffman HJ (1980) Sacral agenesis with progressive neurological deficit. Neurosurgery 7:118–126
Pardou A, Dodion J, Loeb H (1977) Mortality and morbidity in newborns of insulin dependent diabetic mothers. Acta Pediatr Belg 30:165–170
Parisot MJ (1911) Les troubles de la fonction génitale chez les diabétiques: leur pathogénie. Bull Mem Soc Med Hôp Paris 35:95–110
Park SC, Mathews RA, Zuberbuhler JR et al (1977) Down syndrome with congenital heart malformation. Am J Dis Child 131:29–37
Parsons E, Randall LM, Wilder RM (1926) Pregnancy and diabetes. Med Clin N Am 10:679–688
Passarge E (1965) Congenital malformations and maternal diabetes. Lancet 1:324–325
Passarge E, Lenz W (1966) Syndrome of caudal regression in infants of diabetic mothers: observations of further cases. Pediatrics 37:672–675

Pastor X, Domenech P, Jorba JM, et al (1988) Somatometric study in the infant of gestaitonal diabetic mother. In: Weiss PA, Coustan DR (eds) Gestational diabetes. Springer, New York, pp 171–175

Paton DM (1948) Pregnancy in the prediabetic patient. Am J Obstet Gynecol 56:558–560

Patrick SL, Moy CS, LaPorte RE (1989) The world of insulin-dependent diabetes mellitus: what international epidemiological studies reveal about the etiology and natural history of IDDM. Diab Metab Rev 5:571–578

Paterson SJ (1944) Iniencephalus. J Obstet Gynecol Br Emp 51:330–333

Patterson CC, Dahlquist GG, Gyürüs E et al (2009) Incidence trends for childhood type 1 diabetes in Europe during 1989–2003 and predicted new cases 2005–2020: a multicentre prospective registration study. Lancet 373:2027–2033. Epub 2009 May 27

Patterson JW, Lazarow A, Levey S (1949) Alloxan and dialuric acid: their stabilities and ultraviolet absorption spectra. J Biol Chem 177:187–196

Patterson M, Burnstein N (1949) Diabetes and pregnancy: a clinical analysis. Arch Int Med 83:390–401

Pauli RM, Reiser CA (1994) Wisconsin stillbirth service program. II. Analysis of diagnoses and diagnostic categories in the first 1000 referrals. Am J Med Genet 50:135–153

Pavkov ME, Hanson RL, Knowler WC et al (2007) Changing patterns of type 2 diabetes incidence in Pima Indians. Diabetes Care 30:1758–1763

Pavkov ME, Knowler WC, Hanson RL et al (2008) Diabetic nephropathy in American Indians, with special emphasis on the Pima Indians. Curr Diabet Rep 8:486–493

Paxton J (ed) (1987) The Statesman's Year-Book. St. Martin's, New York

Peacock I, Hunter JC, Walford S et al (1979) Self-monitoring of blood glucose in diabetic pregnancy. BMJ 2:1333–1336

Pease JC, Smallpiece V, Lennon GC (1951) Diabetes and pregnancy. BMJ 1(4718):1296–1298

Peck RW, Price DE, Lang GD et al (1991) Birthweight of babies born to mothers with type 1 diabetes: is it related to blood glucose control in the first trimester? Diabetes Med 8:258–262

Peckham CH (1931) Diabetes mellitus and pregnancy. Bull Johns Hopkins Hosp 49:184–201

Pedersen J (1952) Course of diabetes during pregnancy. Acta Endocr 9:342–364

Pedersen J (1954a) Fetal mortality in diabetic pregnancies. Diabetes 3:199–204

Pedersen J (1954b) Weight and length at birth of infants of diabetic mothers. Acta Endocr 16:330–342

Pedersen J (1975) Goals and end-points in management of diabetic pregnancy. In: Camerini-Davalos RA, Cole HS (eds) Early diabetes in early life. Academic, New York, pp 381–391

Pedersen J (1977) The pregnant diabetic and her newborn: problems and management. Munksgaard, Copenhagen

Pedersen J (1979) Congenital malformations in newborns of diabetic mothers. In: Sutherland HW, Stowers JM (eds) Carbohydrate metabolism and the newborn 1978. Springer, Berlin, pp 264–276

Pedersen J, Brandstrup E (1956) Foetal mortality in pregnant diabetics: strict control of diabetes with conservative obstetric management. Lancet 1:607–610

Pedersen J, Mølsted-Pedersen L (1965) Prognosis of the outcome of pregnancies in diabetics: a new classification. Acta Endocr 50:70–78

Pedersen J, Mølsted-Pedersen L (1978) Congenital malformations: the possible role of diabetes care outside pregnancy. Ciba Found Symp 63:265–271

Pedersen J, Mølsted-Pedersen LA, Andersen B (1974) Assessors of fetal perinatal death in diabetic pregnancy: analysis of 1,332 pregnancies in the Copenhagen series, 1946–1972. Diabetes 23:302–305

Pedersen J, Osler M (1958) Development of ossification centres in infants of diabetic mothers. Acta Endocr 29:467–472

Pedersen J, Schondel A (1949) Follow-up examination of children of diabetic mothers. Acta Paediatr Suppl 77:203–204

Pedersen JF, Mølsted-Pedersen L (1979) Early growth retardation in diabetic pregnancy. BMJ 1:18–19

Pedersen JF, Mølsted-Pedersen L (1981) Early fetal growth delay detected by ultrasound marks increased risk of congenital malformation in diabetic pregnancy. BMJ 283:269–271

Pedersen JF, Mølsted-Pedersen L (1985) The possibility of an early growth delay in White's class A diabetic pregnancy. Diabetes 34(2):47–49

Pedersen JF, Mølsted-Pedersen L, Mortensen HB (1984) Fetal growth delay and maternal hemoglobin A_{1c} in early diabetic pregnancy. Obstet Gynecol 64:351–352

Pedersen KK, Hagen C, Sandø-Pedersen SH et al (1994) Infertility and pregnancy outcome in women with insulin-dependent diabetes. An epidemiological study, (In Danish). Ugeskr Laeger 156:6196–6200

Pedowitz P, Shlevin EL (1952) The pregnant diabetic. Bull N Y Acad Med 28:440–453

Pedowitz P, Shlevin EL (1955) The pregnant diabetic patient. Am J Obstet Gynecol 69:395–404

Pedowitz P, Shlevin EL (1964) Review of management of pregnancy complicated by diabetes and altered carbohydrate metabolism. Obstet Gynecol 23:716–729

Pedula KL, Hiller TA, Schmidt MM et al (2009) Ethnic differences in gestational oral glucose screening in a large US population. Ethn Dis 19:414–419

Peel J, Oakley W (1949) The management of pregnancy in diabetics. In: Transactions of the XIIth British Congress of Obstetrics and Gynecology. Austral, London, pp 161–184

Peller S (1923) Die Säulingssterblichkeit nach dem Kriege. I. Wein Klin Wochensch 36:799–801

Peller S (1948) Mortality, past and future. Popul Stud 1:411–456

Penney GC, Mair G, Pearson DW et al (2003) Outcomes of pregnancies in women with type 1 diabetes in Scotland: a national population-based study. BJOG 110:315–318

Penrose LS (1957) The genetics of anencephaly. J Ment Def Res 1:4–15

Perrot LJ, Williamson S, Jimenez JF (1987) The caudal regression syndrome in infants of diabetic mothers. Ann Clin Lab Med 17:211–220

Persson B, Gentz J (1984) Follow-up of children of insulin-dependent and gestational diabetic mothers. Acta Paediatr Scand 73:349–358

Persson B, Hanson U (1993) Insulin dependent diabetes in pregnancy: impact of maternal blood glucose control on the offspring. J Paediatr Child Hlth 29:20–23

Persson B, Gentz J, Möller E (1984) Follow-up of children of insulin dependent (type I) and gestational diabetic mothers: growth pattern, glucose tolerance, insulin response, and HLA types. Acta Paediatr Scand 73:778–784

Persson B, Gentz J, Stangenberg M (1979) Neonatal problems. In: Sutherland HW, Stowers JM (eds) Carbohydrate metabolism in pregnancy and the newborn 1978. Springer, Berlin, pp 376–391

Persson M, Norman M, Hanson U (2009) Obstetric and perinatal outcomes in type 1 diabetic pregnancies: a large, population-based study. Diabetes Care 32:205–209

Petersen MB (1989) Status at 4–5 years in 90 children of insulin-dependent diabetic mothers. In: Sutherland HW, Stowers JM, Pearson DW (eds) Carbohydrate metabolism in pregnancy and the newborn. IV. Springer, New York, pp 353–361

Petersen MB, Pedersen SA, Greisen G et al (1988) Early growth delay in diabetic pregnancy: relation to psychomotor development at age 4. BMJ 296:598–600

Pettitt DJ, Bennett PH, Knowler WC et al (1985) Gestational diabetes mellitus and impaired glucose tolerance during pregnancy: long-term effects on obesity and glucose tolerance in the offspring. Diabetes 34(2):119–122

Pettitt DJ, Knowler WC, Baird HR et al (1980) Gestational diabetes: infant and maternal complications of pregnancy in relation to third-trimester glucose tolerance in the Pima Indians. Diabetes Care 3:458–464

Philipson EH, Kalhan SC, Rosen MG et al (1985) Gestational diabetes mellitus: is further improvement necessary? Diabetes 34(2):55–60

Pijlman BM, de Koning WB, Wladimiroff JW et al (1989) Detection of fetal structural malformations by ultrasound in insulin-dependent pregnant women. Ultrasound Med Biol 15:541–543

Pinget M, Krummel Y, Gandar R et al (1979) Incidence de la maladie diabétique sur l'age de survenue des premières règles. Nouv Presse Med 8:36–64

Pinsky L (1985) Informative morphogenetic variants: minor congenital anomalies revisited. In: Kalter H (ed) Issues and reviews in teratology, vol 3. Plenum, New York, pp 135–170
Piper JM (2002) Lung maturation in diabetes in pregnancy: if and when to test. Semin Perinatol 26:206–209
Piper JM, Langer O (1993) Does maternal diabetes delay fetal pulmonary maturity? Am J Obstet Gynecol 168:783–786
Pirart J (1955) The so-called prediabetic syndrome of pregnancy. Acta Endocr 20:192–208
Pitkin RM, Van Orden DE (1974) Fetal effects of maternal streptozotocin-diabetes. Endocrinology 94:1247–1253
Pitt DB, Findlay II, Cole WG et al (1982) Case report: femoral hypoplasia-unusual facies syndrome. Aust Paediatr 18:63–66
Plauchu M, Pousset G, Chapu H et al (1970) Diabète et grossesse. J Med Lyon 51:169–172
Plehwe WE, Storey GN, Shearman RP et al (1984) Outcome of pregnancy complicated by diabetes: experience with 232 patients in a 4 year period. Diabet Res 1:67–73
Poland BJ, Miller JR, Harris M et al (1981) Spontaneous abortion: a study of 1961 women and their conceptuses. Acta Obstet Gynecol Scand Suppl 102:5–32
Polednak AP (1986) Birth defects in blacks and whites in relation to prenatal development: a review and hypothesis. Hum Biol 58(3):317–335
Pomeranze J, Stone ML, King EJ (1959) The obstetric importance of obesity and "benign" glycosuria in prediagnosis diabetes. Obstet Gynecol 13:181–184
Porter IH, Hook EB (eds) (1980) Human embryonic and fetal death. Academic, New York
Post RH, White P (1958) Tentative explanation of the high incidence of diabetes. Diabetes 7:27–32
Potter EL, Adair FL (1943) Clinical-pathological study of the infant and fetal mortality for a ten-year period at the Chicago Lying-in Hospital. Am J Obstet Gynecol 45:1054–1065
Powell-Griner E (1986) Perinatal death in the United States: 1950–1981. Mon Vit Stat Rep Suppl 34(12):1–16
Powell-Griner E (1989) Perinatal death in the United States: 1981–1985. Mon Vit Stat Rep Suppl 37(10):1–12
Powell-Griner E, Woolbright A (1990) Trends in infant deaths from congenital anomalies: results from England and Wales, Scotland, Sweden, and the United States. Int J Epidemiol 19:391–398
Pradat P (1992a) A case-control study of major congenital heart defects in Sweden: 1981–1986. Eur J Epidemiol 8:789–796
Pradat P (1992b) Epidemiology of major heart defects in Sweden, 1981–1986. J Epidemiol Community Health 46:211–215
Prager R, Ovici A, Liban E et al (1974) Histopathological changes in the placenta of streptozotocin induced diabetic rats. Diabetologia 10:89–91
Pyke DA (1962) Prediabetes. In: Pyke DA (ed) Disorders of carbohydrate metabolism. Lippincott, Philadelphia, pp 95–112
Rahbar S (1968) An abnormal hemoglobin in red cells of diabetics. Clin Chim Acta 22:296–298
Rahbar S, Blumenfeld O, Ranney HM (1969) Studies of an unusual hemoglobin in patients with diabetes mellitus. Biochem Biophys Res Comm. 36:838–843
Rakieten N, Rakieten ML, Hadkarni MV (1963) Studies on the diabetogenic action of streptozotocin (HSC-37917). Canc Chemother Rep 29:91–98
Ramos-Arroyo MA, Rodriguez-Pinilla E, Cordero JF (1992) Maternal diabetes: the risk for specific birth defects. Eur J Epidemiol 8:503–508
Randall LM (1947) Pregnancy associated with diabetes. Am J Obstet Gynecol 54:618–625
Rasmussen SA, Moore CA, Khoury MJ et al (1996) Descriptive epidemiology of holoprosencephay and arhinenecephaly in Metropolitan Atlanta, 1968–1992. Am J Med Genet 66:320–333
Ravussin E (1993) Energy metabolism in obsity. Studies in the Pima Indians. Diabetes Care 16:232–238
Ray JG, O'Brien TE, Chan WS (2001) Preconception care and the risk of congenital anomalies in the offspring of women with diabetes mellitus: a meta-analysis. QJM 94:435–444
Record RG (1961) Anencephalus in Scotland. Br J Prev Soc Med 15:93–105

Reddi AS, Opperman W, Velasco CA et al (1975) Early genetic diabetes in the KK mouse. In: Camerini-Davalos RA, Cole HS (eds) Early diabetes in early life. Academic, New York, pp 4a13–4a25

Reece EA (2010) The fetal and maternal consequences of gestational diabetes mellitus. J Matern Fetal Neonatal Med 23:199–203

Reece EA, Hobbins JC (1986) Diabetic embryopathy: pathogenesis, prenatal diagnosis and prevention. Obstet Gynecol Surv 41:325–335

Reece EA, Homko CJ (2005) Pregnancy outcomes in gestations complicated by type 2 diabetes. Curr Diabet Rep 5:269–270

Reece EA, Winn HN, Smikle C et al (1990) Sonographic assessment of growth of the fetal head in diabetic pregnancies compared with normal gestations. Am J Perinat 7:18–22

Regemorter NV, Dodion J, Druart C et al (1984) Congenital malformations in 10,000 consecutive births in a university hospital: need for genetic counseling and prenatal diagnosis. J Pediatr 104:386–390

Reid M, Hadden D, Harley JM et al (1984) Fetal malformations in diabetics with high haemoglobin A_{1c} in early pregnancy. BMJ 298:1001

Reis RA, DeCosta EJ, Allweiss MD (1950) The management of the pregnant diabetic woman and her newborn infant. Am J Obstet Gynecol 60:1023–1039

Reis RA, DeCosta EJ, Allweiss MD (1952) Diabetes and pregnancy. Thomas, Springfield

Reis RA, DeCosta EJ, Gerbie AB (1958) Pregnancy in the diabetic woman. Am J Obstet Gynecol 76(5):1148–1150

Reis RR (1956) Discussion, in: White et al 1956. pp 68–69

Rerup CC (1970) Drugs producing diabetes through damage of the insulin secreting cells. Pharmacol Rev 22:485–518

Reveno WS (1923) Insulin in diabetic coma, complicating pregnancy. JAMA 81:2101–2102

Richards MR, Merritt KK, Samuels MH et al (1955) Congenital malformations of the cardiovascular system in a series of 6,053 infants. Pediatrics 15:12–32

Rike PM, Fawcett RM (1948) Diabetes in pregnancy. Am J Obstet Gynecol 56:484–493

Ring PA (1961) Congenital abnormalities of the femur. Arch Dis Child 36:410–417

Rizzo G, Arduini D, Romanini C (1991) Cardiac function in fetuses of type I diabetic mothers. Am J Obstet Gynecol 164:837–843

Rizzo TA, Dooley SL, Metzger BE et al (1995) Prenatal and perinatal influences on long-term psychomotor development in offspring of diabetic mothers. Am J Obset Gynecol 173:1753–1758

Rizzo TA, Ogata ES, Dooley SL et al (1994) Perinatal complications and cognitive development in 2- to 5-year-old children of diabetic mothers. Am J Obstet Gynecol 171:706–712

Roach E, DeMyer W, Conneally PM et al (1975) Holoprosencephaly: birth data, genetic and demographic analyses of 30 families. Birth Defects 11(3):294–313

Robert MF, Neff RK, Hubbell JP et al (1976) Association between maternal diabetes and the respiratory-distress syndrome in the newborn. N Engl J Med 294:357–360

Roberts RN, Moohan JM, Foo RL et al (1993) Fetal outcome in mothers with impaired glucose tolerance in pregnancy. Diabet Med 10:438–443

Roccella EJ, Bowler AE, Horan M (1987) Epidemiologic considerations in defining hypertension. Med Clin N Am 71:785–801

Roland JM, Murphy HR, Ball V et al (2005) The pregnancies of women with type 2 diabetes: poor outcomes but opportunities for improvement. Diabet Med 22:1774–1777

Rolland C (1954) Diabetes in pregnancy. Edinb Med J 61:257–272

Roman E, Stevenson AC (1983) Spontaneous abortion. In: Barron SL, Thomson AM (eds) Obstetrical epidemiology. Academic, London, pp 61–87

Ronsheim J (1933) Diabetes and pregnancy. Am J Obstet Gynecol 25:710–714

Rosch C, Steinbicker V (2004) Congenital malformations–etiological factors 20 years after Kalter and Warkany. Reprod Toxicol 18:135–136

Rose BI, Graff S, Spencer R et al (1988) Major congenital anomalies in infants and glycosylated hemoglobin levels in insulin-requiring diabetic mothers. J Perinat 8:309–311

Rosenberg M (1924) Glycosurie, Diabetes und Acidose bei Schwangeren. Klin Wochensch 3:1561–1565

Rosendahl K, Markestad T, Lie RT (1992) Congenital dislocation of the hip: a prospective study comparing ultrasound and clinical examination. Acta Paediatr 81:177–181

Rosenn B, Combs CA, Khoury J et al (1994) Glycemic thresholds for spontaneous abortion and congenital malformations in insulin-dependent diabetes mellitus. Obstet Gynecol 84:515–520

Rosenn B, Miodovnik M, Combs CA et al (1991) Pre-conception management of insulin-dependent diabetes: improvement of pregnancy outcome. Obstet Gynecol 77:846–849

Rosenthal M, McMahan CA, Stern MP et al (1985) Evidence of bimodality of two hour plasma glucose concentrations in Mexican Americans: results from the San Antonio heart study. J Chron Dis 38:5–16

Ross OA, Spector S (1952) Production of congenital abnormalities in mice by alloxan. Am J Dis Child 84:647–648

Roth MP, Dott B, Alembik Y et al (1987) Malformations congénitales dans une série de 66,068 naissances consécutives. Arch Fr Pediatr 44:173–176

Roversi GD, Canussio V, Gargiulo M (1975) Insulin in gestational diabetes. In Camerino-Davalos RA, Coles HS (eds) Early diabetes. Academic Press, New York, pp 469–475

Roversi DG, Gargiulo M, Nicolini U et al (1977) Diabéte de la mère et risque perinatal: reduction du risque perinatal lors de grossesses chez les diabétiques, par la recherche d'un strict équilibre métabolique de la maladie maternelle, 479 cas (1963–1975). Rev Med Suisse Roman 97:401–412

Rowe AW, Gallivan DE, Matthews H (1931) The metabolism in pregnancy. V. The carbohydrate metabolism. Am J Physiol 96:94–100

Rowe BR, Rowbotham CJ, Barnett AH (1987) Pre-conception counselling, birth weight, and congenital abnormalities in established and gestational diabetic pregnancy. Diabet Res 6:33–35

Rowe RD, Freedom RM, Mehrizi A et al (1981) The neonate with congenital heart disease. Saunders, Philadelphia

Rowland TW, Hubbell JP, Nadas AS (1973) Congenital heart disease in infants of diabetic mothers. J Pediatr 83:815–820

Rubin A (1958) Studies in human reproduction. II. The influence of diabetes mellitus in men upon reproduction. Am J Obstet Gynecol 76:25–29

Rubin A, Murphy DP (1958) Studies in human reproduction. III. The frequency of congenital malformations in the offspring of non-diabetic and diabetic individuals. J Pediatr 53:579–585

Ruoff W (1903) Glycosuria gravidarum. Am Med 5:663–665

Rushforth NB, Bennett PH, Steinberg AG et al (1971) Diabetes in the Pima Indians: evidence of bimodality in glucose tolerance distributions. Diabetes 20:756–765

Rushton DI (1985) The nature and causes of spontaneous abortions with normal karyotypes. In: Kalter H (ed) Issues and reviews in teratology, vol 3. Plenum, New York, pp 21–63

Rusnak SL, Driscoll SG (1965) Congenital spinal anomalies in infants of diabetic mothers. Pediatrics 35:989–995

Russell DS (1949) Observations on the pathology of hydrocephalus. MRC Special Report Series No. 265. HMSO, London

Russell HE, Aitken GT (1963) Congenital absence of the sacrum and lumbar vertebrae with prosthetic management. J Bone joint surg 45A:501–508

Russell NE, Foley M, Kinsley BT et al (2008) Effect of pregestational diabetes mellitus on fetal cardiac function and structure. Am J Obstet Gynecol 199:312.e107

Ryan EA, Tobin BW, Tang J et al (1993) A new model for the study of mild diabetes during pregnancy: syngeneic islet-transplanted STZ-induced diabetic rats. Diabetes 42:316–323

Sachon C, Grimaldi A, Bosquet F et al (1994) Grossesse diabétique: bilan et perspective à partir de l'étude de 212 grossesses diabétiques suivies entre 1985 et 1992. Ann Med Intern 145: 391–397

Sadovnik AD, Baird PA (1985) Congenital malformations associated with anencephaly in liveborn and stillborn infants. Teratology 32:355–362

Saint-Hilaire IG (1832–1837) Histoire générale et particulière des anomalies de l'organisation chez l'homme et les animaux: ouvrage comprenant des recherches sur les caractères, la classification, l'influence physiologique et pathologique, les rapports généraux, les lois et les causes des monstruosités, des variétés et vices de conformation, ou traité de tératolgie. Baillière, Paris

Saintonge J, Côté R (1984) Fetal brain development in diabetic guinea pigs. Pediat Res 18:650–653

Saintonge J, Côté R (1983) intrauterine growth retardation and diabetic pregnancy: two types of fetal malnutrition. Am J Obstet Gynecol 146:194–198

Salans LB, Graham BJ (eds) (1982) Proceedings of a task force on animals appropriate for studying diabetes mellitus and its complications. Diabetes 31(Suppl 1):1–102

Salvioli GP, Dallacasa P, Bottiglioni F et al (1976) Prognosi dei figli nati da madri affete da diabete mellito. Min Pediatr 28:212–216

Salzberger M, Liban E (1975) Diabetes and antenatal fetal death. In: Shafrir E (ed) Contemporary topics in the study of diabetes and metabolic edocrinology. Academic, New York, pp 97–102

Sanctis CD (1969) Il neonato di madre diabetica: orientamenti clinico-terapeutici. Min Pediatr 21:2139–2144

Sarnat HB, Case ME, Graviss R (1976) Sacral agenesis: neurologic and neuropathologic features. Neurology 26:1124–1129

Saunders N, Paterson C (1991) Can we abandon Naegele's rule? Lancet 337:600–601

Saugstad LF (1981) Weight of all births and infant mortality. J Epidemiol Community Health 35(3):185–191

Saxén L (1983) Twenty years of study of the etiology of congenital malformations in Finland. In: Kalter H (ed) Issues and reviews in teratology, vol 1. Plenum, New York, pp 73–110

Saxén L, Klemetti A, Härö AS (1974) A matched-pair register for studies of selected congenital defects. Am J Epidemiol 100:297–306

Schaefer UM, Songster G, Xiang A et al (1997) Congenital malformations in offspring of women with hyperglycemia first detected during pregnancy. Am J Obstet Gynecol 117:1165–1171

Schaefer-Graf UM, Buchanan TA, Xiang A et al (2000) Patterns of congenital anomalies and relationship to initial maternal fasting glucose levels in pregnancies complicated by type 2 and gestational diabetes. Am J Obstet Gynecol 182:313–320

Schmid J, Kunz J, Sutter R (1984) Diabetes und Schwangerschaft. Gyn Rund 24:197–209

Schmidt MI, Matos MC, Branchstein L et al (1994) Variation in glucose tolerance with ambient temperature. Lancet 344:1054–1055

Schwalbe E (1906) Die Morphologie der Missbildungen des Menschen und der Tiere. Gustav Fischer, Jena

Schwaninger D (1973) Katamnestische Untersuchungen von Kindern diabetischer Mütter. Schweiz Med Wochensch 103:1130–1134

Schwartz JG, Phillips WT, Blumhardt MR et al (1994) Use of a more physiologic oral glucose solution during screening for gestational diabetes mellitus. Am J Obstet Gynecol 171:685–690

Schwartz M, Schneeweiss J, Bock E (1960) Über perinatale Sterblichkeit von Kindern diabetischer Mütter. Schweiz Med Wochensch 90:751–754

Schwartz ML, Brenner WE (1982) The need for adequate and consistent diagnostic classifications for diabetes mellitus diagnosed during pregnancy. Am J Obstet Gynecol 143:119–124

Schwartz R, Teramo KA (2000) Effects of diabetic pregnancy on the fetus and newborn. Semin Perinatol 24:120–135

Schwartz W, Poulsen HK, Andersen PE (1982) Sirenomelia: the caudal regression syndrome. Mon Kinderheilk 130:565–566

Second International Workshop-Conference on Gestational Diabetes Mellitus (1985) Summary and recommendations. Diabetes 34(2):123–126

Sehgal NN (1976) Pregnancy in diabetic women: a review of five years' experience at the Sacramento Medical Center. W Va Med J 72:81–87

Sekhavat S, Kishore N, Levine JC (2010) Screening fetal echocardiography in diabetic mothers with normal findings on detailed anatomic survey. Ultrasound Obstet Gynecol 35:178–182

Seligman SA (1963) Hazards facing the neonate. Proc Roy Soc Med 56:1019–1021

Sells CJ, Robinson NM, Brown Z et al (1994) Long-term developmental follow-up of infants of diabetic mothers. J Pediatr 125:S9–S17

Selman JJ (1932) The results of glucose tolerance tests in pregnant women. Ohio St Med J 28:184–188

Sentrakul P, Potter EL (1966) Pathologic diagnosis on 2,681 abortions at the Chicago Lying-in Hospital, 1957–1965. Am J Publ Health 56:2083–2092

Sepe SJ, Connell FA, Geiss LS et al (1985) Gestational diabetes: incidence, maternal characteristics, and perinatal outcome. Diabetes 34(2):13–16

Shanberg AM, Rosenberg MT (1989) Partial transposition of the penis and scrotum with anterior urethral diverticulum in a child born with the caudal regression syndrome. J Urol 142:1060–1062

Shands AR, Bundens WD (1966) Congenital malformations of the spine: an analysis of the roentgenograms of 700 children. Bull Hosp Jt Dis 17:110–133

Shapiro S, Schlesinger ER, Nesbitt EL Jr (1965) Infant and perinatal ddeath in the United States. U.S. Government Printing Office, Washington

Sharpe PB, Chan A, Haan EA et al (2005) Maternal diabetes and congenital anomalies in South Australia 1986–2000: a population-based cohort study. Birth Defects Res A 73:605–611

Shea MA, Garrison DL, Tom SK (1971) Diabetes in pregnancy. Am J Obstet Gynecol 111:801–803

Sheffied JS, Butler-Koster E, Casey BM et al (2002) Maternal diabetes and infant malformations. Am J Obstet Gynecol 100:925–930

Shepard TH, Fantel AG, Fitzsimmons J (1989) Congenital defects among spontaneous abortuses: twenty years of monitoring. Teratology 39:325–332

Shepard TH, Fantel AG, Mirkes PE (1988) Collection and scientific use of human embryonic and fetal material: 25 years of experience. In: Kalter H (ed) Issues and reviews in teratology, vol 4. Plenum, New York, pp 129–162

Sheridan-Pereira M, Drury MI, Baumgart R et al (1983) Haemoglobin A_1 in diabetic pregnancy: an evaluation. Ir J Med Sci 152:261–267

Shields LE, Gan EA, Morphy HF et al (1993) The prognostic value of hemoglobin A_{1c} in predicting fetal heart disease in diabetic pregnancies. Obstet Gynecol 81:954–957

Shiota K (1993) Teratothanasia: prenatal loss of abnormal conceptuses and the prevalence of various malformations during human gestation. Birth Defects 29:189–199

Shir MM (1939) Diabetes in pregnancy with observations in 28 cases. Am J Obstet Gynecol 37:1032–1035

Sicree RA, Hoet JJ, Zimmet P et al (1986) The association of non-insulin-dependent diabetes with parity and still-birth occurrence amongst five Pacific populations. Diabet Res Clin Prac 2:113–122

Siddiqi T, Rosenn B, Mimouni F et al (1991) Hypertension during pregnancy in insulin-dependent diabetic women. Obstet Gynecol 77:514–519

Sievers G (1969) Discussion. In: Swinyard CA (ed.) Limb development and deformity: problems of evaluation and rehabilitation. Thomas, Springfield, pp 232–248

Silva IS, Higgins C, Swerdlow AJ et al (2005) Birthweight and other pregnancy outcomes in a cohort of women with pre-gestational insulin-treated diabetes mellitus, Scotland, 1979–1995. Diabet Med 22:440–447

Silverman BL, Rozzo T, Green OC et al (1991) Long-term prospective evaluation of offspring of diabetic mothers. Diabetes 40(2):121–125

Simmons D (2009) Diabetes: diabetes risk after gestational diabetes mellitus. Nat Rev Endocrinol 5:646–648

Simpson JL (1978) Genetics of diabetes mellitus (DM) and anomalies in offspring of diabetic mothers. Sem Perinat 2:383–394

Simpson JL, Elias S, Martin AO et al (1983) Diabetes in pregnancy, Northwestern-University Series (1977–1981). I. Prospective study of anomalies in offspring of mothers with diabetes mellitus. Am J Obstet Gynecol 146:263–270

Simpson JL, Mills JL, Moren A et al (1989) Drug ingestion during pregnancy: infrequent exposure in a contemporary United States sample. Am J Perinat 6:244–251

Sindram IS (1951) De sectio Caesarea bij diabetes mellitus. Ned Tijd Geneesk 95:2686–2694

Singer DB (1984) The placenta in pregnancies complicated by diabetes mellitus. Perspect Pediatr Path 8:199–212

Sípek A, Gregor V, Horacek J et al (2009) Birth defects incidence in children from single and twin pregnancies in the Czech Republic–current data. Article in Czech Ceska Gynekol 74:369–382

Sisson WR (1940) The neonatal problem in infants of diabetic mothers. J Am Med Assoc 115:2040–2044

Skipper E (1933) Diabetes mellitus and pregnancy: a clinical and analytical study (with special observations upon thirty-three cases). QJM 2:353–380

Skyler JS (1989) Diabetes and pregnancy: consensus and controversy. In: Sutherland HW et al (eds) Carbohydrate metabolism in pregnancy and the newborn. IV. Springer, New York, pp 363–372

Slot JB, Sande PL, Terpstra J (1967) Diabetes mellitus and pregnancy. Folia Med Neerl 10:77–84

Small M, Cassidy L, Leiper JM et al (1986) Outcome of pregnancy in insulin-dependent (type 1) diabetic women between 1971 and 1984. QJM 61:1159–1169

Smith DW (1971) Minor malformations: their relevance and significance. In: Hook EB et al (eds) Monitoring, birth defects and environment: the problem of surveillance. Academic, New York, pp 169–175

Smith GV, Smith OW (1935) Further quantitative determinations of prolan and estrin in pregnancy, with especial reference to late toxemia and eclampsia. Surg Gynecol Obstet 61:27–35

Smith R (1994) Promoting research into peer review. BMJ 309:143–144

Smith RS, Comstock CH, Lorenz RP et al (1997) Maternal diabetes mellitus: which views are essential for fetal echocardiography? Obstet Gynecol 90:575–579

Smithells RW, Newman CG (1992) Recognition of thalidomide defects. J Med Genet 29:716–723

Smorenberg-School ME, Heringa GM (1983) Diabetes mellitus en zwangerschap; behandelung en resultaten in de periode 1969–1982. Ned T Geneesk 127:1999–2003

Smorenberg-Schoorl ME, Klomp J, Sluyter AH et al (1970) De behandeling van de diabetische zwangere. Ned T Verlosled 70:341–348

Snell LM, Little BB, Knoll KA et al (1992) Reliability of birth certificate reporting of congenital anomalies. Am J Perinat 9:219–222

Soares JA, Dornhorstt A, Beard RW (1997) The case for screening for gestational diabetes. BMJ 315:737–738

Soler NG, Soler SM, Malins JM (1978) Neonatal morbidity among infants of diabetic mothers. Diabetes Care 1:340–350

Soler NG, Walsh CH, Malins JM (1976) Congenital malformations in infants of diabetic mothers. QJM 45:303–333

Sonek JD, Gabbe SG, Landon MB et al (1990) Antenatal diagnosis of sacral agenesis syndrome in a pregnancy complicated by diabetes mellitus. Am J Obstet Gynecol 162:806–808

Soni AL, Kishan J, Mir NA et al (1989) Cyclopic malformation in infants of diabetic mothers. Ind J Pediatr 56:141–144

Spellacy WN, Miller S, Winegar A et al (1985) Macrosomia–maternal characteristics and infant complications. Obstet Gynecol 66:158–161

Spiegelman M, Marks HH (1946) Age and sex variations in the prevalence and onset of diabetes mellitus. Am J Publ Health 36:26–33

Spiers PS (1982) Does growth retardation predispose the fetus to congenital malformation? Lancet 1:312–313

Spooner EW, Hook, EB, Farina MA et al (1988) Evaluation of a temporal increase in ventricular septal defects: estimated prevalence and severity in northeastern New York, 1970–1983. Teratology 37:21–28

Srinivasan BT, Jarvis J, Khunti K et al (2008) Recent advances in the management of type 2 diabetes mellitus: a review. Postgrad Med J 84:524–531

Stallone LA, Ziel HK (1974) Management of gestational diabetes. Am J Obstet Gynecol 119:1091–1094

Stanley FJ, Priscott PK, Johnston R, Brooks B, Bower C (1985) Congenital malformations in infants of mothers with diabetes and epilepsy in Western Australia, 1980–1982. Med J Aust 143(10):440–442

Steel JM (1988) Preconception, conception, and contraception. In: Reece EA, Coustan DR (eds) Diabetes mellitus in pregnancy: principles and practice. Churchill, New York, pp 601–620

Steel JM, Johnstone FD, Duncan LJ (1980) Abnormal infants of diabetic mothers. Lancet 1:771

Steel JM, Livingstone FD, Smith AF et al (1982) Five years' experience of a "prepregnancy" clinic for insulin-dependent diabetics. BMJ 285:353–356

Steel JM, Johnstone FD, Smith AF et al (1984a) The pre-pregnancy clinic approach. In: Sutherland HW, Stowers JM (eds) Carbohydrate metabolism in pregnancy and the newborn. Livingstone, Edinburgh, pp 75–86

Steel JM, Johnstone SD, Corrie JE (1984b) Early assessment of gestation in diabetics. Lancet 2:975–976

Steel JM, Johnstone FD, Hepburn DA et al (1990) Can prepregnancy care of diabetic women reduce the risk of abnormal babies? BMJ 301:1070–1074

Steel JM, Johnstone FD (1992) Pre-pregnancy clinics for diabetic women. Lancet 340:918–919

Steel JM, Wu PS, Johnstone FD et al (1995) Does early growth delay occur in diabetic pregnancy? Br J Obstet Gynecol 102:224–227

Steer C, Campbell S, Davies M et al (1989) Spontaneous abortion rates after natural and assisted conception. BMJ 299:1317–1318

Stehbens JA, Baker GL, Kitchell M (1977) Outcome at ages 1, 3, and 5 years of children born to diabetic women. Am J Obstet Gynecol 127:408–414

Steindel E, Mohnike A (1971) Über Häufigkeit und Verlauf der schwangerschaften bei Diabetikerinnen und Frauen mit Schwangerschaftsglukosurien in Berlin im Zeitraum von 1963 bis 1970. Dtsch Gesundheit 26:2075–2079

Stengel A (1904) Diabetes as a complication of pregnany. U Penn Med Bull 17:296–299

Stephens JW, Page OC, Hare RL (1963) Diabetes and pregnancy: a report of experiences in 119 pregnancies over a period of ten years. Diabetes 12:213–219

Stern L, Ramos A, Light I (1965) Congenital malformations and diabetes. Lancet 1:1393–1394

Stern MP, Rosenthal M, Haffner SM (1985) A new concept of impaired glucose tolerance: relation to cardiovascular risk. Arteriosclerosis 5:311–314

Stevenson AC, Warnock HA (1959) Observations on the results of pregnancies in women resident in Belfast. I. Data relating to all pregnancies ending in 1957. Ann Hum Genet 23:382–394

Stevenson AC, Johnston HA, Stewart MI et al (1966) Congenital malformations: a report of a study of series of consecutive births in 24 centres. Bull WHO 34:1–127

Stevenson AE (1956) Pregnancy complicated by diabetes mellitus: a review of 119 cases. BMJ 2:1514–1518

Stevenson DK, Hopper AO, Cohen RS et al (1982) Macrosomia: causes and consequences. J Pediatr 100:515–520

Stevenson RE, Jones KL, Phelan MC et al (1986) Vascular steal: the pathogenetic mechanism producing sirenomelia and associated defects of the viscera and soft tissues. Pediatrics 78:451–457

Stocker JT, Heifetz SA (1987) Sirenomelia: a morphological study of 33 cases and review of the literature. Perspect Pediatr Path 10:7–50

Stoll C, Alembik Y, Dott B et al (1992) An epidemiologic study of environmental and genetic factors in congenital hydrocephalus. Eur J Epidemiol 8:797–803

Stone DH (1992) RE "Completeness of the discharge diagnoses as a measure of birth defects in the hospital record." Am J Epidemiol 136:498–499

Strong RM (1925) The order, time and rate of ossification of the albino rat (Mus Norvegicus Albinus) skeleton. Am J Anat 36:313–351

Stroup NE, Edmonds L, O'Brien TR (1990) Renal agenesis and dysgenesis: are they increasing? Teratology 42:383–396

Stubbs SM (1987) Personal communication

Stubbs SM, Doddridge MC, John PN et al (1987) Haemoglobin A_1 and congenital malformation. Diabet Med 4:156–159

Styrud J, Thunberg L, Nybacka O et al (1995) Correlations between maternal metabolism and deranged development in the offspring of normal and diabetic rats. Pediatr Res 37:343–353

Suhonen L, Hiilesmaa V, Teramo K (2000) Glycaemic control during early pregnancy and fetal malformations in women with type 1 diabetes mellitus. Diabetologia 43:79–82

Sulovic V, Lazarevic B, Avramovic D et al (1981) Gestational and pre-gestational diabetes: course and issue of prenancy. Spr Arh Celok Lek 109:1583–1598

Sutherland HW, Pedersen JF, Mølsted-Pedersen L (1981) Treatment of diabetic pregnancy with special reference to fetal growth. In: Van Assche FA, Robertson WB (eds) Fetal growth retardation. Livingstone, Edinburgh, pp 197–207

Sutherland HW, Fisher PM (1982) Fetal loss and maternal glucose intolerance: a retrospective study. Päd Päd 17:279–286

Sutherland HW, Pritchard CW (1986) Increased incidence of spontaneous abortion in pregnancies complicated by maternal diabetes mellitus. Am J Obstet Gynecol 155:135–138

Sutherland I (1949) Stillbirths: their epidemiology and social significance. Oxford Univ, London

Svanteson G (1953) Diabetes mellitus och graviditet. Nord Med 49:533–536

Sybulski S, Maughan BB (1971) Use of streptozotocin as diabetic agent in pregnant rats. Endocrinology 89:1537–1540

Szabó M, Tóth T, Tóth Z et al (1986) Fetal malformation and serum alpha-fetoprotein concentration of diabetic mothers. Zentralbl Gynakol 108:1228–1236

Taeusch HW, Ballard TR, Avery ME (1991) Schaffer and Avery's diseases of the newborn. Saunders, Philadelphia

Takano K, Nishimura H (1967) Congenital malformations induced by alloxan diabetes in mice and rats. Anat Rec 158:303–312

Takano K, Tanimura T, Nishimura H (1965) The susceptibility of the offspring of alloxan-diabetic mice to a teratogen. J Embryol Exp Morph 14:63–73

Takeuchi A, Benirschke K (1961) Renal venous thrombosis of the newborn and its relation to maternal diabetes:report of 16 cases. Biol Neonat 3:237–256

Tallarigo L, Giampietro O, Penno G et al (1986) Relation of glucose tolerance to complications of pregnancy in nondiabetic women. N Engl J Med 315:989–992

Tanigawa K, Kawaguchi M, Tanaka O et al (1991) Skeletal malformations in rat offspring: long-term effect of maternal insulin-induced hypoglycemia during organogenesis. Diabetes 40:1115–1121

Taylor FW (1899) Diabetes mellitus and pregnancy. Bost Med Surg J 140:205–207

Taylor R, Lee C, Kyne-Grzebalski D et al (2002) Clinical outcomes of pregnancy in women with type 1 diabetes(1). Obstet Gynecol 99:537–541

Tchobroutsky C, Breart GL, Rambaud DC et al (1985) Correlation between fetal defects and early growth delay observed by ultrasound. Lancet 1:706

Tchobroutsky C, Vray MM, Altman JJ (1991) Risk/benefit ratio of changing late obstetrical strategies in the management of insulin-dependent diabetic pregnancies: a comparison between 1971–1977 and 1978–1985 periods in 389 pregnancies. Diabet Metab 17:287–294

Tchobroutsky C (1991) Blood glucose levels in diabetic and non-diabetic subjects. Diabetologia 34:67–73

Tegnander E, Eik-Nes SH, Johansen OJ et al (1995) Prenatal examination of heart defects at the routine fetal examination at 18 weeks in a non-selected population. Ultrasound Obstet Gynecol 5:372–380

Temple R, Aldridge V, Greenwod R et al (2002) Association between outcome of pregnancy and glycemic control in early pregnancy in type 1 diabetes: population based study. BMJ 325:1275–1276

Teramo K, Kuusisto AN, Raivio KU (1979) Perinatal outcome of insulin-dependent diabetic pregnancies. Ann Clin Res 11:146–155

Teramoto S, Hatakenaka N, Shirasu Y (1991) Effects of the Ay gene on susceptibility to hydrocortisone fetotoxicity and teratogenicity in mice. Teratology 44:101–106

Tevaarwerk GJ, Harding PG, Milne KJ et al (1981) Pregnancy in diabetic women: outcome with a program aimed at normoglycemia before meals. Can Med Assoc J 125:435–442

Thalhammer O, Lachmann D, Scheibenreiter S (1968) "Caudale Regression" beim Kind einer 18 jährigen Frau mit Prädiabetes. Z Kinderchir 102:346–355

Theile U, Rückel E, Hust U (1985) Kinder diabetischer Eltern–zur Frage von Entwicklungsstörungen während der Schwangerschaft mit besonderer Berücksichtigung des sogenannten Riesenkindes. Z Geburtsh Perinat 189:79–83

Thomson AM, Barron SL (1983) Perinatal death. In: Barron SL, Thomson AM (eds) Obstetrical epidemiology. Academic, London, pp 347–398

Thosteson GC (1953) Diabetes and pregnancy. Harper Hosp Bull 11(6):245–247

Tiisala R, Michelsson K, Wist A (1967) Observations on the perinatal period of infants of diabetic mothers. Ann Paediatr Fenn 13:9–16

Tingle CD (1926) A contribution to the study of the causation of foetal death. Arch Dis Child 1:255–278

Titus RS (1937) Diabetes in pregnancy from the obstetric point of view. Am J Obstet Gynecol 33:386–392

Tochino Y (1987) The NOD mouse as a model of type 1 diabetes. Crit Rev Immun 8:49–81

Todorova K, Mazneikova V, Ivanov S et al (2004) Role of glycemic control and incidence of spontaneous abortions pregnant in women with type 1 diabetes mellitus. in Bulgarian. Akush Ginekol (Sofia) 43:16–23

Tolstoi E, Given WP, Douglas RG (1953) Management of the pregnant diabetic. JAMA 153:998–1002

Towner D, Kjos SL, Leung B et al (1995) Congenital malformations in pregnancies complicated by NIDDM. Diabetes Care 18:1446–1451

Traub AI, Harley JM, Cooper TK et al (1987) Is centralized hospital care necessary for all insulin-dependent pregnant diabetics? Br J Obstet Gynecol 94:957–972

Traub AI, Harley JM, Montgomery DA et al (1983) Pregnancy and diabetes–the improving prognosis. Ulster Med J 52:118–124

Tunçer M, Tunçer M (1981) Congenital malformations and diabetes mellitus. Turk J Pediat 23:157–169

Tuomilehto J, Korhonen HJ, Kartovaara L et al (1991a) Prevalence of diabetes-mellitus and impaired glucose tolerance in the middle-aged population of three areas in Finland. Int J Epidemiol 20:1010–1017

Tuomilehto J, Korhonen HJ, Kartovaara L et al (1991b) Prevention of type 2 diabetes mellitus by changes in lifestyle among subjects with impaired glucose tolerance. N Engl J Med 344:1343–1350

U.S. Bureau of the Census (1960) Historical Statistics of the United States: colonial times to 1957. U.S. Department of Commerce, Washington

Ueda K, Nishida Y, Oshima K et al (1979) Congenital rubella syndrome: correlation of gestational age at the time of maternal rubella with type of defect. J Pediatr 94:763–765

Ullmo S, Vial Y, Di Bernardo S et al (2007) Pathologic ventricular hypertrophy in the offspring of diabetic mothers: a retrospective study. Eur Heart J 28:1319–1325

Ullrich E (1979) Gewusst und/oder nachgeschlagen: kaudale Hypoplasie. Med Akt 5:45

Uriu-Hare JY, Stern JS, Keen CL (1989) Influence of maternal dietary Zn on expression of diabetes-induced teratogenicity in rats. Diabetes 38:1282–1290

Uriu-Hare JY, Stern JS, Reaven GM et al (1985) The effects of maternal diabetes on trace element status and fetal development in the rat. Diabetes 34:1031–1040

Vääräsmäki MS, Gissler M, Ritvanen A et al (2002) Congenital anomalies and first year surveillance in type 1 diabetic births. Diabet Med 19:589–593

Vääräsmäki MS, Hartikainen AL, Anttila M et al (2000) Factors predicting peri- and neonatal outcome in diabetic pregnancy. Early Hum Dev 59:61–70

Vadheim CM (1983) Pregnancy with diabetes: Washington state, 1978–1980. Ph.D. Thesis, Univ of Washington, Seattle, Wa

Vaes G, Meyer R de (1957) Étude histochimique du glycogène utérin chez la lapine: ses variations au cours du diabète alloxanique et sous l'action de la cortisone. Ann Endocr 18:828–840

Vallance-Owen J, Braithwaite F, Wilson JS et al (1967) Cleft lip and palate deformities and insulin antagonism. Lancet 2:912–914

Van Allen DC, Petersen MC, Lin-Dyken DC et al (1995) Delays in diagnosis in children with saral anomalies. Am J Med Genet 55:251–252

Van Allen MI, Brown ZA, Plovie B et al (1994) Deformations in infants of diabetic and control pregnancies. Am J Med Genet 53:210–215

Van Allen MI, Myhre S (1991) New multiple congenital anomalies syndrome in a stillborn infant of consanguinous parents and a prediabetic pregnancy. Am J Med Genet 38:523–528

Van Der Wal KG, Mulder JW (1993) Median lip without holoprosencephaly: case report. Int J Oral Maxillofac Surg 22:39–41

Van Dyke DC, Petersen MC, Lin-Dyken DC, Smith WL (1995) Delays in diagnosis in children with sacral anomalies. Am J Med Genet 55(2):251–252 (No abstract available)

Vangen O, Molne K, Bjøro K (1972) Diabetes mellitus og svangerskap: den perinatale mortalitet ved Rikshospitalitet, Kvinneklinikken, i tiden 1950–1970. T Norske Laegefor 92:1313–1317

Vangen S, Stoltenberg C, Holan S et al (2003) Outcome of pregnancy among immigrant women with diabetes. Diabetes Care 26:327–332

Vasilenko P, Mead JP, Slaughter T et al (1989) Detrimental effects of maternal diabetes on growth and development of offspring in the rat. Diabetes 33:91A

Ventura SJ, Martin JA, Taffel SM et al (1992) Advance report of final natality statistics, 1992. Mon Vit Stat Rep 43(5):1–88

Vercheval M, Hertogh R de, Pampfer S et al (1990) Experimental diabetes impairs rat embryo development during the preimplantation period. Diabetologia 33:187–191

Verheijen EC, Critchley JA, Whitelaw DC et al (2006) Outcomes of pregnancies in women with pre-existing type 1 or type 2 diabetes, in an ethnically mixed population. BJOG 112:1500–1503

Verrotti A, Chiarelli F, Capani F et al (1993) Prediabetes: genetic, immunological and metabolic aspects. Panmin Med 35:179–185

Versiani BR, Gilbert-Barness E, Giuliani LR et al (2004) Caudal dysplasia sequence: severe phenotype presenting in offspring of patients with gestational and pregeststional diabetes. Clin Dysmorphol 13:1–5

Viberti G (1995) A glycemic threshhold for diabetic complications? N Engl J Med 332:1292–1293

Victor A (1974) Normal blood sugar variation during pregnancy. Act Obstet Gynecol Scand 53:37–40

Villumsen AL (1970) Environmental factors in congenital malformations: a prospective study of 9,006 human pregnancies. F.A.D.L.s, Copenhagen

Villumsen AL Zachau-Christiansen B (1963) Incidence of malformations in the newborn in a prospective child health study. Bull Soc Roy Belg Gynecol Obstet 33:95–105

Visser GH, Bedekam DJ, Mulder EJ et al (1985) Delayed emergence of fetal behaviour in type-1 diabetic women. Early Hum Dev 12:167–172

von Noorden C (1910) Die Zuckerkrankheit und ihre Behandlung. Hirschwald. Berlin

Wada M, Iwase M, Wakisaka M et al (1995) A new model of diabetic pregnancy with genetic hypertension: pregnancy in spontaneously hypertensive rats with neonatal streptozotocin-induced diabetes. Am J Obstet Gynecol 172:626–630

Wahabi HA, Alzeidan RA, Bawazeer GA et al (2010) Preconception care for diabetic women for improving maternal and fetal outcomes: a systematic review and meta-analysis. BMC Pregnancy Childbirth 10:63

Wald NJ, Cuckle H, Boreham J et al (1979) Maternal serum alpha-fetoprotein and diabetes mellitus. Br J Obstet Gynecol 86:101–105

Walden RH, Logosso RD, Brennan L (1971) Pierre Robin syndrome in association with combined congenital lengthening and shortening of the long bones: case report. Plast Reconstr Surg 48:80–82

Walker A (1928) Diabetes mellitus and pregnancy. J Obstet Gynecol Br Emp 35:271–281

Wang J, Palmer RM, Chung CS (1988) The role of major gene in clubfoot. Am J Hum Genet 42:772–776

Warburton D, Fraser FC (1964) Spontaneous abortion risks in man: data from reproductive histories collected in a medical genetics unit. Am J Hum Genet 16:1–25

Ward RJ, Readhead SM (1970) The effect of alloxan-induced diabetes on the foetal toxicity of thalidomide, carbutamide and myleran in rats. In: The problems of species difference and statistics in toxicology. Proceedings of the European society for the study of drug toxicity, vol 11. Exerpta Medica Foundation, Amsterdam. pp 151–166

Wareham NJ, O'Rahilly S (1998) The changing classification and diagnosis of diabetes. BMJ 317:359–360

Warkany J (1971) Congenital malformations: notes and comments. Year Book Medical, Chicago

Warkany J (1977) History of teratology. In: Wilson JG, Fraser FC (eds) Handbook of teratology, vol 1. Plenum, New York, pp 3–45

Warkany J (1978) Terathanasia. Teratology 17:187–192

Warkany J, Nelson RC (1941) Skeletal abnormalities in the offspring of rats reared on deficient diets. Anat Rec 79:83–100

Warkany J, Kalter H (1961) Congenital malformations. N Engl J Med 265:993–1001, 1046–1052

Warren S, LeCompte PM (1952) The pathology of diabetes mellitus. Lea & Febiger, Philadelphia

Warrner RA, Cornblath M (1969) Infants of gestational diabetic mothers. Am J Dis Child 117:678–683

Watanabe G, Ingalls TH (1963) Congenital malformations in the offspring of alloxan-diabetic mice. Diabetes 12:66–72

Watson C (1968) A follow-up study of children born to diabetic mothers, with particular reference to frequency of congenital abnormalities. Arch Dis Child 43:746–747

Watson C (1970) Prognosis for infants born to diabetic mothers, with particular reference to the prevalence of congenital abnormalitites. Int J Gynecol Obstet 8:212–213

Watson CM (1973) Late prognosis for children born to diabetic mothers. M.D. Thesis, Univ of London

Weicker H (1963) Klinik und Epidemiologie der Thalidomid-Embryopathie. Bull Soc Roy Belg Gynecol Obstet 33:21–27

Weicker H (1969) Epidemiological and etiological considerations in the increase of limb malformations in Germany. In: Swinyard CA (ed) Limb development and deformity: problems of evaluation and rehabilitation. Thomas, Springfield, pp 225–232

Weijers RN, Bekedam DJ, Oosting H (1998) The prevalence of type 2 diabetes and gestational diabetes mellitus in an inner city multi-ethnic population. Eur J Epidemiol 14:693–699

Weindling AM (2009) Offspring of diabetic pregnancy: short-term outcomes. Semin Fetal Neonatal Med 14:111–118

Weiner CP (1988) Effect of varying degrees of "normal" glucose metabolism on maternal and perinatal outcome. Am J Obstet Gynecol 159:862–870

Weintrob N, Karp M, Hod M (1996) Short- and long-range complications in offspring of diabetic mothers. J Diabetes Complications 10:94–301

Welch P, Aterman K (1984) The syndrome of caudal dysplasia: a review, including etiologic considerations and evidence of heterogeneity. Pediatr Path 2:313–327

Wentzel P, Jansson L, Eriksson UJ (1995) Diabetes in pregnancy: uterine blood flow and embryonic development in the rat. Pediatr Res 38:598–606

West KM (1971) Epidemiology of diabetes. In: Fajans SS, Sussman KE (eds) Diabetes mellitus: diagnosis and treatment. American Diabetes Association, New York, pp 121–126

West KM (1975) Substantial differences in the diagnostic criteria used by diabetes experts. Diabetes 24:641–644

West KM, Wulff JA, Reigel DG et al (1964) Oral carbohydrate tolerance tests. Arch Int Med 113:641–648
Wheller JJ, Reiss R, Allen HD (1990) Clinical experience with fetal echocardiography. Am J Dis Child 144:49–53
White BM, Beischer NA (1990) Perinatal death in the infants of diabetic women. Aust N Z J Obstet Gynecol 30:323–326
White P (1935) Pregnancy complicating diabetes. Surg Gynecol Obstet 61:324–332
White P (1946) Pregnancy complicating diabetes. In: Joslin EP et al (eds) The treatment of diabetes mellitus. Lea & Febiger, Philadelphia, pp 769–784
White P (1949) Pregnancy complicating diabetes. Am J Med 7:609–616
White P (1950) Diabetes in pregnancy. Trans Int Cong Obstet Gynecol 4:382–387
White P (1952) Pregnancy complicating diabetes. In: Joslin EP et al (eds) The treatment of diabetes mellitus. Lea & Febiger, Philadelphia, pp 676–698
White P (1965) Pregnancy and diabetes, medical aspects. Med Clin N Am 49:1015–1024
White P (1971) Pregnancy and diabetes. In: Marble A et al (eds) Joslin's diabetes mellitus. Lea & Febiger, Philadelphia, pp 581–598
White P (1974) Diabetes in pregnancy. Clin Perinat 1:331–347
White P (1978) Classification of obstetric diabetes. Am J Obstet Gynecol 130:228–230
White P, Gillespie L, Sexton L (1956) Use of female sex hormone therapy in pregnant diabetic patients. Am J Obstet Gynecol 71:57–69
White P, Hunt H (1943) Pregnancy complicating diabetes. J. Clin Endocr Metab 3:500–511
White P, Koshy P, Duckers J (1953) The management of pregnancy complicating diabetes and of diabetic mothers. Med Clin N Am 39:1481–1496
White P, Titus RS, Joslin EP et al (1939) Prediction and prevention of late pregnancy accidents in diabetes. Am J Med Sci 198:482–492
Whiteford ML, Tolmie JL (1996) Holoprosencephaly in the west of Scotland. J Med Genet 33:578–584
Whitehouse FW, Lowrie WL, Hodgkinson CP (1956) Diabetes and pregnancy. J Mich St Med Soc 55:1211–1217
Whitely JM, Adams TW (1952) Diabetes and pregnancy. West J Surg 60:98–107
Whitely JM, Adams TW, Parrott MH (1953) Diabetes and pregnancy. West J Surg 61:439–447
Whittaker PG, Aspillaga MO, Lind T (1983) Accurate assessment of early gestational age in normal and diabetic women by serum human placental lactogen concentration. Lancet 2:304–305
Whittle MJ, Anderson D, Lowensohn RI et al (1979) Estriol in pregnancy. VI. Experience with unconjugated plasma estriol assays and antepartum fetal heart rate testing in diabetic pregnancies. Am J Obstet Gynecol 135:764–772
Widness JA, Cowett RM, Coustan DR, Carpenter MW, Oh W (1985) Neonatal morbidities in infants of mothers with glucose intolerance in pregnancy. Diabetes 34(Suppl 2):61–65
Wiener HJ (1924) Diabetes mellitus in pregnancy. Am J Obstet Gynecol 7:710–718
Wilcox AJ, Russell IT (1983) Perinatal mortality: standardizing for birthweight is biased. Am J Epidemiol 118(6):857–864
Wilcox AJ, Weinberg CR, O'Connor JF et al (1988) Incidence of early loss of pregnancy. N Engl J Med 319:189–194
Wilder RM, Parsons E (1928) Treatment of diabetes during pregnancy. Col Med 25:372–382
Wilkerson HL (1959) Pregnancy and the prediabetic state. Ann N Y Acad Sci 82:219–228
Wilkerson HL, O'Sullivan JB (1963) A study of glucose tolerance and screening criteria in 752 unselected pregnancies. Diabetes 12:313–318
Wilkerson HL, Remein QR (1957) Studies of abnormal carbohydrate metabolism in pregnancy: the significance of impaired glucose tolerance. Diabetes 6:324–329
Willhoite MB, Bennert HW, Palomaki GE et al (1993) The impact of preconception counseling on pregnancy outcomes: the experience of the Maine Diabetes in Pregnancy Program. Diabetes Care 16:450–455
Williams EC, Wills L (1929) Studies in blood and urinary chemistry during pregnancy: blood sugar curves. QJM 22:493–505

Williams JJ (1930) Obstetrics. Appleton, New York
Williams JW (1909) The clinical significance of glycosuria in pregnant women. Am J Med Sci 137:1–26
Williger VM (1965) Fetal outcome in the diabetic pregnancy. Am J Obstet Gynecol 94:57–60
Wilmshurst JM, Kelly R, Borzyskowski M (1999) Presentation and outcome of sacral agenesis: 20 years' experience. Dev Med Child Neurol 41:806–812
Wilson GN, Howe M, Stover JM (1985) Delayed development sequences in rodent diabetic embryopathy. Pediatr Res 19:1337–1340
Wilson JG (1960) Factors involved in causing congenital malformations. Bull N Y Acad Med 36:145–157
Wilson JG (1973) Environment and birth defects. Academic, New York
Wilson JS, Vallance-Owen J (1966) Congenital deformities and insulin antagonism. Lancet 2:940–941
Wolfe RR, Way GL (1977) Cardiomyopathies in infants of diabetic mothers. Johns Hopkins Med J 140:177–180
Wolff E (1948) La science des monstres. Gallimard, Paris
Woolf B (1947) Studies on infant mortality. B J Soc Med 2:73–125
World Health Organization (1977) Recommended definitions, terminology and format for statistical tables related to the perinatal period and use of a new certificate for cause of perinatal deaths. Acta Obstet Gynecol Scand 56:247–253
World Health Organization (1985) Diabetes mellitus: report of a WHO study group. Tech Rep Ser 727. WHO, Geneva
World Health Organization Multinational Project for Childhood Diabetes Group (1991) Familial insulin-dependent diabetes mellitus (IDDM) epidemiology: standardization of data from the DIAMOND Project. Bull WHO 69:767–777
Worm M (1955) Menstruation und Fertilität bei Diabetes mellitus. Zentralbl Gynak 77:886–893
Worm M (1960) Behandlung, Geburtsleitung und Ergebnisse bei 300 Entbindungen diabetischer Frauen. In: Prenatal care. Noordhoff, Groningen, pp 140–145
Wren C, Birrell G, Hawthorne G (2003) Cardiovascular malformations in infants of diabetic mothers. Heart 89:1217–1220
Wrenshall GA, Hetenyi G, Feasby WR (1962) The story of insulin: forty years of success against diabetes. Indiana Univ, Bloomington
Wright AD (1984) Diabetes in pregnancy. In: Natrass M, Santiago JV (eds) Recent advances in diabetes. Chuchill Livingstone, Edinburgh, pp 239–254
Wright AD, Nicholson HO, Pollock A et al (1983) Spontaneous elnell and diabetes mellitus. Postgrad Med J 59:295–298
Yamashita Y, Kawano Y, Kuriya N et al (1996) Intellectual development of offspring of diabetic mothers. Acta Paediatr 85:1192–1196
Yang J, Cummings EA, O'connell C et al (2006) Fetal and neonatal outcomes of diabetic pregnancies. Obstet Gynecol 108:644–650
Yankauer A (1990) What infant mortality tells us. Am J Publ Health 80:653654
Ylinen K, Aula P, Stenman UH et al (1984) Risk of minor and major fetal malformations in diabetics with high haemoglobin A_{1c} values in early pregnancy. BMJ 289:345–346
Ylinen K, Raivio K, Teramo K (1981) Haemoglobin A_{1c} predicts the perinatal outcome in insulin-dependent diabetic pregnancies. Br J Obstet Gynaecol 88:961–967
Yssing M (1975) Long-term prognosis of children born to mothers diabetic when pregnant. In: Camerini-Davalos RA, Cole HS (eds) Early diabetes in early life. Academic, New York, pp 575–586
Yudkin JS, Alberti KG, McLarty DG et al (1990) Impaired glucose tolerance. BMJ 301:397–401
Zachau-Christiansen B, Villumsen AL, Sinkbaek SA (1962) Antihistaminpraeparater og graviditet. Ugeskr Laeg 124:1843–1844
Zanardo V, Pesenti P, Mittiga SM et al (1983) Embriofetopatia nei nati di madri con diabete gravidico e di madri con diabete insulino-dependente. Pediatr Med Chir 5:185–188
Zarowitz H, Moltz A (1966) Management of diabetes in pregnancy. Obstet Gynecol 27(6):820–826

Zarzycki W, Zieniewicz M (2005) Reproductive disturbances in type 1 diabetic women. Neuro Endocrinol Lett 26:733–738

Zazworsky D, Bolin JN, Gaubeca VB (2006) Handbook of diabetes management. Springer, New York

Zilliacus H (1950) Pregnancy and diabetes mellitus. Acta Endocr 4:63–78

Zusman I, Ornoy A (1986) The effect of maternal diabetes and high sucrose diets on the intrauterine development of rat fetuses. Diabet Res 3:153–159

Index

H. Kalter, *A History of Diabetes in Pregnancy*,
DOI 10.1007/978-94-007-1557-8, © Springer Science+Business Media B.V. 2012

CPSIA information can be obtained at www.ICGtesting.com
Printed in the USA
LVOW102212060312

271948LV00004B/94/P